Chronic
Wound Care

For Mosby:

Senior Commissioning Editor: Sarena Wolfaard
Project Development Manager: Claire Wilson
Project Manager: Derek Robertson
Design: Judith Wright

Chronic Wound Care

A problem-based learning approach

Edited by

Moya J Morison BA BSc(Hons) MSc PhD PGCE RGN
Professor of Health and Nursing, School of Social and Health Sciences,
University of Abertay, Dundee, UK

Liza G Ovington PhD CWS
Ovington & Associates Inc, Pittsburgh, USA

Kay Wilkie BSc MN PhD RN RM NDNCert DipNursStuds
Lecturer, School of Nursing and Midwifery, University of Dundee, UK

Foreword by
Christine J Moffatt
Professor of Nursing, Centre for Research & Implementation of Clinical Practice,
Thames Valley University, London

and
Peter J Franks
Professor of Health Sciences, Centre for Research & Implementation of Clinical
Practice, Thames Valley University, London

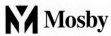 Mosby

EDINBURGH LONDON NEW YORK OXFORD PHILADELPHIA ST LOUIS SYDNEY TORONTO 2004

Mosby
An affiliate of Elsevier Limited

First published 2004
    Reprinted 2005 (twice), 2006 (twice), 2007

ISBN 13: 978 0 7234 3235 7
ISBN 10: 0 7234 3235 X

British Library Cataloguing in Publication Data
A catalogue record for this book is available from the British Library

Library of Congress Cataloguing in Publication Data
A catalogue record for this book is available from the Library of Congress

Notice
Medical knowledge is constantly changing. Standard safety precautions must be followed, but as new research and clinical experience broaden our knowledge, changes in treatment and drug therapy may become necessary appropriate. Readers are advised to check the most current product information provided by the manufacturer of each drug to be administered to verify the recommended dose, the method and duration of administration, and contraindications. It is the responsibility of the practitioner, relying on experience and knowledge of the patient, to determine dosages and the best treatment for each individual patient. Neither the Publisher nor the editors assume any liability for any injury and/or damage to persons or property arising from this publication.

The Publisher

ELSEVIER   your source for books,
journals and multimedia
in the health sciences

www.elsevierhealth.com

Working together to grow
libraries in developing countries

www.elsevier.com | www.bookaid.org | www.sabre.org

ELSEVIER   BOOKAID   Sabre Foundation
International

The
publisher's
policy is to use
paper manufactured
from sustainable forests

Printed in China

CONTENTS

CONTRIBUTORS

Denis Anthony
Professor of Nursing Informatics, Head of Research, School of Nursing & Midwifery, De Montfort University, Leicester, UK

Tami de Araujo
Resident, Department of Dermatology, University of Miami/Veterans Administration Medical Center, Florida, USA

Janice M Beitz
Associate Professor, Director of Certificate and Distributive Learning Programs, La Salle University School of Nursing, Philadelphia, USA

Ysabel Bello
Assistant Professor, Department of Dermatology, University of Miami, USA

Janice Cameron
Clinical Nurse Specialist Wound Healing, Department of Dermatology, Oxford Radcliffe Hospitals NHS Trust, Oxford, UK

Dorothy B Doughty
Emory University WOC Nursing Education C, The Emory Clinic, Atlanta, USA

Mary Dyson
Visiting Professor, Department of Physical Therapy and Rehabilitation Sciences, Kansas University Medical Center, Kansas City, KS, USA

David Eisenbud
Managing Partner, Millburn Surgical Associates, Millburn, New Jersey, USA

William J Ennis
Medical Director, Wound Treatment Program, Advocate Christ Hospital and Medical Center, IL, USA

Ana Falabella
Assistant Professor, University of Miami Department of Dermatology, Florida, USA

Don R Fishman
Clinical Assistant Professor of Surgery, University of Illinois, USA

Yvonne Franks
Head of Nursing and Clinical Services, Outpatient and Diagnostic Service, Queen Mary's Hospital, London, UK

Jane Harris
School of Nursing and Midwifery, University of Dundee, UK

Cathy Tomas Hess
Wound Care Strategies Inc., Harrisburg, PA, USA

N Blair Hughes
Director, FMH Advanced Skin and Wound Care Center, MD, USA

Robert S Kirsner
Department of Dermatology, University of Miami/Veterans Administration Medical Center, Florida, USA

Susan McLaren
Faculty of Healthcare Sciences, University of Kingston, UK

David M McNaughton
Director, Pain Management Research Centre, University of Abertay, Dundee, UK

Patricia Meneses
Research Director, Wound Program Advocate Christ Medical Center, Illinois, USA

Christine J Moffatt
*Professor of Nursing, Centre for Research &
Implementation of Clinical Practice,
Thames Valley University, London*

Moya J Morison
*Professor of Health and Nursing, School of Social and
Health Sciences, University of Abertay, Dundee, UK*

Heather Newton
*Nurse Consultant Tissue Viability, Practice
Development Department, Royal Cornwall Hospitals
NHS Trust, Truro, UK*

Sheila M Nimmo
*Lecturer in Nursing, Associate Director of Pain
Management Research Centre, Institute for Health
Studies, University of Abertay, Dundee, UK*

Jane Nixon
*Deputy Head of Unit, Northern and Yorkshire Clinical
Trials and Research Unit, University of Leeds, UK*

Liza G Ovington
*President, Ovington & Associates Inc, Pittsburgh,
USA*

Linda Russell
*Tissue Viability Nurse Specialist, Queen's Hospital,
Burton-on-Trent, UK*

Steven Salzman
*Clinical Assistant Professor, Advocate Christ Medical
Center, Illinois, USA*

Gregory Schultz
*Department of Obstetrics and Gynecology, University
of Florida, USA*

Mick Smith
*Associate Professor, Departments of Geography,
Environmental Studies and Philosophy,
Queen's University, Kingston, Ontario, Canada*

Catharine Spence
*School of Nursing and Midwifery, University of
Dundee, Kirkcaldy, UK*

Nancy A Stotts
*Professor, School of Nursing, University of California,
San Francisco, USA*

Nancy Tomaselli
*Premier Health Solutions, Cherry Hill, New Jersey,
USA*

Wesley N Valdes
*Wound Care Fellow, Advocate Christ Medical Center,
Illinois, USA*

Kay Wilkie
*Director of Learning and Teaching, School of Nursing
and Midwifery, University of Dundee, UK*

FOREWORD

Wound care is a major health problem that affects many patient groups and consumes vast resources – it impacts on many aspects of patients' lives, frequently leading to a deterioration in quality of life. The past 20 years have seen major advances in the care of patients with different types of wounds. The publication of *Chronic Wound Care* is timely as it incorporates up-to-date clinical information from both national and international authors and uses a problem-based learning approach to integrate theory and practice.

Problem-based learning (PBL) allows students to learn through real life situations relevant to their clinical area. The reflective case studies in this book facilitate this process and encourage students to explore new ideas and to challenge the basis of their practice. This book recognises that people have very different learning needs, and that much attention must be placed on how students apply their knowledge. Most importantly, through integrated learning PBL aims to bridge the gap between theory and practice, leading to real improvements in clinical practice.

The international health care arena is rapidly working towards evidence-based practice. The adoption of evidence-based wound care has led to major benefits to patients, health professionals and health services. There is a vast amount of literature in this area, and a need to identify up-to-date sources of information – this book has a very valuable chapter on assisting students in this process, together with useful material on accessing key websites.

The editors of *Chronic Wound Care* combine clinical wound care expertise with sound educational approaches to learning. We believe that this book will be an invaluable resource for pre- and post-registration students, teachers and practitioners. We congratulate the editors on this excellent publication.

Christine J Moffatt, Peter J Franks
2004

ACKNOWLEDGEMENTS

No enterprise such as this is undertaken without a personal cost to those involved, both directly and indirectly. It is a tribute to the contributors that each has seen this complex undertaking through to its conclusion. We would like to extend our warmest thanks to them for their outstanding contributions and encouragement. Special thanks are also extended to all the families and friends of those involved for their support and forbearance while this work was undertaken.

MM, LO, KW, 2004

Introduction

CHAPTER

1

A new approach to learning how to care for patients with wounds

Moya J Morison

INTRODUCTION

The care of patients with wounds is a commonly encountered responsibility for nurses, doctors and allied health professionals in most care settings and with many patient groups, from neonates to care of the elderly. Although a number of excellent teaching programmes have been developed by specialist centres, on the whole, wound care tends to be underrepresented on the undergraduate curriculum, and in the UK opportunities for continuing professional and specialist practice development are fragmented.

There are a number of possible explanations for this at a strategic level, which have not yet been fully researched. These include:

- lack of a nationally recognized core curriculum for wound care
- lack of a nationally recognized qualifications framework in this speciality
- lack of suitably qualified teachers in the subject
- lack of suitable, high-quality learning resources.

In the US, many of these problems have been overcome by the development of accredited programmes, such as the Wound Ostomy and Continence Nurses Society (WOCN) programmes.

At a practical level, there are concerns that undergraduate and diplomate programmes:

- devote insufficient time to the subject
- rely too heavily on didactic teaching approaches
- are not interactive enough

- provide learning opportunities and assessment methods that do not sufficiently mirror the situations that clinicians will encounter in real life
- pay insufficient attention to fostering clinical reasoning and problem-solving skills.

As is described in Chapter 2, problem-based learning (PBL) is a valuable means for overcoming these deficiencies. PBL is now described as *the* alternative to 'traditional' curriculum design for tertiary education, satisfying all of the requirements for optimal learning.

This chapter describes how PBL can be used in undergraduate and postgraduate programmes, as well as for individual, independent learning. This approach is suitable for both specialist practitioners and for generalists who encounter patients with wounds during routine practice. It is suitable for novices, ideally under the supervision of a clinically based mentor, and for experienced practitioners, who realize that learning is a life-long process. The value of this approach is that it acknowledges that individuals can have very different learning needs.

NEW APPROACHES TO TEACHING AND LEARNING IN WOUND CARE

Learning through problem solving is an everyday process that has enabled the human species to survive and to evolve in an ever-changing world. Problems can drive the search for new knowledge by stimulating research questions and scientific inquiry (Margetson 1993). However, the traditional model of teaching and learning fails to capitalize on this natural learning process because in a typical curriculum knowledge is presented first, often by teaching staff from different disciplines, and problem-solving exercises are used later with the aim of encouraging students to apply information (Glen & Wilkie 2000).

Hallmarks of quality in learning

One of the most influential concepts to emerge in relation to student learning is Entwistle's (1988) distinction between deep and superficial approaches to learning.

Deep learning
This is characterized by the student's ability to:

- examine arguments critically
- look for patterns and underlying principles
- relate ideas to previous knowledge and experience.

The underlying intention of the student is to gain understanding. Research has shown that students who adopt a deep approach to learning also tend to act strategically. They put a consistent effort into studying, they manage their time effectively, they find appropriate materials for studying and are generally highly organized.

Superficial learning
This is characterized by the student who:

- studies without reflection
- treats the course as though it is composed of unrelated facts

- memorizes facts and procedures
- finds difficulty in making sense of new ideas.

The underlying intention is to cope with course requirements. These students are less focused, and generally less well organized.

Factors affecting students' approaches to learning

Educational research has shown that a student's approach to learning is influenced by many factors, including the nature of the teaching, the learning activities provided, the assessment procedures adopted and the personal qualities of the teacher (Entwistle 1994). Deep learning is more likely when:

- the teacher:
    - o inspires an interest in the subject
    - o is enthusiastic and empathetic
    - o demonstrates the relevance of the learning to the student's perceived needs
    - o gives a coherent overview of the subject, and
    - o gives clear explanations of concepts, when required
- the learning activities give the student practice in developing their understanding and applying knowledge to real-life situations
- the assessment methods require the student to demonstrate understanding and the ability to solve problems, rather than simply to repeat factual information.

PBL facilitates deep learning by emphasizing the importance of these issues.

The emergence of PBL

The impetus for PBL came in the 1980s from employers who observed that students on placements and newly qualified graduates could not apply knowledge effectively in real-life situations. An unintended consequence of the traditional *knowledge–problem–solution* sequence is that it can foster superficial rather than deep learning, with students studying to pass examinations rather than seeking real understanding for themselves (Sadlo 1995). A PBL curriculum has a different philosophy, which puts the responsibility for learning squarely onto the student. It entails a *problem–knowledge and understanding–solution* structure and, from the very beginning of a course, students work on scenarios that they will be expected to manage successfully once professionally qualified. The scenarios trigger in students both a need and a desire for relevant knowledge.

Although the recent history of PBL dates back to the setting up of a PBL course in medicine at McMaster University, Ontario, in the mid-1960s, its antecedents are much older and reflect the tutorial system still utilized at Oxford University, which dates back to medieval times. PBL has now spread from medical courses to other health professions, including nursing, dentistry and professions allied to medicine. The key educational objectives of PBL, as it applies to health care are:

- the acquisition of an integrated body of knowledge related to commonly encountered health problems
- the development and application of problem-solving skills
- the learning of clinical reasoning skills.

THE USE OF PBL IN THE CONTEXT OF TEACHING WOUND CARE TO UNDERGRADUATE AND POSTGRADUATE STUDENTS

The integration of theory with practice in the clinical setting has been seen as problematic in relation to the teaching of both nurses and doctors (Harden et al 1999, Hislop et al 1996). The Dearing and Garrick Reports of the National Committees of Enquiry into Higher Education, published in 1997, emphasized the value of flexible, self-directed approaches to learning in preference to traditional teacher-centred, subject-based methods. PBL is an attractive strategy for programmes that have a practice element because learning is integrated and contextualized (Wilkie & Burns 2003). As is illustrated in Chapter 5, patient assessment and care planning requires the application of knowledge from many different disciplines. Providing high-quality teaching and learning in this context requires teachers to:

- help students to perceive the relevance of different types of knowledge and to develop an interest in the syllabus
- provide a syllabus that encourages depth and avoids excessive rote learning
- encourage students to be more independent, purposeful and reflective in their approach to studying
- select text books and other learning resources that stimulate deep learning
- provide opportunities for discussion and collaborative working on realistic patient problems
- build in opportunities for exploring difficult concepts
- design assignments that encourage and reward critical thinking and reflection, and offer some flexibility in the choice of topics.

An example of how a PBL approach might be used in practice is illustrated in Box 1.1, in the context of facilitating pre-registration nursing students to learn more about the prevention and treatment of pressure ulcers. Although often regarded as 'basic' care, the case presented here is challenging, involving a number of quality assurance and management-related issues, as well as some very important clinical topics.

APPROACHES TO USING THIS BOOK

PBL is an attractive strategy for use in all wound-care programmes as learning is integrated and contextualized. So far, however, most textbooks in this field have tended to take a somewhat didactic approach, even when case studies have been included and have been recognized as providing important opportunities for learning (Morison 2001). Appropriate case studies are an invaluable aid to teaching clinical problem solving (Dowd & Davidhizar 1999) and it is no accident that the case studies are brought to the fore in the present book.

Different approaches to the use of PBL are explored in Chapter 2. The present book can be a valuable resource whether the approach taken to teaching the subject is 'pure' PBL, a hybrid approach, or where a more traditional approach is being taken. Its strengths lie in fostering skills that enable the reader to access knowledge from many sources and to solve the complex clinical problems that they will encounter in practice.

Box 1.1
An example of the use of a PBL approach to teaching wound care

During their undergraduate training, student nurses are presented with a case study involving an elderly woman, Mrs Smith, who has developed extensive pressure ulcers while in a nursing home following a stroke (Fig. 1.1). Mrs Smith is subsequently admitted to hospital in an attempt to heal the ulcers. In a situation where care has clearly been suboptimal, students will be highly motivated to evaluate the possible causes of the wound and they will be able to discuss many relevant factors, based on their earlier clinical experiences. They might speculate about the nature and extent of the tissue damage and about their reactions to having to cope with such a malodorous wound. The patient's relatives are threatening to sue the nursing home for negligence. Issues of professional accountability, quality assurance, and patient and carer education could well arise.

Students explore with their tutor the information that they will need to develop a plan of care. The learning objectives are decided upon by the students themselves. Topics selected by them could include: the structure and function of normal skin, the risk factors and causes of pressure ulcers, ways to assess the wound itself, the effects of nutrition on wound healing, the management of pain, possible local treatments for the ulcer (and the research evidence for their effectiveness), the indications for surgical intervention, and infection control.

Students then direct their own learning using a diversity of resources, which can include the 'resource' chapters (Chapters 6–20) in this book.

The group then meets again to enable members to share their recently found knowledge and to discuss new insights. The tutor will challenge their appreciation of the clinical significance of their new knowledge.

At every stage, students are active learners, autonomous and responsible for their own learning, with the tutor acting both as facilitator and as a safety net to ensure that the learning objectives are met.

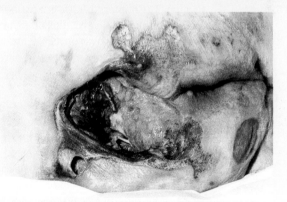

Figure 1.1
Extensive pressure area damage in an elderly woman following a stroke.

This text can be used by teachers as the basis of interactive small group work, in both higher education and practice settings, whether or not a PBL approach is being taken in the programme as a whole. It can also be used by healthcare professionals for individual, independent learning. It is suitable both for novices (ideally under the supervision of a clinically based mentor) and for experienced practitioners who realize that learning is a life-long process.

In the classroom

Developing suitable PBL materials can be a very time-consuming activity (Wilkie & Burns 2003). The scenarios presented in Section 2 are grouped according to the wound type. Teachers can review the scenarios and match them to the learning needs of students at particular stages in their education and training. Once the basic principles of patient assessment and care planning have been established, it can be useful to include ethical issues (Chapter 19) and practice development (Chapter 20). Case studies can be modified and multistage case studies developed by teaching staff so that topics can be explored in more breadth and depth (Box 1.2). Following a patient's progress over time also adds realism, and can make students aware of the consequences of the avoidable and unavoidable complications that can arise.

Students work in small groups with a facilitator to gain knowledge and acquire problem-solving skills. Problems are presented in the context in which they are most likely to be encountered and students are asked to:

1. clarify terms and concepts not readily understood
2. define the problem
3. analyse it
4. generate learning issues
5. collect information – outside of the tutorial group
6. report back to the group and to synthesize the new information.

Section 3 (Chapters 6–20) is a valuable resource for students to tap into, but should merely be regarded as one starting point to finding further information (see Chapter 4). Other sources of information and advice include societies and groups that specialize in wound care (Box 1.3), as well as conferences and specialist journals.

By the individual based in clinical practice

Reflection is an important skill for enhancing and improving practice. The identification of learning needs is often triggered by challenging cases encountered in real life. It is fully acknowledged that everyone's learning needs will be different. Individuals are therefore encouraged to read Chapter 3 first, which illustrates how it is possible to identify and clarify learning needs for oneself. Ways of systematically finding information to answer the questions identified are described in Chapter 4. Chapter 5 gives a coherent overview of issues relating to patient assessment and care planning. Chapters 6–20 provide a useful overview of key issues, such as nutrition, dressing selection and pain management, and these chapters might, in themselves, trigger new questions and should stimulate further enquiry.

Individuals with a special interest in a clinical topic might prefer to begin by reading the relevant chapters and then testing their understanding by applying

Box 1.2
An example of
a four-stage PBL
scenario

This scenario presents a sequence of events for the same patient. Students are encouraged to use the PBL process to work through each stage of Sharon's history. In each of the stages the student is asked to assume the identity of Sharon's named nurse.

Stage One

Sharon is an 18-year-old who developed septicaemia following meningococcal infection. Extensive purpuric lesions over all of her skin, particularly on the extremities and face, have left her with tissue necrosis of varying degrees on all of her limbs (Fig. 1.2).

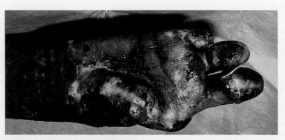

Figure 1.2
Extensive tissue necrosis following meningococcal infection.

Stage Two

Three weeks later, Sharon requires amputation of several fingers from both hands, and of her right leg below the knee.

Stage Three

Sharon spends 3 months in hospital for skin grafting and hand surgery to promote optimum function. She is then discharged but has to spend time away from home to have her leg prosthesis fitted and to attend rehabilitation to encourage her to walk.

Stage Four

Sharon is readmitted for a repeat skin graft to her right knee (Fig. 1.3) and to surrounding areas, using stored skin. She has numerous superficial wounds on

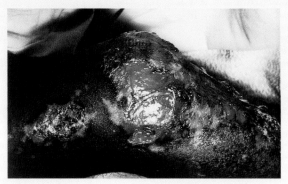

Figure 1.3
The previous graft to the knee has failed.

continued

Box 1.2 continued

her knees and elbows (Fig. 1.4). Many of these areas have been grafted – with varying degrees of success. On admission, Sharon is angry and depressed. Her mother admits that she is finding things difficult. Her marriage is under pressure, in part because of attending to Sharon's hygiene needs and daily wound dressing changes. Fearful of infection, she has limited visits from Sharon's friends. Angry, isolated and in pain, Sharon has subjected her mother to intense psychological pressure and verbal outbursts. Independently, they complain that they are receiving conflicting information and advice from different professionals in the multidisciplinary team responsible for Sharon's care.

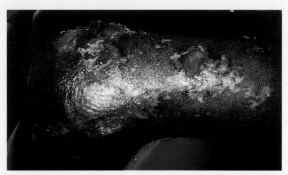

Figure 1.4
Numerous superficial wounds.

Box 1.3 *Other sources of information and opportunities for networking*

Cochrane Wounds Group
Health Sciences Research
Seebohm Rowntree Building
University of York
York YO10 5DD, UK
Website: www.cochranewounds.org

European Pressure Ulcer Advisory Panel (EPUAP)
Wound Healing Institute
Department of Dermatology
The Churchill Hospital
Old Road
Headington
Oxford OX3 7LJ, UK
e-mail: EuropeanPressureUlcerAdvisPanel @compuserv.com

The Tissue Viability Society (TVS)
Glanville Centre
Salisbury District Hospital
Salisbury SP2 8BJ, UK
Website: www.tvs.org.uk

Wound Care Society
PO Box 170
Hartford
Huntingdon PE29 1PL, UK
Website: www.woundcaresociety.org

Wound, Ostomy and Continence Nurses Society (WOCN)
WOCN National Office
4700 W. Lake Ave
Glenview, IL 60025, USA
Website: www.wocn.org

the insights gained to the relevant case studies. This is a more traditional approach but it can be a useful way of consolidating existing knowledge as well as identifying further learning needs.

CONCLUSION

Although it is now widely accepted that healthcare provision should be evidence based, approaches to fostering high-quality teaching and learning in wound care have tended to lag behind the evidence provided by educational research. The arguments for using a PBL approach in this context are compelling.

The present text can be used as the basis of interactive small group work, in both higher education and practice settings, or it can be used by healthcare professionals for independent learning. Its strengths lie in fostering skills that enable the reader to access knowledge from many sources and to solve complex clinical problems. It should therefore be regarded as a springboard to encouraging self-directed, life-long learning in an ever-changing and clinically challenging field.

REFERENCES

Dowd S B, Davidhizar R 1999 Using case studies to teach clinical problem solving. Nurse Educator 24(5):42–46

Entwistle N J 1988 Styles of learning and teaching. David Fulton, London

Entwistle N J 1994 Teaching and the quality of learning. CVCP, London

Glen S, Wilkie K (eds) 2000 Problem-based learning in nursing: a new model for a new context? Macmillan Press, London

Harden R M, Crosby J R, Davis M H 1999 An introduction to outcome-based education. Medical Teacher 21:7–14

Hislop S, Inglis B, Cope P et al 1996 Situating theory in practice: student views of theory and practice in Project 2000 nursing programmes. Journal of Advanced Nursing 23:171–177

Margetson D B 1993 Understanding problem-based learning. Educational Philosophy and Theory 25(1):40–57

Morison M (ed) 2001 The prevention and treatment of pressure ulcers. Mosby, Edinburgh

National Committee of Enquiry into Higher Education (the Dearing Report) 1997 Higher Education in the Learning Society, NCHIE, London

National Committee of Enquiry into Higher Education (the Garrick Report) 1997 Higher Education in the Learning Society: Report of the Scottish Committee, NCHIE, London

Sadlo G 1995 Problem-based learning. Tertiary Education News 5(6):8–11

Wilkie K, Burns I 2003 Problem-based learning: a handbook for nurses. Palgrave Macmillan, Basingstoke

FURTHER READING

Glen S, Wilkie K (eds) 2000 Problem-based learning in nursing: a new model for a new context? Macmillan Press, London

Rideout E 2001 Transforming nurse education through problem-based learning. Jones and Bartlett, Boston, MA

Wilkie K, Burns I 2003 Problem-based learning: a handbook for nurses. Palgrave Macmillan, Basingstoke

2

What is problem-based learning?

Kay Wilkie

CHAPTER CONTENTS

INTRODUCTION

This chapter provides an introduction to problem-based learning (PBL), highlighting the reasons for its increasing use as a learning and teaching strategy. PBL promotes learning by encouraging students to engage with material presented in the form of scenarios, which present a problem. Students work together in small groups to try to resolve the problem. The problem-based approach differs from other learning and teaching strategies, such as problem-solving, in that students are presented with the problem *first*. Knowledge is acquired and developed as a consequence of trying to find a solution to the problem. PBL originated in medical education in North America in the 1960s. From there its use has spread to many other countries and disciplines. As the method has grown in popularity, it has been altered and adapted to meet the needs of the various programmes, professions and cultures that have adopted it. The number of problem-based healthcare programmes has increased rapidly over the past decade. Although it is used mainly in courses that prepare students for occupations that have a vocational element, such as engineering and health care, it is also employed in a diversity of other courses, such as English literature and ballet.

What, then, is PBL and why is it regarded by many educationalists as an attractive and appropriate strategy?

TERMINOLOGY

Barrows, one of the 'founding fathers' of PBL, commented in 1986 that there were almost as many forms of PBL as there were courses. Sometimes the adaptations in PBL have led to the relabelling of the strategy, for example as context-based learning (CBL) or enquiry-based learning (EBL). Some of these variations adhere to the principles of PBL whereas others do not, even although they continue to be called 'PBL'. In other instances, the PBL strategy remains but it has been relabelled because the course organizers have disliked the term 'problem', claiming that patients or clients should not be considered as problems. This book uses the term PBL because it is the original term and continues to be the most widely used. The 'problems' presented in the book should be seen as being problems, situations or challenges for the student to explore, and should not be interpreted as implying 'problem clients' or 'problem patients'.

THE ORIGINS OF PBL

The development of PBL as a learning and teaching strategy is usually credited to the Faculty of Health Sciences at McMaster University, Hamilton, Ontario. The originators at McMaster, however, point out that some of their inspiration for PBL came from the use of cases in medical education pioneered by Case Western University in the early 1960s, and also from the work of Dewy in the 1930s, the tutorial system at Oxford University in medieval times and even from the teachings of Socrates. The impetus for the development of PBL at McMaster came from increasing dissatisfaction with subject-based teaching methods such as lectures. The disadvantages of lectures include inhibition of student interaction with teachers and presenting each subject as a discrete area. In clinical practice, students are expected to draw together elements from each of the subject areas, such as anatomy, pathophysiology and pharmacology, and to apply them to individual patients. Individual subjects were perceived to have a hierarchical order, thus the underlying assumption was that students could not be introduced to disease processes until they had studied all of the normal anatomy and physiology. However, students reaching the clinical years of the programme had often forgotten the material that had been taught in the earlier years. A further difficulty was the rapid advance in medical science. Even where students were taught the most up-to-date information available, it could be anticipated that much of it would be obsolete within a few years of their qualification. Incorporating recent changes in diagnosis and treatment methods into traditional curricula raised problems with timetabling and sequencing. Staff at McMaster therefore sought a strategy that would integrate and contextualize the various subject areas, allow patient-centred teaching to be introduced early in the programmes and provide students with the skills to keep abreast of current changes in medicine. The result was problem-based learning (Neufeld & Barrows 1974).

PBL was adopted rapidly by other American medical schools and spread to medical schools in Australia and Europe. The experiences of medicine education were transferred to other vocational programmes, for example occupational therapy, nursing, engineering, law and architecture. PBL has been recommended as a strategy for healthcare professional education by institutions such as the World Health Organization (WHO 1993) and the World Bank (1993). The Report of the UKCC Commission for Nursing and Midwifery Education (UKCC 1999) recommended the use of PBL as a strategy to assist with the integration of theory with practice in nursing programmes. More recently, PBL has been applied successfully in courses as diverse as mathematics, English literature and ballet; it is also used in both primary and secondary school education. Although originally devised as a small-group technique, the strategy has been employed effectively by individual students in open, distance and e-learning (Price 2000, Rogerson 2003).

THE PBL PROCESS

The problem-based strategy is interactive. It allows students to discuss and explore issues that they perceive as relevant to them, it integrates and contextualizes their learning, it promotes evidence-based practice and it helps to develop the lifelong learning skills essential to functioning in the ever-changing climate of health care. PBL has as an added bonus that both students and facilitators report it to be enjoyable.

In the original PBL format, students work in small groups (ideally five to eight people) with a tutor or facilitator. Staffing and accommodation constraints in nurse education have resulted in the use of groups of up to 12 (groups with more than 12 members are too big for the PBL process to function effectively) and the development of problem-based materials in an open-learning format (such as this book). Barrows (1988) stated that the role of the facilitator is to assist students in identifying their learning needs, to keep the PBL process moving, to ensure that all students are involved and to probe students' understanding. However, Schmidt (1994) found that many students have the ability to work without the constant attention of a facilitator. The student group is presented with a problem that requires a solution. Problems are based on real patients/clients and mirror the situations that students will encounter in practice. The PBL process consists of a series of stages: engaging with the material presented in the problem, identifying the issues, defining individual learning needs, undertaking the learning and applying the learning to the original problem to create a solution. Wilkie (2002) likened the process to that of an orchestra performing (Table 2.1).

Examining the trigger material

The first step in the PBL process consists of examining the 'trigger'. 'Triggers' are material that is intended to stimulate learning. They come in a variety of formats (Box 2.1) to stimulate discussion.

Included with the trigger is often a statement to indicate the situation in which the student is placed, e.g. named nurse, nurse specialist. If the students are qualified staff they might be asked to apply the situation as it might arise in their everyday work. Some PBL scenarios might include a PBL task such as creation of a care pathway or compilation of a discharge plan. Students should take time to consider the trigger material and, when working in groups, they should ensure that they all have a similar understanding of the trigger. Students using PBL in an open, distance or electronic setting might want to discuss the trigger with others on the programme or with colleagues or they might brainstorm the issues, have a short break and then look at the trigger again. Occasionally, students will have difficulty in identifying issues from the trigger. In this situation it might be useful to consider feelings or responses to the trigger. Some triggers can be upsetting, some can appear trivial or silly at first glance. Expressing these feelings can help with identifying topics for discussion.

Table 2.1
The music of PBL

Stage in the performance	What happens
Tuning up: introductory session	The phase following the issue of the trigger. The initial silence is broken as students, in twos and threes, begin to seek clarification from each other about the trigger and situation
	Students working with open or distance material read the material several times, noting concepts that seem important
Overture: introductory session	Students begin to compare ideas. Themes that will be identified as learning issues start to be heard, much like an operatic overture, in which fragments of the main musical themes are heard for the first time
	Students with open or distance material, brainstorm and begin to note themes and make links
The performance: introductory session/ intermission	The individual themes are expanded and developed. Previous learning is applied and new learning needs identified
	Students seek the required new learning (intermission)
Finale: feedback session	The new learning is applied to and integrated with existing learning and tested against the original scenario for fit – does it provide an evidence-based solution or improvement to the original situation?

Box 2.1 _Examples of PBL triggers_	• **Paper cases**, e.g. case notes, referral letters, charts, nursing notes, discharge summaries. • **Photographs/pictures/story boards**, e.g. pictures of patients over time, nurses in a range of settings, wound stages, classical paintings such as battle scenes. • **Music**, e.g. classical, popular. • **Equipment**, types of wound dressings, cleansing solutions. • **Games**, snakes and ladders, with ladders as elements promoting wound healing and snakes as factors that inhibit healing. • **Literature/poetry**, e.g. from Romeo and Juliet 'he jests at scars that never felt a wound' Shakespeare. • **Videos**. • **Simulated patients/clients/carers**, who can give histories and who can be given a simulated wound. • **Simulators**, e.g. sacral pressure ulcer simulator.

Identifying learning needs and seeking out the evidence

When the situation has been discussed, students then clarify the issues to be explored. Prior learning is noted and applied at this point. Students have the opportunity to share any personal previous learning with the group and to relate it to the problem under consideration. Following exploration of the problem, learning needs are identified, often being formulated as questions to be answered. The resulting work is divided among the group members through negotiation within the group. Students then seek out the evidence to supply the answers. This can be undertaken individually or by two or three students if the topic is large and does not lend itself to subdivision. Dividing the workload across a number of students allows more material to be searched and brought back to the group than could be undertaken by a single student alone. To achieve the identified learning, students need to identify their learning needs (Chapter 3) and to develop literature-searching skills (Chapter 4).

Formulating a solution

Learning is brought back to the group, integrated and applied to the problem to create a resolution. During this discussion students are expected to challenge the material and to justify their findings.

THE PHILOSOPHY UNDERPINNING PBL

Using PBL might require a shift in beliefs about how learning is best achieved.

The foundationalist perspective

Many subject-based courses adopt a foundationalist perspective, which views knowledge as being fixed. Transmission of knowledge is seen as being one-way, from teacher to student. Subjects are treated as sequential, with some being given higher status than others. The philosophy is that learning about certain topics cannot begin until others have been covered. The motivation for learning is often to pass tests or to meet assignments. As a result, material can be poorly learned and quickly forgotten. This style of learning is sometimes referred to as 'surface learning' (Marton & Säljö 1976).

The coherentist perspective

In contrast, PBL adopts a coherentist view of knowledge (Margetson 1991), which sees knowledge as ever-changing. Learning is regarded as part of society and as occurring in a variety of settings, not restricted to being enrolled on a course. Everyone is seen as possessing some relevant knowledge. Teachers are not portrayed as all-knowing or as having all of the answers. Subjects are learned and assigned importance in accordance with the needs of the problem situation. In vocational programmes this belief allows practice issues to be raised from the start of a programme. The theory is that learning takes place for learning's sake and is not motivated solely by the need to pass examinations. It is therefore more likely to endure. This type of learning can be referred to as deep learning (Marton and Säljö 1976).

Applying the coherentist perspective through PBL
PBL was originally devised as a learning philosophy that was applied across the whole curriculum. The entire curriculum was structured around problem scenarios from the beginning. Lectures were reduced to a minimum, often

offered at student request on given topics. The McMaster undergraduate medical programme reduced lectures on anatomy and physiology from 1000 hours to nil. Other resources were developed to support student learning. In addition to library facilities, and in later years computer databases and internet access, resources included laboratories, statutory and voluntary agencies and contact numbers for expert practitioners. PBL is potentially a resource-intensive strategy. This attribute has led educational institutions to look at alternative ways of designing problem-based curricula (Box 2.2).

The mainly anecdotal evidence published on these uses of PBL suggests that while they can be successful, there are potential pitfalls. Where PBL is used in only part of a programme, students might be unfamiliar with the technique. Lack of understanding of the process of PBL by both students and teachers can cause the module to be poorly evaluated, often being seen as a 'soft option'. Alternatively, PBL can be perceived as too difficult by students used to a traditional teaching delivery that directs them to what has to be learned. Initially, the lack of teacher direction in PBL can lead to feelings of insecurity in students because they might be uncertain that they are learning the 'right' material. Alternatively, students who welcome the opportunity to identify their own learning needs might be dissatisfied on their return to subject-based teaching, where they are guided to learn what the teacher thinks that they should learn. Care is also required if PBL is adopted for a single strand within a curriculum. PBL is well suited to topics that require integration of material from a variety of sources. If the topic is too narrowly defined, PBL might not allow students sufficient scope for application of knowledge, leading to boredom.

In nursing and midwifery programmes, PBL is commonly utilized as one of several teaching strategies. Programmes are organized around problems but 'fixed resources' are provided in the form of lectures, skills workshops and open learning. If this design is utilized, the curriculum delivery team must ensure that the fixed resources do not simply provide all of the material that students should be addressing through PBL. Where double teaching of material occurs, students can lose interest and fail to develop the lifelong learning skills required for professional life. Some organizations claim to use PBL as an 'integrator'. The students are given scenarios that draw on material from a range of taught subjects. If this style of PBL is employed, the scenarios should trigger new learning. Where new learning is not required, this strategy becomes problem-solving rather than problem-based, and therefore students will not gain the benefits associated with PBL.

Box 2.2 *Some designs for problem-based curricula*	<ul><li>**'Pure' format PBL**, can reduce the overall amount of teacher contact. Many institutions have found that it requires increased teaching input.</li><li>**Parallel-track PBL**, PBL option offered to around 20% of the intake. Runs concurrently with the subject-based curriculum.</li><li>**Single-strand PBL**, PBL used in specific parts of a programme, for example a single module, or term, or for a specific subject.</li><li>**Hybrid PBL**, PBL used with other teaching strategies.</li></ul>

Currently, there is no single agreed definition of PBL. In a study on the use of PBL in four different institutions and disciplines, Savin-Baden (2000) identified five models of PBL used within curricula to meet different needs. These ranged from PBL for epistemological competence to PBL for critical contestability. The models were not specific to any discipline or institution. Savin-Baden claimed that, whereas the choice of model might relate to the overall aims of the programme, factors such as assessment strategies and facilitator beliefs about student learning and its purpose influenced the form of PBL chosen. Thus, several of the identified models might be in use at any one time in a given curriculum. The debate continues among the many proponents of PBL, who are agreed on one issue – problem-based learning is a valuable and enjoyable strategy.

STRENGTHS OF PBL

PBL has many strengths, including the promotion of adult learning styles, learning in context, the currency of learning, student centredness, the ability to handle complexity, the development of critical thinking and other transferable skills, and increased flexibility.

Learning styles

PBL reflects the principles of adult learning. Knowles (1978) identified that adults learn cumulatively as they acquire growing familiarity with a topic. Learning takes place where it is relevant to the students' own aims and goals and where students have the opportunity to identify for themselves what they need to learn. Adult learning is fostered by having opportunities to think through what has been learned, to test the new learning to find out how well material has been learned and to apply the new learning. Most of us can identify with these concepts. Learning a foreign language is easier and better remembered when we have a reason for learning it, such as a holiday. We decide which language we need to learn and try it out on fellow learners and friends. Using the newly learned language on holiday reinforces the learning and creates new learning. Commonly used words such as 'hello', 'please', 'thank you' and the names of food and drink are thus more easily learned, for example, than the names of parts of the body. PBL operates in a similar way. Scenarios are based on situations that will commonly be encountered in practice, such as the care of an elderly immobile patient with a pressure sore (Chapter 14). Students identify what they already know about a situation and what they will need to learn to improve the situation for the patient or client. They then find the evidence, bring it back and test their learning within the group. Experience in practice allows the learning to be applied. Application in practice creates new learning that may be relevant to another situation. This builds up a body of professional knowledge and the skills required to keep the knowledge base up to date with current research.

Learning in context

Learning is also more effective when it takes place in context. Car maintenance, for example, is learned better by working through specific elements, such as oil changing or spark-plug cleaning, than by beginning with the theory of the internal combustion engine. By the end of the course, participants will have built up an understanding of the workings of the internal combustion engine through cumulative learning. PBL promotes learning in context. In a subject-based curriculum, care of a patient with a venous leg ulcer, for example, might be taught through lectures or workshops. These focus on separate aspects: normal anatomy and physiology of the vascular system in the lower limb, pathophysiology of peripheral vascular disease and chronic venous hypertension, psychology of chronic illness, sociology of the sick role plus the necessary nursing skills such as Doppler monitoring and health education (Chapter 15). These subjects might be taught at different points in the curriculum. When nurses encounter a patient with a leg ulcer, they have to pull together all of this knowledge from the various memorized compartments. In a problem-based curriculum, the students would be presented with the problem of caring holistically for a patient with a leg ulcer. They have to decide what they will need to know. Their learning is organized to fit the context in which it will be used in practice. Previous knowledge, such as the physiology of blood flow to the lower limb and the importance of patient-centred education, can be recognized and incorporated into learning about leg ulcers.

Currency of learning

PBL is claimed to offer benefits relating to current and updateable knowledge, retention of knowledge and improved communication skills. There is little empirical evidence to indicate that students from problem-based programmes perform better than students from subject-based programmes in examinations. There is, however, some evidence to support the concept of improved retention of knowledge and the development of lifelong learning skills. Studies by Norman and Schmidt (1992) found that graduates from problem-based medical programmes could recall more information in the years after graduation than those who had graduated from more traditional programmes. In a study of Canadian medical graduates, Shin et al (1993) discovered that those who had undertaken problem-based programmes had more up-to-date knowledge in the years after graduation than those who had undertaken subject-based courses.

Student centredness

Student-centred learning places the ownership of and the responsibility for learning with the student (Rogers 1969). Learning is self-initiated and the learner also has responsibility for evaluating the results. Unlike problem-solving approaches, where students are presented with problems *after* they have had some teaching input, PBL operates by presenting students with the problem *before* they have undertaken learning. The approach is highly student-centred because students have to identify what they need to learn, rather than being told what they ought to learn. Although the scenario is created by teaching staff, students have the freedom to select the topics that they want to explore. Unlike lectures, in which the material is chosen by the teacher and is aimed towards a broad spectrum of the class, PBL can be tailored to the individual needs of the students. In pre-registration nursing programmes, for example, students come from a variety of backgrounds. Some students have just left high school, others might have been care assistants. PBL allows the school leavers to focus more on nursing skills while allowing those who have been out of formal education for some time to give more attention to aspects such as physiology. The application and integration of individual learning to the PBL scenario benefits all the students in the group. Students have the opportunity to share their experience with other members of the group.

Barrows (1988) pointed out that few students arrive on courses completely without knowledge. This can be particularly beneficial when teaching those who already possess a first-level degree or qualification and who also have professional experience on which to draw. This belief, coupled with the coherentist view of knowledge, allows students to begin to address practice issues from an early point in the programme. As knowledge is related to individual student needs, there is no requirement to wait until students have been taught about one subject before introducing another. Students can be given a problem related to, for example, a diabetic patient who has developed a foot ulcer, with no prior learning about the structure and function of the pancreas. Students will identify that they need to learn about insulin production and control in order to resolve the situation.

In addition to deciding what should be learned, students also have control over the organization of PBL sessions, deciding how long should be spent on discussion of each of the topics raised, even when breaks should be taken. The division of work is also discussed and decided by the group, as is the method of presenting material.

Handling complexity

PBL is particularly useful for dealing with problems that are complex and might not have a clear-cut solution. Such problems mirror the types of situations that students are likely to meet in practice situations. Evidence presented to the English National Board for Nursing, Midwifery and Health Visiting (1998) indicated that PBL was effective in assisting students to deal with complex situations. The PBL approach differs from other learning and teaching approaches in that there is no single 'right' answer. Students are not expected to reach a preset answer devised in advance by the facilitator. Students often produce acceptable solutions to problems that have not been identified by the facilitator.

Critical thinking

PBL is claimed to promote critical thinking. Glen (1995) pointed out that critical thinking is a complex concept that is further compounded when linked with the complexities of nursing. She argues that, as the nature of health care is changing constantly and will vary according to context, students need to develop critical thinking skills that will enable them 'to formulate well-thought-through but always tentative views of their own on contentious health issues' (p 175). Through addressing problems, questioning and considering alternative solutions, students begin to develop the skills required for critical thinking. In PBL, material brought back to the group is integrated with the material brought by the other members. Students are required to justify the application of their intervention. Through challenge from peers and discussion, group members begin to develop the skills necessary to make an informed judgement about material and the choices made.

Transferable skills

Although the PBL process promotes the learning of content, it also has the potential to provide experience of skills that are difficult to teach by other methods. These include team-working skills, literature-searching skills and skills required in nursing, such as care planning, interviewing and assessment. The problem scenarios can be designed to include some of these skills. Where

PBL is run through small groups, the team members have to learn to work with each other. This involves the development of sound communication skills. Students need to ensure that all members of the group understand what is presented. Team-working includes ensuring that everyone has an equal share of the workload and that the same members do not consistently do most of the work. Members are expected to manage the group in situations where work is not produced or if there is disharmony between members. Working in this way promotes skills that will be required when working within a nursing or multi-disciplinary team.

Flexibility

PBL is flexible and allows curricula to be tailored to meet the needs of the environment in which students will work. A community nursing scenario, for example, might focus on caring for a terminally ill patient, a problem that could be encountered worldwide. In the UK or USA, provision of social support might be identified as an issue, whereas in South Africa a major issue could be access to fresh water. New scenarios can be written to reflect recent advances in healthcare technology and treatments, such as gene therapy, or a change in epidemiology, such as the increase in tuberculosis. There is no need to rewrite the curriculum totally or to radically alter timetables but rather to adapt them to meet local needs.

DRAWBACKS TO PBL

Although the PBL strategy has many strengths that make it attractive to nurse education, there are also some disadvantages. As mentioned above, PBL is resource intensive. Increased group size and the use of open learning material help to offset the need for facilitators, but the need for access to resources such as books, journals and the worldwide web remains. To be effective, PBL requires a particular pedagogical stance, namely that students are capable, active learners who can be trusted to take responsibility for their own learning. Although at first glance this might seem a reasonable belief, many students and teachers come from a background where the control of learning lies with the teacher, and students expect to be told what to learn and how to learn it. Having the freedom to decide one's own learning needs can be frightening and create uncertainty about what should be learned. Other disadvantages relate to teaching roles because staff can feel that they are undervalued and have lost their status as 'experts' when PBL is implemented. The authors of this book believe that teacher expertise is retained in developing trigger materials that will stimulate learning and in facilitating learning by providing guidance.

EVALUATING PBL AND ASSESSING THE STUDENT

Any process that seeks to measure the effectiveness of PBL must match the PBL process. Traditional, time-limited examinations do not fit well with PBL. When students have identified their own learning needs it is difficult to test what they have actually learned. This might be one reason why students from PBL programmes do not perform any better in examinations than students from subject-based programmes. They do not, however, perform any worse (Albanese 2000). Traditional PBL assessments such as the triple-jump exercise, are too time consuming for most nursing programmes (Taylor & Marks-Maran 2000).

Assignments based around problems, such as care studies and projects, fit well with PBL. Portfolios, which include evidence of learning opportunities along with a reflective account of the learning that has taken place, also match the PBL process. They are, however, time-consuming to grade. Use of information technology makes it possible for the portfolio to be built up and modified online, allowing for continuous review by facilitators.

Although facilitators can evaluate the performance of students in PBL groups, PBL is a student-centred process and reflection by students on their learning of both factual knowledge and the processes involved in learning is, possibly, the most effective form of evaluation.

CONCLUSION

PBL is interactive, relevant and real. It integrates subject areas, contextualizes learning and promotes learning for its own sake. Under student control, it provides opportunities for new ideas to be explored and challenged, thus providing increased understanding. Problem-based learning has the potential to develop sound communication skills and critical-thinking skills. PBL has the potential to develop the lifelong learning skills required by healthcare professionals in the twenty-first century. The strategy is particularly applicable to learning in relation to wound care.

REFERENCES

Albanese M 2000 Problem-based learning; why curricula are unlikely to show little effect on knowledge or clinical skills. Medical Education 34(9):729–738

Barrows H S 1986 A taxonomy of problem-based learning methods. Medical Education 20:481–486

Barrows H S 1988 The tutorial process. Southern Illinois University School of Medicine, Springfield, IL

English National Board for Nursing, Midwifery and Health Visiting 1998 Developments in the use of an evidence and/or enquiry-based approach in Nursing, Midwifery and Health Visiting Programmes of Education. ENB, London

Glen S 1995 Developing critical thinking in higher education. Nurse Education Today 15:170–176

Knowles M 1978 The adult learner: a neglected species. Gulf Publishing Co, Houston, TX

Margetson D 1991 Problem-focused education and the question of theory and practice, with special reference to some university courses. Unpublished PhD Thesis, University of Tasmania

Marton F, Säljö J 1976 On qualitative differences in learning. I. Outcome and process. British Journal of Educational Psychology 46:4–11

Neufeld V R, Barrows H S 1974 The McMaster Philosophy: an approach to medical education. Journal of Medical Education 49:1040–1050

Norman R, Schmidt H G 1992 The psychological basis of problem-based learning: a review of the evidence. Academic Medicine 67(9):557–565

Price B 2000 Introducing problem-based learning into distance learning. In: Glen S, Wilkie K (eds) Implementing problem-based learning in nursing. Macmillan, Basingstoke

Rogers C 1969 Freedom to learn. Merrill, Columbus, OH

Rogerson E (2003) The role and facilitation of problem-based learning in a distance learning programme leading to the award of Bachelor of Nursing. PhD Thesis, University of Dundee

Savin-Baden M 2000 Problem-based learning in higher education: Untold stories. Open University Press/SRHE, Buckingham

Schmidt H G 1994 Resolving inconsistencies in tutor expertise research: does lack of structure cause students to seek tutor guidance? Academic Medicine 69(8):656–662

Shin J H, Haynes B, Johnston M E 1993 Effect of problem-based, self-directed undergraduate education on life-long learning. Canadian Medical Association Journal 146(6):969–976

Taylor B, Marks-Maran D 2000 Assessment in problem-based learning. In: Glen S, Wilkie K (eds) Implementing problem-based learning in nursing. Macmillan, Basingstoke

UKCC 1999 Fitness for practice. The report of the Commission for Nursing and Midwifery Education. UKCC, London

WHO 1993 Increasing the relevance of education for health professionals. WHO, Geneva

Wilkie M C K 2002 Actions, attitudes and attributes: developing facilitation skills for problem-based learning. Unpublished PhD thesis, Coventry University

World Bank 1993 World development report 1993: investing in health. Oxford University Press, Oxford

FURTHER READING

Boud D, Feletti G (eds) 1997 The challenge of problem-based learning, 2nd edn. Kogan Page, London

Duch B J, Groh S E, Allen D E (eds) 2001 The power of problem-based learning. Stylus, Sterling, VA

Rideout E 2001 Transforming nursing education through problem-based learning. Jones and Bartlett, Boston, MA

Wilkie K, Burns I 2003 Implementing PBL: a handbook for nurses. Palgrave Macmillan, Basingstoke

3

Identifying your learning needs

Moya J Morison

CHAPTER CONTENTS

INTRODUCTION

This chapter aims to help you to identify your learning needs in relation to the case studies presented in Section 2. The chapter is intended for use both by individuals who are studying alone and by groups who have decided to use a problem-based learning approach. For those working in groups, this will involve coming to a shared understanding of the issues before organizing the workload associated with finding the answers to the issues identified. The skills involved are an important component of continuing professional development and reflective practice. Ultimately, it is up to you to decide what you need to learn and how you are going to achieve it.

PRACTICE IN IDENTIFYING YOUR LEARNING NEEDS

This chapter is centred around a number of activities that will give you practice in identifying your learning needs. It is a useful guide to the types of questions to ask yourself when working on the cases given in Section 2.

Activity 1 *Identifying your learning needs*	Read the case study in Box 3.1. Assume that you have just encountered this patient for the first time and that you have been given the responsibility for assessing, planning, implementing and evaluating her care.
	Question 1. What are the key issues that you will need to address?
	Question 2. Which of these issues are immediate and which are medium and longer term?

Hint: Jot down your ideas in any order, as they come to you, and then attempt to reorganize them. What questions might you ask yourself when presented with a patient such as this?

| **Box 3.1** **An introduction to Mrs Rudetsky** | Mrs Rudetsky is 50 years old and has a large ulcer on her right leg (Fig. 3.1). She is clinically obese and a non-insulin-dependent diabetic. She has complained of pain in her leg, especially at dressing changes, and this has yet to be resolved. She has become unpopular with the community nurses because of her abrupt manner and they have adopted a rota system to share the responsibility for her care, which includes daily dressing changes. |

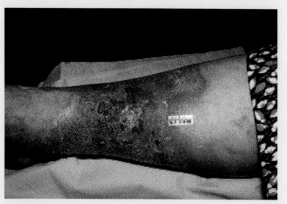

Figure 3.1
A leg ulcer in an obese 50-year-old woman

Commentary on Activity 1
The issues that you have identified can probably be grouped under three broad headings:
1. knowledge
2. skills
3. attitude.

Two scenarios related to Mrs Rudetsky are presented below. The first considers the learning needs of Community Nurse Green, who is a novice in relation to leg ulcers, and the second the learning needs of Community Nurse McMasters, a more experienced nurse. Where would you position yourself – are you a novice, an expert, or somewhere in between? Compare the needs that you have identified with the scenarios below.

The learning needs identified by Community Nurse Green, who has little or no experience of caring for a patient with a leg ulcer

Knowledge

1. Assessing the underlying cause of the leg ulcer:
  - What are the most common causes of leg ulcers?
  - How can I decide the cause of Mrs Rudetsky's leg ulcer? What assessment methods should I use?
  - Might I need to refer Mrs Rudetsky for a specialist assessment? What criteria should I use to decide whether a referral is needed?

2. Local wound assessment and management:
  - The wound bed looks unhealthy. How can I tell whether the wound is healing or not?
  - How should I dress it?

3. Pain assessment and management:
  - How can I assess Mrs Rudetsky's pain?
  - Is it due to the dressing adhering? If so, how does this affect my choice of dressing?
  - How can her pain best be managed?

4. Factors delaying healing:
  - Could Mrs Rudetsky's diabetes be affecting the healing process? If so, how?
  - What influence is Mrs Rudetsky's obesity likely to have on the healing process?

Skills

Assessment and bandaging skills:
  - Is it safe to apply a compression bandage to Mrs Rudetsky's leg? (answering this question involves both knowledge and skill in the assessment process)
  - Should I take any special precautions when bandaging Mrs Rudetsky's leg, because she is diabetic?

Attitude

Feelings, attitudes and their consequences:
  - What are my feelings towards this patient, whom other nurses have labelled as abusive, lazy and non-compliant with treatment?
  - What influence might any negative feelings have on the quality of care that I give?

The learning needs identified by Community Nurse McMasters, who has more experience of caring for patients with leg ulcers

Knowledge

1. Assessing the underlying cause of the leg ulcer:
  - This looks like a 'classic' venous ulcer, but how can I be sure?
  - What vascular assessments have already been undertaken and when? What do they suggest? What would indicate that it would be prudent to reassess Mrs Rudetsky's peripheral vascular problems?

2. Local wound assessment and management:
  - Should we be using a pre-existing local wound assessment tool to enable us to assess and monitor Mrs Rudetsky's leg ulcer more systematically? What tools are in existence? Which one might be most appropriate for Mrs Rudetsky?

continued

(continued)

    – A number of new wound dressing products has recently come on the market. What are their performance characteristics? What would be best in Mrs Rudetsky's case?

3. Pain assessment and management:
    – Are the pharmacological methods of pain management currently being used the most effective?
    – Is there a place here for also trying some non-pharmacological methods? What are the options? What could we try first?

4. Factors delaying healing:
    – Who else is currently involved in Mrs Rudetsky's diabetic care? Who is liaising between the different agencies involved and how well is this liaison working in practice? Are there any models in existence for best practice in relation to interagency working?
    – Mrs Rudetsky's obesity is recorded in the nursing notes but could she also be deficient in any micronutrients? How could we assess this?

Skills
Assessment and bandaging skills:
- Because of her diabetes, I am particularly concerned about Mrs Rudetsky's peripheral circulation. How can I assess this in the clinic? I have little experience with diabetic patients. Is there anyone with these skills locally who can supervise my practice until I feel confident and can demonstrate that I am competent?
- I am concerned about the sub-bandage pressures that I am achieving when I bandage Mrs Rudetsky's leg – I may be applying too much pressure, which is hazardous, or I may be applying insufficient pressure to have a therapeutic effect. How can I measure the pressures that I am actually achieving? Might my colleagues benefit from exploring these practical issues too? Who can help us to address these practical learning needs?

Attitude
Feelings, attitudes and their consequences:
- Is there such a thing as 'the unpopular patient' and if so what are the consequences for the patient, and for their professional and lay carers?
- How can I help the 'team' to develop a more therapeutic relationship with Mrs Rudetsky?
- How important is it that we ensure continuity of care? How have other nurses overcome the problems that we are facing with the organization of Mrs Rudetsky's care?

PEOPLE'S LEARNING NEEDS ARE DIFFERENT

Clearly, the learning needs of a nurse who already has considerable experience of caring for patients with leg ulcers are different from the needs of a novice in this area, as illustrated above. However, even the 'expert' in tissue viability is likely to have some learning needs, whether these relate to keeping up to date with the latest wound care dressing products, the therapeutic use of more experimental treatments such as growth factors, the use of adjuvant therapies such as low intensity light laser, or the best ways to organize a service.

A central tenet of PBL is that *you* decide what you need to know, not the authors of this book! This book is merely a springboard to deeper learning.

TRANSLATING YOUR LEARNING NEEDS INTO ANSWERABLE QUESTIONS

The next step is to translate your learning needs into answerable questions. A preliminary search of easily accessible literature might reveal further practice-related questions that will need to be addressed, and could even trigger the need for you to reconsider your priorities.

Activity 2
Refining your learning needs

When you have identified your learning needs from Activity 1 look at them again.

Question 1. Are your questions clear?
Question 2. Do you know exactly what you are looking for?

Commentary on Activity 2
It is well worth clarifying your questions at this point, as this will save you considerable time when searching for information from electronic databases and other sources (Chapter 4).

Activity 3
Identifying further, related questions

Using the learning needs that you have identified for yourself in Activities 1 and 2, identify the chapters in this book that could be a useful starting point in your journey for new knowledge. Then chose one chapter which looks particularly relevant to your needs.

Question 1. To what extent does this chapter meet your needs?
Question 2. Has reading this chapter raised more questions that you should consider in relation to Mrs Rudetsky's care?
Question 3. Might you need to change your priorities when planning Mrs Rudetsky's care?

Commentary on Activity 3

Reading a chapter in a textbook can be a very useful introduction to key issues but any book, by its very nature, is unlikely to be completely up to date for very long, as there is a burgeoning of new knowledge in the wound-care domain. You might also have highly specific questions that are beyond the scope of this book. In either case, it is very useful to be able to access for yourself the latest research and other information from bibliographic databases and the worldwide web. How to search systematically for this information is the subject of the next chapter (Chapter 4).

SUMMARY

A problem-based approach to learning requires that you identify your own learning needs, which can be triggered by specific patient problems. An exploration of a particular issue can raise more questions than it answers and might cause you to reconsider your priorities. Learning is thus an iterative process of problem identification and refinement. It can be likened to a road without an ending, but with a number of recognizable milestones upon the way.

FURTHER READING

Glen S, Wilkie K (eds) 2000 Problem-based learning in nursing: a new model for a new context? Macmillan Press, London

Rideout E 2001 Transforming nurse education through problem-based learning. Jones and Bartlett, Boston, MA

Wilkie K, Burns I 2003 Problem-based learning: a handbook for nurses. Palgrave Macmillan, Basingstoke

Finding information

Denis Anthony

CHAPTER CONTENTS

INTRODUCTION

A problem-based approach to learning often involves accessing a range of material from many different sources (see Chapter 2). Some sources might be readily accessible, for example the chapters in this book. Finding material from other sources is not always so simple and requires special skills.

This chapter is a guide to locating information from such sources as the worldwide web, subject directories, online library catalogues and bibliographic databases. The chapter also includes information on accessing resources such as newsgroups, e-mail lists, the websites of charitable organizations and international, intergovernmental sites. At the end of the chapter there are a number of useful links to facilitate your own searches. As you will discover, searching for a textbook is a very different exercise from searching for an academic article.

The chapter includes examples of worked problems, together with problem scenarios for you to work through for yourself. You might find it useful to have access to a computer while you work through this chapter. Although the chapter assumes little prior knowledge, it nevertheless provides a useful overview for those who already have some experience of searching the literature.

WEB SEARCHES

The worldwide web (WWW or web) is a massive collection of linked information, located in computers across the globe. The information is displayed as 'web pages' or simply 'pages'. A web browser is a program, such as Netscape or Internet Explorer, that allows you to access the web. You will almost certainly have such a program installed on your personal computer (PC) if you bought it in the last few years. If you have access to a computer at work, it too should have a web browser. To gain entry to the web from your PC might also require a modem; most new computers have modems as standard. The final requirement is an internet provider. This is a company that provides you with a telephone link from your PC to the 'servers' that store the information you require. The examples shown in this chapter use Windows 2000 and Internet Explorer, but you should find that your computer display looks very similar to the figures illustrated here.

Getting started

Start by opening your web browser to access the 'home page' on your computer. This is a 'default' page, which can be reset to another page of your choice. Near the top of the page you will see the address (sometimes called uniform resource locator or URL), which is its unique reference. For example, http://www.library.dmu.ac.uk is the address (URL) for the De Montfort University library. If you know the URL of a page, typing it into the address space, and then clicking on the Go button to the right of it, or hitting the Return key on the keyboard, will take you straight to that page.

Search engines

The web is very large, therefore it can be difficult to know where relevant and useful information is located. Fortunately, there are methods to assist you, including programs that search for specified information. These programs are called 'search engines'. Yahoo and Lycos are examples of search engines. Each search engine has its strengths and weaknesses, and so some programs have been developed to use several of these search engines together, for example Google and Copernic. These take a little longer to run but give access to more web pages.

SEARCH STRATEGIES

Searching all of the web is a good way to find sites or pages when you do not know any sites at all. Once you have identified a good site, this might point you to others because many sites have 'links' to other sites of a similar type. This can save a lot of time. Furthermore, if the site you are looking at is of a high quality (e.g. it presents information about a professional body, university, a large charity or government organization) then the list of links is *likely* to be relevant and of high quality.

   The problem with web searching is that you will inevitably locate a lot of irrelevant material, and much material of dubious quality. To overcome this you will need to use your critical judgement to evaluate the pages you locate. An excellent discussion of quality assurance of web-based material can be found on www.nursing-standard.co.uk/archives/vol11-45/ol-art.htm.

Simple searching

As noted above, if you use a simple search you will probably find much irrelevant information. Initially, you might find it difficult to find a good quality site and you will miss most academic articles because these are indexed elsewhere. You will need to develop strategies that will allow you to find relevant, high-quality material quickly. Searching can be achieved by using:

- 'any word' entered
- only those pages where 'all words' are found
- the 'exact phrase'.

You will get very different results from each type of search, as illustrated below.

Search for any word

Suppose you want to find information on leg ulcers. If you use the 'Search for any word' method you will get all pages with any of the words entered, so you will get all pages with 'ulcer' and this will include, for example, stomach ulcers. Similarly, you will get all pages with the word 'leg'. Usually, you will find this is a poor method of searching. It will give you too many pages, most of which will not be relevant. This is only a good method if there are several very specific words that will be found on relevant pages but probably not elsewhere.

Search for all words

If you search using 'Search for all words' then you will get a more refined search, as here only files with both 'leg' and 'ulcer' will be located. This is a middle path between searching for the exact phrase and searching for any word. You will still get some irrelevant pages, but far fewer than searching for any word. You will get more pages than searching for the exact phrase, some of which might be highly relevant.

Using exact phrase

If you use the exact phrase you will only get pages where the phrase 'leg ulcers' occurs, and thus a page with 'venous ulcer' or even 'leg ulcer' (singular not plural) will not be found. This is a very useful search method if there is a phrase that will probably be in any page you may want, but you might still miss many relevant pages.

Figure 4.1 shows how the number of web pages on leg ulcers and risk assessment decreases as the search is refined.

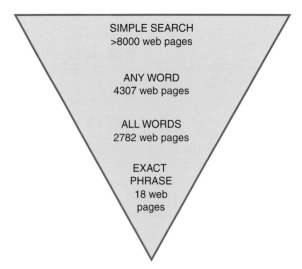

Figure 4.1
The influence of the search strategy on the number of web pages found in a search for information about risk assessment and leg ulcers

In most search engines you can refine your search much more precisely. In particular, you might be able to use 'Boolean operators', which are described in the section on 'Advanced Searching' a little later in this chapter.

APPLYING A SEARCH STRATEGY WHEN SEEKING INFORMATION IN THE CONTEXT OF PBL

The example illustrated in Box 4.1 shows how a simple search strategy can be employed when a PBL approach is adopted.

Box 4.1
Jyoti needs information for her mother, who has a leg ulcer

Scenario
Jyoti's mother has a leg ulcer. She speaks Gujerati and a little English. Jyoti speaks fluent Gujerati and English.

Jyoti's identified learning needs
Jyoti wants to identify some general resources on leg ulcers, ideally in Gujerati so that her mother can read them, or at least in English so that she is better able to explain the condition to her mother.

Learning activity
Jyoti uses the web search tool Copernic (www.copernic.ac.uk) and initially looks for 'patient information'. She finds some useful general sites but none of them immediately suggest they have multilingual information. She then accesses Patient UK (via Copernic), which gives an alphabetical list of conditions and includes leg ulcers. She also finds some information sheets from the Tissue Viability Society.

Another search on Copernic using simply 'Gujerati' gave a set of links that included the NHS Direct site (www.nhsdirect.nhs.uk), which does have patient information in many languages but there is nothing on leg ulcers.

Solution
Jyoti has found part of what she wanted – that is, information on leg ulcers – but not in a language that her mother can read.

Comment
One of the problems with web searching is that new sites take time to be indexed. There is a new site that deals with multilingual patient information: mypil.com (Fig. 4.2). Mypil does not yet have any information on leg ulcers but in due course this will probably appear.

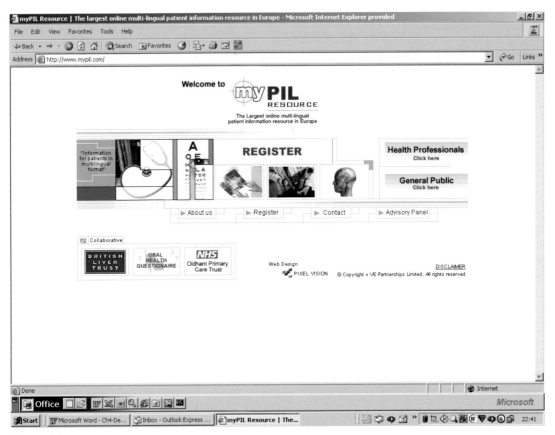

Figure 4.2
Mypil. com

You might now like to work through the problem illustrated in Box 4.2 for yourself.

Box 4.2 **Tissue viability in orthopaedic nursing**	**Scenario** As a qualified nurse on an orthopaedic ward, you want to locate clinically useful sites relating to tissue viability.

Identified learning needs
Identify your learning needs.
Remember that these might include web-searching skills in addition to tissue viability related to orthopaedic patients.

Learning activity
Try using Copernic or another search engine such as Google (www.google.com) to meet your learning needs. You will find a list of useful websites at the end of this chapter.

Comment
If you found the Tissue Viability Society site (TVS on www.tvs.org.uk) you will have noticed a list of links to other wound sites, in particular the World Wide Wounds (WWW) site (www.smtl.co.uk/World-Wide-Wounds), which has lists of relevant sites. The TVS site gives some really useful patient information sheets and the WWW site has some practical papers explaining how to treat wounds with various dressings.

Subject directories

Searching the web can be very time consuming. However, some sites act as directories, with links to other sites for a given subject. For health workers there is a hierarchy of such sites, starting with BIOME for biological sciences, which contains OMNI (www.omni.ac.uk) for medicine and health and NMAP (http:nmap.ac.uk) for nursing and the therapies (Fig. 4.3) The advantage of subject directories is that they provide a focused list of sites because the entries are made by humans who know the field, rather than by computer programs searching websites indiscriminately. The entry for leg ulcers on NMAP is shown in Fig. 4.4.

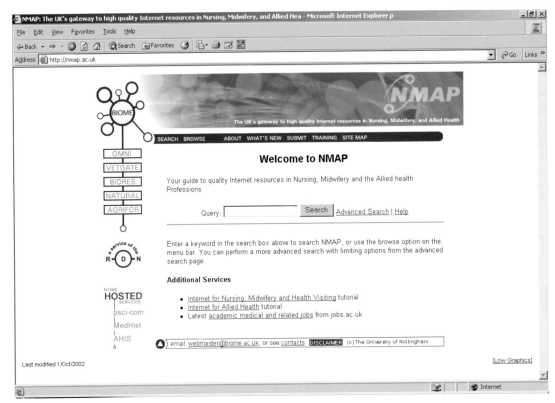

Figure 4.3
NMAP home page

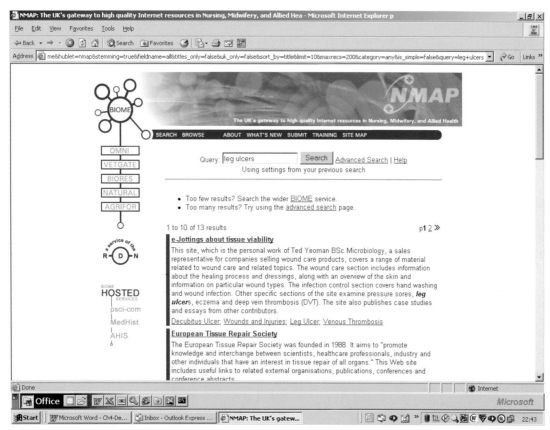

Figure 4.4
Leg ulcers on NMAP

ONLINE LIBRARY SEARCHING

If you want to locate a textbook in your library, you might have access to an online catalogue or database. Most, if not all, universities have such a catalogue, many based on the OPAC system. You can search with a title, an author's name or simply for books on a certain subject. An example of a search for a textbook is illustrated in Box 4.3.

Box 4.3
Margaret would like to find a textbook on the nursing management of chronic wounds

Scenario
Margaret is a recently appointed, hospital-based tissue viability nurse. When attending a conference she hears mention of a book by Moya Morison on chronic wounds.

Identified learning needs
Margaret would like to find Moya Morison's book so that she can review it, to see whether it will meet her practice needs.

Learning activity
She looks for Moya Morison's book but finds that it is not listed in her local library. Rather than give up, she thinks about trying other university libraries,

continued

**Box 4.3
continued**

but this is inefficient. She decides to use COPAC (www.copac.ac.uk). She selects one of three menu options, Author search, because she knows the author. This gives a list of titles for this author and any other author of the same name. Fortunately, Morison is not a very common spelling variant and several of Moya's books appear at the top of the screen. Clicking on the top item gives the libraries that hold this textbook. Margaret selects the nearest library showing the details on this holding.

Solution

Margaret can now contact the nearest library holding Moya's book and check whether there are reciprocal lending rights.

BIBLIOGRAPHIC DATABASES

You will probably be familiar with CD-ROM databases like Medline and CINAHL. These and many others are also available online. You might have access to these via your organization using Athens authentication, but some are available freely to anyone with access to the internet, for example PubMed (Fig. 4.5) gives access to Medline, a massive database of healthcare articles dating back to 1966. You might be less familiar with some other very helpful databases, for

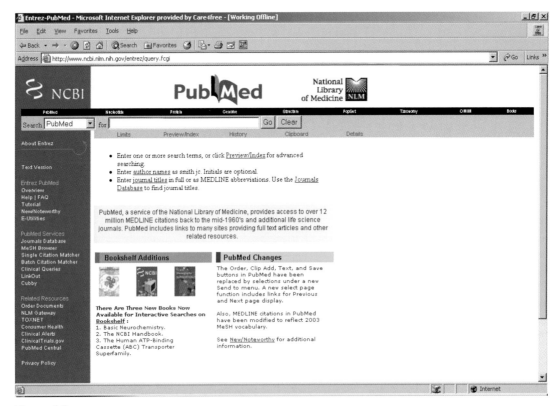

Figure 4.5
PubMed

example the Bath Information Data Service, which is a collection of academic databases including educational research (ERIC) and the Social Science collection. These might not seem directly relevant to wound care but for specific projects you could find these and other databases very helpful, especially where there is an educational or social component.

You should ask your local librarian about the databases to which you can have access and if you can be given an Athens password. Athens is a system whereby you can access many databases and other services to which your organization has access, online with one password. Only articles in journals indexed by the database provider will be given. There will be a 'start date', that is a month and year from which the journals have been indexed. If you are looking for material published earlier than this you will not find it.

With bibliographic searching you can locate a mass of relevant literature very quickly. However, you need to identify relevant keywords. If you are not specific you will get too much unfocused material. Narrowing down your search needs careful consideration to avoid missing relevant studies.

You might now like to try the following problem, summarized in Box 4.4, for yourself.

Box 4.4
Ethnicity and leg ulcers

Scenario
You have been told informally by a colleague that there are few African Americans with venous leg ulcers. You want to confirm whether there is any evidence for this observation.

Identify learning needs
What are your learning needs? Remember that 'learning' is not restricted to gathering facts. Finding out how to do something (like using databases) is also learning.

Comment
You probably accessed Medline and CINAHL for 'leg ulcers' and 'ethnic groups'.

How many articles did you find? At the time of writing, we found little published information on the subject, but that does not necessarily mean that the information is not in existence. We simply might not have been clever enough to find it. Your next step could be to discuss the question with a subject expert, who might have access to the 'grey' literature, or to request information through e-mail lists or newsgroups, as discussed later in this chapter.

FULL TEXT SEARCHING

Sometimes you can access a whole article online, often in portable document format (PDF). PDF files are exact copies of the printed journal articles. You need additional software, Acrobat Reader, to see these PDF files, but this is available free on www.acrobat.com via the web. This service is increasingly offered via online databases such as Medline and CINAHL. Thus you might be able to access the article in full for free if your organization has a subscription, or purchase the article online using a credit card if not. You can also browse the contents of several nursing journals using, for example, Ingenta (Fig. 4.6).

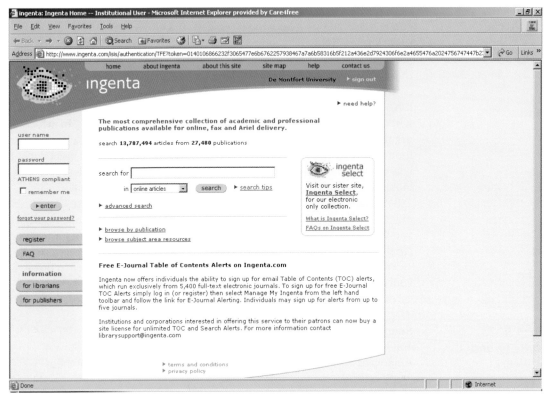

Figure 4.6
Ingenta

OTHER ELECTRONIC INFORMATION SOURCES

In addition to the worldwide web and computerized databases, several other resources can be accessed electronically. PBL requires you to think laterally and to explore a range of information sources, therefore you might find some of the following resources useful.

E-mail lists

When a company or organization uses a mailing list, one copy of an advertising flyer is sent to all people on the list. In general you do not elect to join the list nor, typically, do you have the opportunity to have your name removed. An e-mail list is like a mailing list, but in most e-mail lists you can automatically join or leave the list by sending an e-mail message to a special e-mail address called the listserver address.

E-mail lists help in obtaining information because there is a captive audience of people interested in a given subject. Thus you can ask questions. For example, if you wanted to know about ethnicity and the aetiology of leg ulcers (see Box 4.4), someone on the list might know. You need to be careful that you are sending appropriately targeted messages. It is not helpful to ask if anyone has references on 'wound care', as this is far too large an area for anyone to be able to respond to you fully, but you might ask members what books they have found useful as a source of reference on the subject.

There is no universal and complete list of e-mail lists, so locating relevant lists can be difficult. Some sites have (incomplete) lists, for example on www.jiscmail.ac.uk are the UK academic lists run by JISC, including many for nursing and medicine, and one for PBL. You will also find here instructions on how to join or leave a list, how to send an e-mail to the list, archives of the list and information on what the list is for. There are currently none for wound care but there are many relevant to nurses who deal with wounds, for example DIST-NURSE for district nurses. Another list of lists is at www.topica.com which has many lists for topics of interest to nurses and midwives.

USENET newsgroups

A resource underused by nurses is USENET newsgroups. These are similar to e-mail lists but not all messages are automatically sent to your mailbox. You can elect to view a newsgroup and you can then see the subjects of messages. You can therefore read those that you choose. Newsgroups for nursing such as sci.med.nursing can be accessed.

Personal e-mail

In many journal articles, authors give their e-mail addresses. You can use these if you want to follow-up on an article or ask for more recent work on the subject.

Grey literature

Not all information on a subject is in published peer-reviewed research journals. Some useful material might be in reports, such as the internal reports of an organization. This is called the 'grey' literature. By its nature it is less easy to locate because it is often not indexed, and certainly not in bibliographic data-bases. Various organizations will have lists of documents that you can access. For example, your local library might house a collection of student works such as theses, which were never published but might contain useful information.

NGOs, charities and professional bodies

You might want to access specialized knowledge within certain organizations. Targeting these organizations will be very useful to you. The Tissue Viability Society (www.tvs.org.uk) and the Royal College of Nursing (RCN, on www.rcn.org.uk) are two groups with relevant information. The former has excellent patient information leaflets and the latter has some clinical guidelines for leg ulcers and pressure ulcers. If you want to search for clinical guidelines there are some excellent sites, for example SIGN on www.sign.ac.uk, which has relevant guidelines for wound care, including 'Management of diabetic foot disease' and 'The care of patients with chronic leg ulcer'.

An e-mail or telephone call to organizations like these could save you a lot of time, provided you have a relevant, focused query.

International and intergovernmental sites

If you want international data, many organizations have relevant information and often web sites. For example, www.icn.ch is the International Council of Nurses site; www.who.int is the site for the World Health Organization; www.unsystem.org is the United Nations site; and www.europa.eu.int is the site for the European Union.

Systematic reviews online

There are sites that deal with systematic reviews of the literature. If you can locate a relevant systematic review you can save yourself a lot of time. The

University of York has an excellent site for healthcare reviews (see www.york.ac.uk/inst/crd), including many on wound care written by nurses.

The Cochrane collaboration is an international group that indexes reviews and other evidence-based information. Cochrane allows you to search across a number of databases, including full reviews (ideal if they exist, because you can get the full item online), references (useful, but you have to then locate the item), economic evaluations and so forth (Fig. 4.7). An example of the use of the Cochrane database in relation to pressure sore risk assessment is illustrated in Box 4.5.

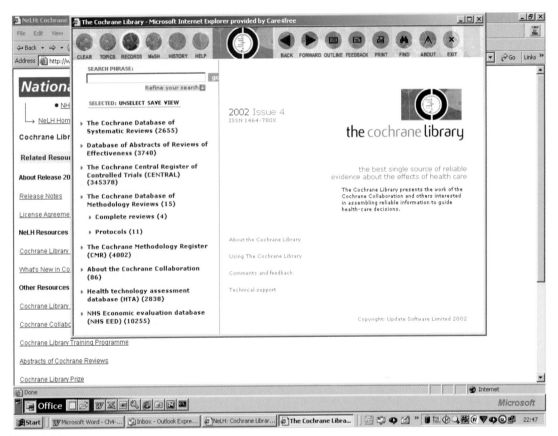

Figure 4.7
The Cochrane Library

Box 4.5
Susan needs information on pressure ulcer risk assessment methods

Scenario
Susan is a Charge Nurse in an elderly-care ward. She wants to introduce a pressure ulcer risk assessment scoring system to the ward to enable her staff to match pressure-relieving mattresses and cushions to the patients most at risk.

Identification of learning needs
Susan is aware of the existence of several risk assessment tools, including those by Waterlow, Braden and Norton – this represents previous learning identified – but she wants to know if there is any evidence to suggest which of these is the most appropriate for use in her care setting – this is the new learning required.

Learning activity
She accesses Cochrane and searches for 'risk assessment' and 'decubitus ulcer', by combining two previous searches. This yields one hit in complete reviews and 21 hits in references. The item she finds under 'complete reviews' is a review of mattresses and cushions. In its reference list she finds some articles of more relevance.

Solution
Susan now has sufficient articles for critique to help her to decide which assessment tool is most suitable for her patients.

ADVANCED SEARCHING

In many databases, and in some search engines (for example Copernic) it is possible to search in a more sophisticated way than simply typing in a word or phrase. One common method is to use Boolean operators. Boolean operators are typified by AND, OR, EXCEPT, etc. Parentheses are used to group search methods together. Double quotation marks are used to show that an exact match is needed. A search thus may be:

> ethnicity AND ("leg ulcer" OR "leg ulcers")

The use of capitals here is conventional and merely identifies the operators. The search would locate all articles (or pages if on the web) with either the singular or plural ('ulcer' or 'ulcers') but only where the word 'ethnicity' is also found.

Other search engines use the plus sign (+) rather than AND. The Boolean operators can be very helpful for focusing your search when one of the parameters (such as 'leg ulcers') is associated with a very extensive literature. Search engines are being continually improved. Many now prompt you towards the use of AND and OR or will ask if you want the terms combined or left separately for the search.

TRADITIONAL LIBRARY SEARCH

Although this chapter is about obtaining information online, not all material is available online, referenced in online databases or necessarily even published, therefore you should not forget your local library. The use of bibliographic databases typically helps with identifying literature from a variety of journals, however, in some cases, manually searching through specific journals might be at least as helpful and will bring you up to date with the most recently published work. Situations where this is useful include issues highlighted by the media or by a recently published report, or for specialized journals that might not be indexed by your database provider. If full text articles are available at your library you might be able to conduct 'hand' searching online.

SUMMARY

The advantages and disadvantages of different methods of accessing information are shown below in Table 4.1.

Table 4.1
The advantages and disadvantages of a number of methods for information searching

Method	Advantages	Disadvantages	Example
Online library searching	Able to find any book in your library	You might not have this text, although COPAC will let you know where else it might be	De Montfort library www.library.dmu.ac.uk
Web searches	Finds enormous numbers of pages, including individual unpublished material	Finding relevant material can be difficult. Quality of material needs to be assessed	Copernic www.copernic.ac.uk
Bibliographic databases	Finds all articles indexed by database	Finds none that are not in indexed journals	CINAHL biomed.niss.ac.uk (needs a password)
Full text searching	You do not need to go to the library to see the article	It might cost you	Ingenta, accessible from BIDS www.bids.ac.uk
E-mail lists	Very rapid response to requests for information	Not guaranteed to get any response	Nurse-uk Nurse-uk@jisc.ac.uk
USENET newsgroups	Same as e-mail lists but your e-mail box does not fill up	Same as e-mail lists but you might need additional software	Sci.med.nursing
Personal e-mail	Able to speak to the expert	The expert might not reply	Danthony@dmu.ac.uk (chapter author)
Grey literature	Able to locate information that might not be in published journals	You need to know where to look	RCN newsletter
Hand-searching journals	Highly focused search	Time consuming	*Journal of Wound Care*
Systematic reviews and clinical guidelines	Typically very high-quality work	There might not be a systematic review or guidelines. They are expensive to create	York CRD www.york.ac.uk/inst/crd SIGN www.sign.ac.uk

Table 4.1—cont'd

Method	Advantages	Disadvantages	Example
NGOs, inter-governmental, international and other organizations	Focused on issues relevant to the organization, with expertise in these areas	Might show bias	Europa (EU site) www.europa.eu.int
Subject directories	Access to relevant focused material	Misses useful material on (for example) personal homepages	NMAP nmap.ac.uk

SOME USEFUL LINKS

Some useful links are given below. Other sources of information and opportunities for networking are given in Box 1.3.

General

- World Wide Wounds: www.smtl.co.uk/World-Wide-Wounds/Common/Links.html
- OMNI on www.omni.ac.uk is a generic health site, but has items on decubitus ulcer.
- Pressure Sore Web Forum: www.medicaledu.com/pressure_sore_forum
- Venous Stasis Ulcer Web Forum: www.medicaledu.com/venous_stasis_forum
- Wound and Skin Care Links: members.tripod.com/~DianneBrownson/wound_skin.html Dianne Brownson's 'wound and skin' links – other healthcare links too.
- Wound Care Information Network www.medicaledu.com
- Wound Care Web Forum medicaledu.com/wound_care_forum

Guidelines

- The NHS Centre for Reviews and Dissemination at York, in particular look at www.york.ac.uk/inst/crd/ehc21.htm
- Scottish Intercollegiate Guidelines Network (SIGN) guidelines located at www.sign.ac.uk
- RCN guidelines at www.rcn.org.uk/servicecs/promote/clinical/clinical_guidelines.htm
- Clearing House of guidelines at www.guidelines.gov/index.asp

Organizations

- Wound Care Institute www.woundcare.org
- Tissue Viability Society www.tvs.org.uk
- Wound Healing Society wizard.pharm.wayne.edu/woundsoc/WHS.HTM
- The Surgical Materials Testing Laboratory on www.smtl.co.uk/. This has a resource centre on www.smtl.co.uk/WMPRC/index.html. Part of the SMTL is World Wide Wounds (Wound Management, Woundcare and Dressings on the Internet) on www.smtl.co.uk/World-Wide-Wounds/index.html. These contain articles available only on the internet, and abstracts of recent articles in the printed press.

A framework for patient assessment and care planning

Moya J Morison

CHAPTER CONTENTS

INTRODUCTION

Acute and chronic wounds are commonly encountered among patients in both hospital and community settings and can easily develop into complex lesions of the skin and underlying tissues with inappropriate care, as many of the case studies in Section 2 illustrate. Complications are especially common among patients who are elderly, malnourished, immune compromised, immobile, and those with altered levels of consciousness. High-risk groups include critically injured survivors of major trauma, patients who have undergone lengthy surgery, those with spinal cord injuries, the terminally ill and patients in intensive care, of whatever age.

As with all aspects of patient care, the findings from an ongoing process of assessment should form the basis for rational decision making. However, in the case of wound care, it is all too easy for the assessment process to focus on the wound itself, to the detriment of wider issues. Throughout this book it is suggested that it is essential that the emphasis be shifted from the wound towards *the patient with a wound* and to acknowledge the environmental and social factors that might be influencing the healing process.

This change in emphasis reflects the trends in health care, since the 1960s, towards:

- a more holistic, client-centred approach, which takes cognisance of social, psychological and spiritual aspects of health and well being, as well as physical factors
- client empowerment, which acknowledges the individual's rights to autonomy and self-determination and moves away from the paternalistic notion that 'the healthcare professional knows best'.

This chapter aims to provide a framework for patient assessment and care planning that is in keeping with this perspective and with the problem-based (PBL) approach to wound care. A central aim of PBL is the integration and application of knowledge such as the physiology of wound healing (Chapter 6), the diagnosis and management of wound infection (Chapter 7), the selection of appropriate dressings and cleansing agents (Chapter 8), the use of physical therapies such as laser and ultrasound (Chapter 9), dermatological aspects of wound healing (Chapter 10), nutritional support (Chapter 11), pain management (Chapter 12) and health promotion (Chapter 13). Knowledge and issues specific to leg ulcers, pressure ulcers and other chronic wounds, and wounds associated with trauma are the focus of Chapters 14–17. Psychological, social and ethical issues are emphasized in Chapters 18 and 19, and practice development issues are discussed in Chapter 20. These chapters merely provide a jumping-off point for the individual to acquire new knowledge that is appropriate to specific clinical situations.

This chapter is based around two case studies and includes a number of activities relating to patient assessment and care planning. Some of the activities are at the more directive end of PBL. The aim is to give the reader a coherent overview of the multidimensional aspects of caring for patients with wounds and insights into the strengths and limitations of some of the assessment tools available.

Activity 1 **Assessing a patient and planning care**	A case study illustrating the plight of a frail elderly woman who is admitted to hospital from a care home for the assessment of her leg ulcers is given in Box 5.1.
	Question 1. After reading this case study carefully identify your own learning needs (you might like to look back to Chapters 1 and 3 for guidance on how to set about this).
	Question 2. What additional assessments do you propose to undertake?
	Question 3. Devise a care plan for this woman, based on the information that you already have.

Box 5.1
Case study of an 80-year-old woman with leg ulcers

Betty Brown is 80 years old and has just been admitted to hospital from the local care home for the assessment of her leg ulcers (Fig. 5.1). On arrival she is found to have been doubly incontinent. She has a medical history of anaemia and chronic obstructive airways disease.

According to her notes, four-layer compression-bandage therapy was commenced 3 months earlier in an attempt to heal the leg ulcers. However, these have become more extensive and sloughy. Betty says that she is very distressed by the intense pain that she experiences on dressing changes. The notes record that she is given paracetamol 500 mg 10 min beforehand but that this appears to be having little effect in alleviating her suffering.

On initial assessment, Betty is found to have several other ulcers including a sloughy stage 3 sacral pressure ulcer and superficial stage 2 pressure ulcers on both of her elbows. Her skin is extremely dry and fragile. The accompanying notes from the care home state that she has had a poor appetite recently. She is 5 ft 6 inches (1.68 m) tall and weighs 8 stone (51 kg).

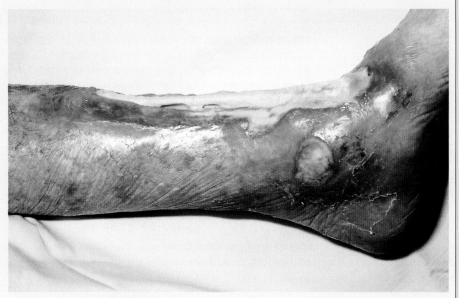

Figure 5.1
An 80-year-old woman with extensive leg ulceration

Her closest living relative is a daughter, aged 55, who lives 30 miles away, but she stopped visiting 6 months ago saying that her mother is abusive and completely uninterested in her wider family. The care home gives a different story, saying how distressed the old lady is that she never sees her grandchildren. Betty confides in the nurse who is admitting her that she feels that she has little left to live for. She is apathetic and has ceased to take any interest in her appearance and personal hygiene.

A MODEL TO FACILITATE PATIENT ASSESSMENT AND CARE PLANNING

The basic principles of caring for a patient with a wound have been known for several centuries. The surgeon Ambrose Paré lived in France in the sixteenth century and articulated the principles that form the basis of much medical and surgical practice today. He stressed the importance of removing the cause of the wound, local wound debridement, the application of a dressing, developing a sound nutritional plan, treating any underlying disease and psychological support. These same principles apply today.

A conceptual schema to aid with patient assessment and care planning is illustrated in Fig. 5.2. This model is in two parts. The first stresses the importance of removing the immediate and any underlying causes of the wound, removing or alleviating more general causes of delayed healing, optimizing the local wound environment and preventing further tissue breakdown, such as the development of one or more pressure sores. The overall aims are to save life, to prevent avoidable (perhaps life-threatening) complications and to promote wound healing. The second part looks at the patient more holistically and encourages the healthcare professional to consider the consequences of the wound for the individual's quality of life, both now and in the future, the optimum setting for care, ways of maximizing patient and carer involvement, and the need for long-term rehabilitation. These dimensions are clearly interconnected and focusing on the wound to the detriment of the whole person is likely to be counterproductive, especially in the longer term, when the responsibility for rehabilitation and health promotion is likely to shift increasingly to the patient and his or her carers.

Activity 2 *Using a conceptual framework to facilitate holistic patient assessment and care planning*	Using Fig. 5.2 as a guide, review the assessments proposed and the care plan that you devised for Betty Brown in Activity 1. *Question 1.* How comprehensive was your initial assessment? Are there any obvious omissions from the assessments that you had planned to carry out? *Question 2.* How holistic was the care that you had planned? *Question 3.* Would you now do anything differently, or consider changing your priorities?

Conceptual frameworks reflect the values, beliefs and perspectives of their authors and vary in their usefulness.

Activity 3 *Exploring other conceptual frameworks*	Do you know of any other published frameworks to facilitate patient assessment and care planning? (you might like to look back to Chapter 4 if you want to explore this further). *Question 1.* What dimensions do these tools have in common and how do they differ? *Question 2.* What are the advantages and drawbacks of using a conceptual framework that is specific to a particular category of wound, such as leg ulcers or pressure ulcers?

ASESSMENT   AIMS OF THE CARE PLANNED

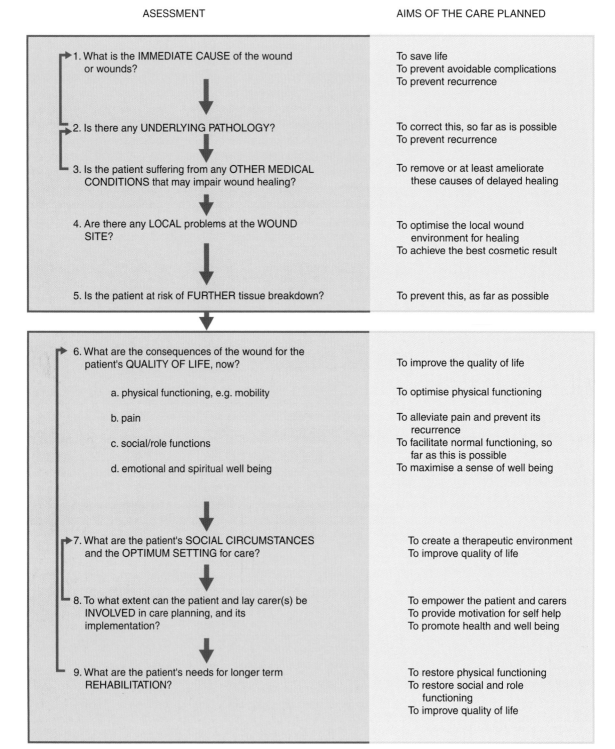

1. What is the IMMEDIATE CAUSE of the wound
   or wounds?

   To save life
   To prevent avoidable complications
   To prevent recurrence

2. Is there any UNDERLYING PATHOLOGY?

   To correct this, so far as is possible
   To prevent recurrence

3. Is the patient suffering from any OTHER MEDICAL
   CONDITIONS that may impair wound healing?

   To remove or at least ameliorate
       these causes of delayed healing

4. Are there any LOCAL problems at the WOUND
   SITE?

   To optimise the local wound
       environment for healing
   To achieve the best cosmetic result

5. Is the patient at risk of FURTHER tissue breakdown?

   To prevent this, as far as possible

6. What are the consequences of the wound for the
   patient's QUALITY OF LIFE, now?

   To improve the quality of life

   a. physical functioning, e.g. mobility

   To optimise physical functioning

   b. pain

   To alleviate pain and prevent its
       recurrence

   c. social/role functions

   To facilitate normal functioning, so
       far as this is possible

   d. emotional and spiritual well being

   To maximise a sense of well being

7. What are the patient's SOCIAL CIRCUMSTANCES
   and the OPTIMUM SETTING for care?

   To create a therapeutic environment
   To improve quality of life

8. To what extent can the patient and lay carer(s) be
   INVOLVED in care planning, and its
   implementation?

   To empower the patient and carers
   To provide motivation for self help
   To promote health and well being

9. What are the patient's needs for longer term
   REHABILITATION?

   To restore physical functioning
   To restore social and role
       functioning
   To improve quality of life

Figure 5.2
A model to facilitate patient assessment and care planning

The sections that follow look at the components of the framework illustrated in Fig. 5.2 and draw out some general principles, with further reference to Betty Brown's case (Box 5.1).

What is the immediate cause of the wound?

The immediate cause of a wound could be avoidable or unavoidable, and it might be highly significant and important in itself or relatively trivial, as illustrated in Table 5.1. What is important is that the immediate cause of a wound is sought and, where possible, rectified so that the wound is prevented from recurring.

A good example is a diabetic foot ulcer, which can be triggered by ill-fitting footwear. As discussed in Chapter 15, the consequences of wound infection for the diabetic patient can be devastating, perhaps even necessitating amputation. Checking a diabetic person's footwear and encouraging individuals and their carers to inspect the feet every day for the signs of even the most minor trauma can help to prevent recurrence.

As a second example, a surgeon might be very reluctant to create a myo-cutaneous flap to repair a defect resulting from a sacral pressure ulcer in a paraplegic patient if that patient is likely to return to a setting where insufficient care has been taken in the past to provide an appropriate pressure-relieving bed or chair. Such lack of care could very quickly undo the surgeon's work.

Table 5.1
Examples of the immediate causes of wounds

Wound type	Examples of the immediate 'cause'
Leg ulcers	Minor trauma of any kind
Diabetic foot ulcers	Ill-fitting footwear, falling asleep too close to the fire
Pressure ulcers	Inappropriate patient support surface (bed or chair)
Scalds to a young child	Lack of supervision in the kitchen
Major industrial accident	Breaches in the health and safety regulations in the workplace

Activity 4
Some practical and ethical issues associated with assessing the immediate causes of a wound

Return to the case study in Box 5.1.

Question 1. What are the likely causes of Betty Brown's pressure ulcers? (see Chapter 14).

Question 2. It is 1 month later and Betty is about to be discharged back to her care home. Do you propose to raise the issue of pressure ulcer prevention with the care home staff; if so, how? (You might wish to turn to Chapter 19, which gives an overview of ethical issues).

Question 3. What other ethical issues can you identify?

The dilemma is often deciding whether a situation is in fact amenable to change, and also where one's professional responsibility ends.

Is there any underlying pathology?

Identifying the underlying pathology of a wound is of paramount importance to planning appropriate care. The underlying pathology might be complex, as with leg ulceration, where differential diagnosis is imperative and where inappropriate care could precipitate the need for amputation.

**Activity 5
Assessing the underlying pathology of a wound**

Return to the case study in Box 5.1.

Question 1. How would you assess the underlying pathology of Betty Brown's leg ulcers?

Question 2. On assessment you discover that Betty is suffering from both chronic venous hypertension in her lower limbs and significant peripheral vascular disease (her ankle/brachial pressure index is 0.5). Devise a care plan to promote the healing of her leg ulcers.

Is the patient suffering from any other medical conditions that might impair healing?

Wound healing is likely to be impaired by a number of concurrent medical conditions such as diabetes mellitus and circulatory and respiratory disorders. It is the variety of factors that can lead to delayed healing that makes patient assessment and care planning so challenging (Fig. 5.3).

Those factors amenable to correction need to be addressed as part of a comprehensive care plan, for example, malnutrition is a factor that can be highly amenable to improvement.

Malnutrition

Malnutrition is a commonly encountered problem, both for hospitalized patients and for debilitated patients living at home. Although it can lead to delayed wound healing of both acute and chronic wounds, nutritional assessment and support are often overlooked. Optimizing the patient's nutritional status is an important goal of care planning (see Chapter 11).

Increasing age

Wound healing in the neonate and in the elderly is qualitatively different from that in a young and fit adult. With increasing age, the barrier functions of the skin are altered, there is reduced sensory perception and the individual is increasingly susceptible to trauma. These factors need to be given particular attention, both in relation to skin care (Chapter 10) and pressure ulcer prevention (Chapter 14).

Are there any local problems at the wound site?

Accurate and ongoing assessment of the wound site and of the surrounding skin is essential to planning the most appropriate local wound management, and to evaluating its effectiveness (see Chapters 8 and 10). Clear and accurate documentation of the findings is essential to ensuring that any abnormal changes are picked up quickly and that appropriate therapeutic action is taken, as well as ensuring continuity of care. It is also important to be able to recognize when healing is progressing well – that is, to be able to recognize the clinical appearance of healthy granulation tissue and epithelium.

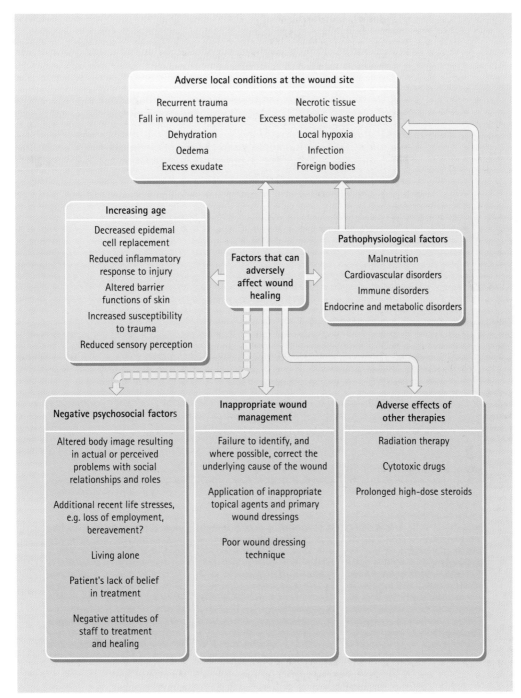

Figure 5.3
Factors that can adversely affect wound healing

Charting wound healing

There are several published wound assessment charts, three of which are featured in this chapter. They are intended to be an aid to the accurate recording of the most important parameters.

Open wounds. The wound assessment chart illustrated in Fig. 5.4 is intended to be used for wounds healing by secondary intention. These include chronic open wounds, such as pressure ulcers and leg ulcers, and surgically 'clean' wounds that are left open, such as excised pilonidal sinuses. The author of this tool advocates tracing the wound, either weekly or more frequently if significant changes in size are observed.

A second assessment tool, which is specific to pressure ulcers, is illustrated in Fig. 5.5.

Activity 6 **Assessing open** **wounds**	Turn back to Fig. 1.1 in Box 1.1, which illustrates pressure area damage in Mrs Smith, an elderly lady who has recently suffered a stroke. *Question 1.* Assess her wounds using each of the assessment tools illustrated in Fig. 5.4 and 5.5. *Question 2.* What problems have you encountered in assessing these wounds? *Question 3.* What indications are there that these wounds are not healing optimally? *Question 4.* What are the advantages and disadvantages of each tool? *Question 5.* Have you used or do you know of any other tools in use in clinical practice that would be suitable in this case? *Question 6.* How do these tools compare? *Question 7.* How could you set about assessing the validity and reliability of these tools for measuring wound healing?

Surgically closed wounds. For surgically closed wounds, the early identification of postoperative wound infection is vital to preventing complications that can be life-threatening (see Chapter 7). Charting healing can aid with the early identification of complications (Fig. 5.6).

The age and 'cleanliness' of the wound, and events in the operating theatre, all have an important bearing on whether a wound infection develops later. In a wound healing by primary intention, the first sign of infection might be spreading erythema, perhaps accompanied by pain, oedema and an elevated body temperature. Complete wound dehiscence can be dramatic and is a serious complication requiring immediate intervention. Partial wound breakdown is more common and occurs where an isolated pocket of infection discharges through the suture line.

Wound measurement techniques

Decreases in wound surface area and volume can be useful indicators of healing. There are many methods of measurement ranging from highly technical, computerized systems to more basic techniques. However, as you will have dis-

Type of wound (e.g. pressure ulcer, venous leg ulcer) _

Location _ _ _ _ _ _ _ _ _ _ _ _ _ _ _ _ How long has wound been open? _ _ _ _ _ _ _ _ _

General Patient factors which may delay healing (e.g. malnourished, diabetes, chronic infection)
_ _

Allergies to wound care products _

Previous treatments tried (comment on success/problems) _ _ _ _ _ _ _ _ _ _ _ _ _ _ _ _ _

Special aids in current use (e.g. pressure relieving bed, compression bandage) _ _ _ _ _ _ _ _
_ _

TRACE THE WOUND WEEKLY, OR MORE FREQUENTLY IF SIGNIFICANT CHANGES ARE OBSERVED,
ANNOTATING TRACING WITH NATURE OF WOUND BED, ORIENTATION OF WOUND,
POSITION/EXTENT OF SINUSES AND UNDERMINING OF SURROUNDING SKIN.

All other parameters should be assessed at *every* dressing change and changes documented.

Wound factors/Date				
1 NATURE OF WOUND BED				
a. healthy granulation				
b. epithelialization				
c. slough				
d. black/brown eschar				
e. other (specify)				
2 EXUDATE				
a. colour				
b. type				
c. approximate amount				
3 ODOUR				
Offensive/some/none				
4 PAIN (SITE)				
a. at wound site				
b. elsewhere (specify)				
5 PAIN (FREQUENCY)				
Continuous/intermediate/only at dressing changes/none				
6 PAIN (SEVERITY)				
Patient's score (0-10)				
7 WOUND MARGIN				
a. colour				
b. oedema?				
8 ERYTHEMA OF SURROUNDING SKIN				
a. present				
b. maximum distance from wound (mm)				
9 GENERAL CONDITION OF SURROUNDING SKIN				
e.g. dry eczema				
10 INFECTION				
a. suspected				
b. wound swab sent				
c. confirmed (specify organism)				

WOUND ASSESSED BY: _

Figure 5.4
Open wound assessment chart

NAME: _____

Complete the rating sheet to assess pressure ulcer status. Evaluate each item by picking the response that best describes the wound and entering the score in the item score column for the appropriate date.

LOCATION: Anatomical site. Circle, indentify right (R) or left (L) and use 'X' to mark site on body diagrams:

_____ Sacrum & coccyx   _____ Lateral ankle
_____ Trochanter   _____ Medial ankle
_____ Ischial tuberosity   _____ Heel   _____ Other site

SHAPE: Overall wound pattern; assess by observing perimeter and depth.
Circle and *date* appropriate description:

_____ Irregular   _____ Linear or elongated
_____ Round/oval   _____ Bowl/boat
_____ Square/rectangle   _____ Butterfly _____ Other shape

Item	Assessment	Date	Date	Date
		Score	Score	Score
1. Size	1 = Length x width < 4 cm^2 2 = Length x width 4–16 cm^2 3 = Length x width 16.1–36 cm^2 4 = Length x width 36.1–80 cm^2 5 = Length x width > 80 cm^2			
2. Depth	1 = Nonblanchable erythema on intact skin 2 = Partial-thickness skin loss involving epidermis &/or dermis 3 = Full-thickness skin loss involving damage or necrosis of subcutaneous tissue; may extend down to but not through underlying fascia; &/or mixed partial- & full-thickness &/or tissue layers obscured by granulation tissue 4 = Obscured by necrosis 5 = Full-thickness skin loss with extensive destruction, tissue necrosis, or damage to muscle, bone or supporting structures			
3. Edges	1 = Indistinct, diffuse, none clearly visible 2 = Distinct, outline clearly visible, attached, even with wound base 3 = Well defined, not attached to wound base 4 = Well defined, not attached to base, rolled under, thickened 5 = Well defined, fibrotic, scarred or hyperkeratotic			
4. Undermining	1 = Undermining < 2 cm in any area 2 = Undermining 2–4 cm involving < 50% wound margins 3 = Undermining 2–4 cm involving > 50% wound margins 4 = Undermining > 4 cm in any area 5 = Tunnelling &/or sinus tract formation			
5. Necrotic tissue type	1 = None visible 2 = White/grey nonviable tissue &/or nonadherent yellow slough 3 = Loosely adherent yellow slough 4 = Adherent, soft, black eschar 5 = Firmly adherent, hard, black eschar			
6. Necrotic tissue amount	1 = None visible 2 = < 25% of wound bed covered 3 = 25–50% of wound covered 4 = > 50% and < 75% of wound covered 5 = 75–100% of wound covered			
7. Exudate type	1 = None or bloody 2 = Serosanguineous: thin, watery, pale red/pink 3 = Serous: thin, watery, clear 4 = Purulent: thin or thick, opaque, tan/yellow 5 = Foul purulent: thick, opaque, yellow/green with odour			

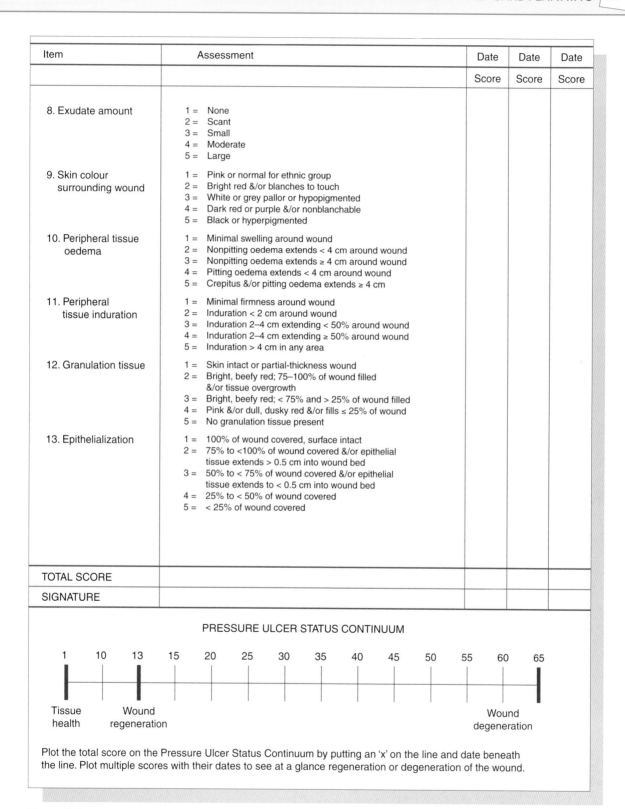

Item	Assessment	Date	Date	Date
		Score	Score	Score
8. Exudate amount	1 = None 2 = Scant 3 = Small 4 = Moderate 5 = Large			
9. Skin colour surrounding wound	1 = Pink or normal for ethnic group 2 = Bright red &/or blanches to touch 3 = White or grey pallor or hypopigmented 4 = Dark red or purple &/or nonblanchable 5 = Black or hyperpigmented			
10. Peripheral tissue oedema	1 = Minimal swelling around wound 2 = Nonpitting oedema extends < 4 cm around wound 3 = Nonpitting oedema extends ≥ 4 cm around wound 4 = Pitting oedema extends < 4 cm around wound 5 = Crepitus &/or pitting oedema extends ≥ 4 cm			
11. Peripheral tissue induration	1 = Minimal firmness around wound 2 = Induration < 2 cm around wound 3 = Induration 2–4 cm extending < 50% around wound 4 = Induration 2–4 cm extending ≥ 50% around wound 5 = Induration > 4 cm in any area			
12. Granulation tissue	1 = Skin intact or partial-thickness wound 2 = Bright, beefy red; 75–100% of wound filled &/or tissue overgrowth 3 = Bright, beefy red; < 75% and > 25% of wound filled 4 = Pink &/or dull, dusky red &/or fills ≤ 25% of wound 5 = No granulation tissue present			
13. Epithelialization	1 = 100% of wound covered, surface intact 2 = 75% to <100% of wound covered &/or epithelial tissue extends > 0.5 cm into wound bed 3 = 50% to < 75% of wound covered &/or epithelial tissue extends to < 0.5 cm into wound bed 4 = 25% to < 50% of wound covered 5 = < 25% of wound covered			
TOTAL SCORE				
SIGNATURE				

PRESSURE ULCER STATUS CONTINUUM

1   10   13   15   20   25   30   35   40   45   50   55   60   65

Tissue health   Wound regeneration   Wound degeneration

Plot the total score on the Pressure Ulcer Status Continuum by putting an 'x' on the line and date beneath the line. Plot multiple scores with their dates to see at a glance regeneration or degeneration of the wound.

Figure 5.5
The Pressure Sore Status tool

Nature of operation _

Wound site _   Date of operation _ _ _ _ _ _ _ _ _ _

Method of closure _

Drains: (a) type _ _ _ _ _ _ _ _ _ _ _ _ _ _ _ _ _ _ _   (b) site _ _ _ _ _ _ _ _ _ _ _ _ _ _ _ _ _

SPECIAL INSTRUCTIONS FROM THE SURGEON _

_ _

General patient factors that may delay healing (e.g. obese, chronic chest infection) _ _ _ _ _ _ _ _

_ _

Allergies to wound care products _

Chart the following factors at *every* dressing change. If there is marked erythema, trace this and
note if erythema spreads.

Wound factors/Date				
1 EXUDATE				
a. amount: heavy/moderate/minimal/none				
b. type				
c. colour				
2 ERYTHEMA OF SURROUNDING SKIN				
a. around stitches only				
b. extending beyond a				
c. maximum distance from the wound edge (mm)				
3 OEDEMA Severe/moderate/minimal/none				
4 HAEMATOMA Severe/moderate/minimal/none				
5 PAIN (SITE)				
a. at wound itself				
b. elsewhere (specify)				
6 PAIN (FREQUENCY) Continuous/intermittent/only at dressing changes/none				
7 PAIN (SEVERITY) Patient's score (0-10)				
8 ODOUR Offensive/some/none				
9 INFECTION				
a. suspected				
b. wound swab sent				
c. confirmed (specify organism)				

WOUND ASSESSED BY: _

Figure 5.6
Assessment chart for surgically closed wounds

covered for yourself in Activity 6, many problems arise when attempting to measure wounds accurately, by whatever means. These include problems relating to:

- **Defining the wound's boundary** – This is observer dependent and so is prone to inaccuracy.
- **Wound flexibility** – Wounds where there is undermining of the skin edge or where the wound is large or deep can be difficult to measure with precision and are capable of changing their appearance significantly according to the position of the patient.
- **The natural curvature of the human body** – Not all currently available measuring devices take this into account.

Measuring area.   There are a number of techniques available for measuring the area of a wound. These include tracing and photography.

Tracing is one of the simplest and most popular methods of assessing the area of a wound. Trace the outline of the wound margin on to a clear plastic sheet using an indelible-ink marker. Commercially available plastic measuring tools are available (Fig. 5.7). Grids can be used to facilitate the calculation of the area in square centimetres. Tracings can be transferred to the patient's notes and annotated to include the nature of the wound bed, the extent of undermining of the surrounding skin and the position of the wound relative to other structures. The calculation of wound area can be undertaken using a computer linked to a camera or hand-held scanner. This is a faster and more accurate method than attempting to count centimetre squares on a grid, as these might be incomplete where the grid straddles both the wound and intact tissue.

Photography is a commonly used approach to wound measurement. A ruler is placed next to the wound and a photograph taken from a standard distance. Although it is prone to inaccuracy, this might be the only practical option for wounds in difficult sites, and it does allow for progress to be evaluated over time, if the photograph is always taken from the same angle.

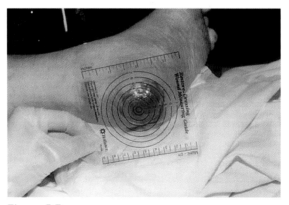

Figure 5.7
The acetate is in place for wound tracing

Measuring volume. Deep wounds with undermined areas are a common phenomenon in patients with pressure ulcers, and in many other wounds left to heal by secondary intention. In these situations it is important to be able to evaluate a wound's progress on a regular basis with some degree of accuracy. However, measurement of the wound area alone might give little indication of the healing that is occurring in the wound bed, which might be accompanied by a significant decrease in the volume of the wound as a whole. The process of granulation is usually accompanied by significant wound contraction as healing progresses.

| **Activity 7**
Assessing the volume of an open wound | To date, no one system can be used quickly, easily and cheaply to assess wound volume accurately.

Question 1. Identify the methods currently available for measuring the volume of open wounds.
Question 2. Compare these methods for: (i) accuracy; (ii) inter-rater reliability; (iii) ease of use; (iv) cost.
Question 3. Which approach would you choose in each of the following circumstances, if cost was not an issue:
  (i) for a randomized controlled clinical trial of the efficacy of a wound dressing in the healing of grade 4 pressure ulcers, in a hospital setting?
  (ii) for clinical use in a hospital setting?
  (iii) for clinical use in a patient's home?
Question 4. In practice, which methods are available to you in the home or hospital setting? |

Optimizing the local wound environment

Over the last 20 years there has been a proliferation of new wound dressing products and the use of new approaches to facilitating wound healing such as the use of ultrasound, laser and vacuum-assisted closure.

Wound dressings and cleansing agents. The issues associated with creating the optimum local environment for healing through the use of cleansing agents and the application of dressings is discussed in Chapter 8. Where the wound contains devitalized tissue, debridement is usually indicated to remove a medium for infection, to enable the true extent of tissue damage to be assessed, and to facilitate uncomplicated healing. Wounds should be cleansed, as necessary, using minimal mechanical force. Irrigation can be useful for cleaning a cavity ulcer. The place of antiseptics in wound management has been the subject of intense debate and certain historical approaches, such as the use of larval therapy and honey, are experiencing a resurgence of interest and are being re-evaluated for both efficacy and clinical effectiveness. Of the new generation products, growth factors are currently stimulating intense interest, because of their potential to actively stimulate wound healing by modulating endogenous repair processes.

The use of physical modalities.   Other therapies that are proving of value today include hyperbaric oxygen therapy, pulsed electromagnetic energy (PEME) therapy, vacuum-assisted wound closure, and ultrasound. The merits, indications and contraindications for these therapies are discussed in Chapter 9. Although many of the published studies involve only a limited number of cases, these physical modalities provide exciting possibilities for the future and deserve closer attention and evaluation now, especially for intractable wounds.

Is the patient at risk of further tissue breakdown?

Every effort should be made to optimize the condition of the patient's skin and to prevent avoidable tissue breakdown. A review of approaches to assessing a patient's risk of developing pressure ulcers, and the evidence for different methods of prevention and treatment are fully discussed in Chapter 14. In essence, it is important to assess the risk of one or more pressure ulcers developing and to develop a plan of care on admission, and whenever there is a significant change in the patient's condition, which includes:

- maximizing mobility and activity
- planning for patient positioning, transferring and turning
- providing the patient with an appropriate support surface when in bed or a chair
- optimizing the condition of the patient's skin (see Chapter 10)
- dealing with wider issues, such as malnutrition (see Chapter 11).

What are the consequences of the wound for the patient's quality of life?

The model to facilitate a holistic approach to patient assessment and care planning, illustrated in Fig. 5.2, emphasizes the importance of gaining a good understanding of the consequences of the wound from the patient's perspective, both currently and in the longer term. Quality of life is a multidimensional construct, which includes physical, social, emotional and spiritual dimensions.

Physical functioning

There are a number of well-validated tools to assess physical functioning, such as the ability to mobilize and to carry out normal activities of daily living including attending to personal hygiene and dressing. In patients with acute or chronic wounds these abilities can be compromised.

Activity 8
Assessing physical functioning

Question 1. In the context of your current work, do you use any tools to assess physical functioning in your patients?

Question 2. Have these tools been validated, and if so for which care group?

Question 3. What are the advantages and the 'costs' of a systematic process for assessing physical functioning?

Question 4. Reflect on the psychological and social consequences of physical disability for a patient of your choice (see Chapter 18, once you have thought this through).

Question 5. For the same patient, what are the consequences for care planning and for longer term rehabilitation, where this is realistic, and to what extent can the patient be involved in setting goals and monitoring them (see Chapter 13)?

Pain

Pain is a common and often underestimated problem for patients with wounds and inadequately managed pain can lead to sleep disturbance, irritability, anxiety and depression. Pain is a complex phenomenon that is influenced only in part by the degree of tissue injury or disease, as described in Chapter 12.

Activity 9 **The assessment** **and management** **of pain**	Return to the case study at the beginning of this chapter (Box 5.1). *Question 1.* How would you assess Betty Brown's pain? *Question 2.* What would you do about it?

Possible causes of pain at the wound site are summarized in Box 5.2.

Box 5.2 **Possible causes of** **pain at the wound** **site and at** **dressing changes** *(based on Morison et al* *1997, p. 75)*	If the patient complains of pain at the wound site, or experiences pain at dressing changes, consider the following questions: **A. Pain at the wound site** 1. Is the wound infected? Look for clinical and systemic signs of infection (Chapter 7). 2. Is any overlying conforming or compression bandage too tightly applied? Has the bandage slipped? Are there tight bands of constriction overlying the wound or over any nearby bony prominence? 3. Is there underlying ischaemia? For example, in a patient with severe peripheral vascular disease even small open wounds can be very painful and there might be rest pain in the limb (Chapter 15). **B. Pain at dressing changes** 1. Is the dressing adhering, causing tissue trauma on removal? Even low-adherent dressings can adhere to the wound if they are left in place for too long, especially if exudate strikes through the dressing and then dries out. Fresh bleeding on dressing removal is an obvious sign of trauma. 2. If prescribed analgesia has been used, has it had sufficient time to become effective when it is anticipated that a dressing change might be painful? Consult your pharmacist if you are unsure how long an analgesic takes to become effective. 3. Is the most painless method of dressing removal being employed? Removal of adhesive dressings or the surgical tape used to hold it in place can be very painful if removed against the lie of any hair present. Removing dressings and tapes in line with the hairs is usually less painful and releasing the adhesive bond of adhesive dressing facilitates easy removal. If a dressing has adhered to the wound bed it should be gently soaked off, not ripped off 'quickly'. 4. Is a cleansing solution being used that could cause an irritant tissue response, such as a hypochlorite? (Chapter 8)?

continued

Box 5.2
continued

5. Does the nurse lack empathy? Is the nurse underestimating the significance of the wound to the individual (Chapter 18)?
6. Is the most appropriate dressing type being used for this wound? Modern dressing materials provide a range of functions and provide a variety of wound environments (Chapter 8). Choose the most appropriate for the wound.

Social and role functions

Acute and chronic wounds can have both short- and longer-term consequences for the individual in terms of their relationships with others and the performance of their normal social roles of 'husband', 'wife', 'mother', 'friend' or 'work colleague' (see Chapter 18). Wounds can lead to short- or longer-term loss of independence, and they can lead to financial hardship if they affect the individual's ability to carry on their normal work. A young otherwise fit man who loses a leg in a motor cycle accident could lose his job, have more restricted recreational opportunities and suffer from loss of self-esteem and altered body image. Even a relatively minor injury can have devastating consequences for anyone whose work involves highly developed psychomotor skills, such as a musician or a surgeon. Assessing the consequences of a wound for the individual is therefore a very important component of both short-term care and longer-term rehabilitation, and might involve many other members of the multidisciplinary team such as physiotherapists and occupational therapists.

Emotional and spiritual well-being

The cause of a wound and its physical and social consequences can have a direct bearing on the patient's feelings both about the wound and about themselves, as described in Chapter 18.

Activity 10
Assessing emotional and spiritual well-being

It is not common for a formal assessment to be made of a patient's emotional and spiritual well-being, in the context of wound care.

Question 1. Can you think of any circumstances when this might be a very important component of patient assessment and care planning?
Question 2. What preformulated tools exist for assessing these dimensions of quality of life?
Question 3. Which of these tools might be of use to you in a clinical practice setting?

What are the patient's social circumstances and the optimal setting for care?

A patient's social circumstances and the setting for care can have a profound effect on that person's physical, emotional and social well-being. Hospitalization might be essential for patients following trauma or planned surgery because of the specialist facilities and expertise required, but care is likely to be costly, both to the provider and to individuals, who might suffer major disruption to their normal life. Care at home is usually associated with more freedom for the individual and often easier access for family and friends, but facilities are more restricted, as is access to health-related services and advice. Deciding on the optimum time to discharge a patient from hospital can be more difficult than it might seem because there is usually some degree of risk associated with this, especially in the short term. Discharge planning and the organization of home-care support services prior to discharge is therefore very important. For some patients, a return to their own home will never be possible and arrangements will need to be made for long-term care, which can have deleterious consequences for the individual's quality of life and require major adjustments both for the individuals and for their carers.

To what extent can the patient and lay carer be involved in care planning and its implementation?

A client-centred approach is characterized by shared responsibility, mutuality and client autonomy.

The patient's central role

Many patients with wounds might seem to healthcare professionals to have little motivation to help themselves. As Betty Brown's case illustrates (Box 5.1), chronic wounds often develop at a time when patients are least able to help themselves because of illness or disability and, when a chronic wound is slow to heal, people can come to believe that they are helpless to influence the situation in a positive way. However, in a client-centred approach, which fully acknowledges the individual's rights to autonomy and self-determination, the healthcare professional and the client share responsibility for care planning and the focus shifts from the individual's deficits to facilitating the client's potential for self help. The principles of patient education, ways of creating a therapeutic environment for learning, and maximizing the patient's commitment and involvement in care are discussed in detail in Chapter 13.

Involving the patient's family and lay carers

A task that is often neglected is the education and support of family and lay carers. Educational programmes should be structured, organized and comprehensive, and made available to family or care givers as well as to patients (Chapter 13).

Activity 11
Involving the patient's family in assessment and care planning

Refer back to the case of Betty Brown (Box 5.1). It is not uncommon for family relationships to break down when a person becomes old and debilitated and actually needs the family's care and support the most.

Question 1. How would you attempt to involve Betty's family in her care?
Question 2. What other agencies might usefully be involved?

Seeing the patient in a wider social context

Although the focus of this chapter is predominantly on the individual, there are many hints in the literature to suggest that society's view of health and health care, and the attitudes of family members, friends and healthcare professionals in the local community have an impact on the nature of the individual's experience of a wound. As illustrated in Fig. 5.8, individuals are members of families, who are in turn embedded within a local community, set in a wider society. The term 'system' describes 'an integrated whole' in which the parts are interconnected with one another in a complex web of relationships (Fig. 5.8). Systems theory is reflected in a number of models of nursing such as Neuman's systems model, where the client is seen as a unique individual, decision making is shared and diversity is valued and respected. Family systems theory underpins the move towards the practice of family nursing in the home.

The aim of care planning should be to take a holistic approach to understanding the unique context within which each individual's wound is to be managed, and to understanding the interaction of a multiplicity of variables on many system levels.

What are the patient's needs for rehabilitation? Rehabilitation involves restoration of the individual's physical and social functioning, so far as this is possible, and as such builds on all of the dimensions of patient assessment and care planning discussed so far.

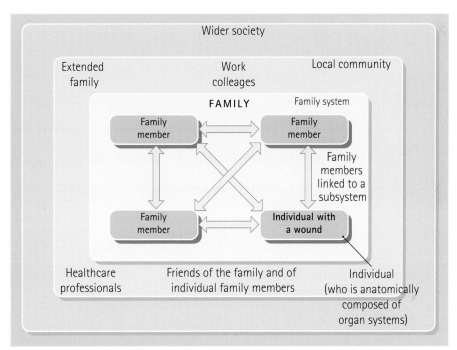

Figure 5.8
A conceptualization of the individual, embedded with a family, set in a local community and encompassed by a wider society

Activity 12 *Developing a long-term care plan*	Review the care that you have planned for Betty Brown so far (Box 5.1 and the related activities). *Question 1.* What are your long-term goals for Betty? *Question 2.* What other professionals will need to be involved in implementing this care plan?

THE IMPLEMENTATION OF EVIDENCE-BASED PRACTICE AND MULTIDISCIPLINARY CARE PLANNING

There are many published examples of the tremendous benefits that can arise from the implementation of evidence-based practice guidelines within organizations. Specialists in tissue viability clearly have an important role to play as advanced practitioners, researchers and educators, liaising effectively with other professionals such as physiotherapists, dieticians and occupational therapists and promoting best practice (Chapter 20).

CONCLUSION

Wounds can have a significant impact on an individual's quality of life, including physical and social functioning and the performance of normal social roles. Wounds are often accompanied by pain and discomfort, lowered self-esteem and altered body image and, for some patients complications such as sepsis, can be life-threatening.

A systematic and holistic approach to patient assessment and care planning is essential for the delivery of care that is effective and that meets the needs of individuals and their families. The use of a conceptual framework can facilitate the adoption of a holistic, client-centred approach and can shift the emphasis from the wound towards the patient with a wound.

FURTHER READING

Wound care

Bryant R A 2000 Acute and chronic wounds: nursing management, 2nd edn. Mosby, St Louis, MO

Hollinworth H 2002 How to alleviate pain at wound dressing changes. Nursing Times 98(44):51–52

Mear J, Moffatt C 2002 Bandaging technique in the treatment of venous ulcers. Nursing Times 98(44):44–46

Morison M (ed) 2001 The prevention and treatment of pressure ulcers. Mosby, Edinburgh

Samad A et al 2002 Digital imaging versus conventional contact tracing for the objective measurement of venous leg ulcers. Journal of Wound Care 11(4):137–140

Seal D V et al 2000 Skin and wound infection: investigation and treatment in practice. Martin Dunitz, Andover

Williams L 2002 Assessing patients' nutritional needs in the wound-healing process. Journal of Wound Care 11(6):225–228

Clinical effectiveness and professional issues

Chambers R, Boath E 2001 Clinical effectiveness and clinical governance made easy, 2nd edn. Radcliffe Medical Press, Oxford

Gomm R, Davies C 2000 Using evidence in health and social care. Sage, London, in association with the Open University

Guyatt G, Rennie D (eds) 2001 Users' guide to the medical literature: a manual for evidence-base clinical practice. AMA Press, Washington DC

Moulin M 2002 Delivering excellence in health and social care: quality, excellence and performance measurement. Open University Press, Buckingham

Taylor B J 2000 Reflective practice: a guide for nurses and midwives. Open University Press, Buckingham

<table>
<tr><td>PART **1**</td><td># Pressure ulcers</td></tr>
</table>

PART **1** Pressure ulcers

Yvonne Franks

Case study 1:
A 62-year-old diabetic man with a pressure ulcer on his heel

A 62-year-old man is admitted to the limb rehabilitation ward in preparation for undergoing a series of daily adjustments to the artificial limb of his right leg in the following week. He had an above-knee amputation 10 years previously, at the age of 52, as a consequence of peripheral vascular disease. He is an insulin-dependent diabetic. He was widowed 4 years ago and, by his own admission, 'has not been looking after himself too well'. His admission is seen by staff as an opportunity to assess him more holistically and to engage the multidisciplinary team in planning his longer-term care.

On initial assessment it is observed that he has a pressure ulcer on the outer aspect of his left heel (Figs CS 1.1 and 1.2). He has been dressing this himself for some months using gauze padding.

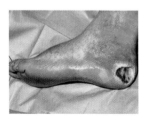

Figure CS 1.1
A pressure ulcer in a diabetic man with peripheral vascular disease

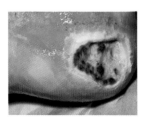

Figure CS 1.2
The pressure ulcer as seen on initial assessment

Case study 2:
A 75-year-old woman who developed a sacral pressure ulcer following knee replacement surgery

A 75-year-old woman has been a resident of a nursing home, in a country setting, for some time. She has many friends and is known for her eccentricities. She had a lively social life in the home, taking an active part in activities including gentle fitness sessions until she developed a sacral pressure ulcer (Fig. CS 2.1) following a period in hospital for knee replacement surgery.

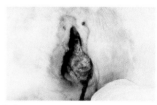

Figure CS 2.1
A sacral pressure ulcer that developed in an elderly woman following orthopaedic surgery

Her stay in hospital had been prolonged by an MRSA infection of her surgical wound, which had required her to be nursed in isolation. Naturally slim, the period of reduced mobility following the orthopaedic surgery was accompanied by a marked reduction in her dietary intake.

Case study 3:
An elderly woman who developed extensive pressure area damage following a stroke
See Box 1.1 and Figure 1.1 (p 7 in Chapter 1).

PART 2

Ulcers of the leg and foot

Ysabel Bello and Ana Falabella

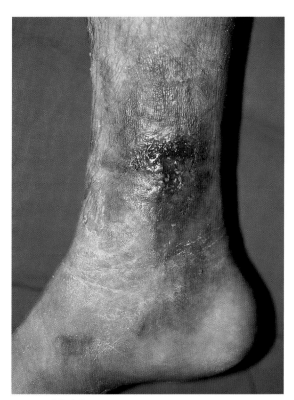

Figure CS 4.1
A leg ulcer on the right medial malleolus

Case study 4:
A 42-year-old man with an ulcer on the right medial malleolus
A 42-year-old man presents with an ulcer on the right medial malleolus, which has been open for almost 2 years. He has a history of recurrent leg swelling and aching at the end of the day. His past medical history includes hypertension, diabetes mellitus and right ankle closed fracture. His medications included glipizide and antihypertensives. His ulcer had been treated with mupirocin ointment, non-adherent dressing and compression stockings for several months. It then was treated with non-adherent dressing and Unna boot bandage plus self-adherent wrap (Duke's boot) weekly for 1 month without improvement. His job required him to stand for over 8 hours a day. He stated that his pain had markedly increased during the 2 weeks prior to his visit.

On physical examination there was pitting oedema on the right leg up to the knee. He had an ulcer with irregular margins, measuring 3.2 × 3.6 cm and 0.4 cm deep over the right medial malleolus. The wound bed was covered with granulation tissue and fibrinous slough (Fig. CS 4.1). There was a heavy amount of serous drainage, and the periwound skin was macerated, warm and erythematous. Hyperpigmented patches and woody induration of the periwound skin were noted. Varicosities were observed on the medial aspect of the right leg. The pulses were palpable and strong. His ankle brachial pressure index was 1.0.

Case study 5:
A 38-year-old man with a leg ulcer that had been open for 9 years
A healthy 38-year-old man presents with a recurrent painful ulcer on the left lower extremity, which had been open for 9 years. He had been treated with multilayer compression bandage systems and

different categories of dressings, including hydrogel dressing, foam dressing, collagen dressing and cadexomer iodine, according to the wound characteristics. He had been treated with skin equivalents on several occasions. The ulcer bed improved but the ulcer failed to heal. The patient was very compliant with compression and leg elevation. His past medical history was unremarkable. His medications included ibuprofen for leg ulcer pain.

On physical examination, he had an ulcer located on the left medial malleolus measuring 4.5 × 5.3 cm with irregular margins (Fig. CS 5.1). The ulcer was superficial and the wound bed was completely covered with tissue, beefy red and granular in appearance. A moderate amount of serous exudate was present. No oedema was observed. The periwound skin was hyperpigmented and surrounded by woody induration. Oedema was not present. Pulses were present. His ankle brachial pressure index was 1.0.

Duplex evaluation of the left lower extremity demonstrated venous insufficiency involving the common femoral, the common great and lesser saphenous, as well as the profunda and popliteal veins. A wound culture reported abundant *Escherichia coli* and *Proteus mirabilis* sensitive to levofloxacin. Osteomyelitis, infection of soft tissues by atypical mycobacteria and fungal infection were ruled out. A biopsy reported dermal chronic inflammation with vascular proliferation and hemorrhage, suggesting venous dermatitis. There was no evidence of malignancy. His complementary laboratory studies including cell blood count, factor V Leiden, protein C and protein S, cryoglobulins, cryofibrinogens, anticardiolipin antibodies and lupus anticoagulant were within normal limits.

The patient was treated with oral levofloxacin 500 mg daily for 7 days. Wound care included cadexomer iodine dressing, non-adherent dressing, conforming bandage, and self-adherent wrap, to be changed daily for 1 week. The patient was hospitalized for the performance of an autologous split thickness skin graft (Fig. CS 5.2).

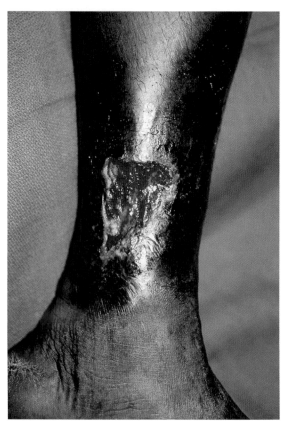

Figure CS 5.1
A leg ulcer on initial presentation

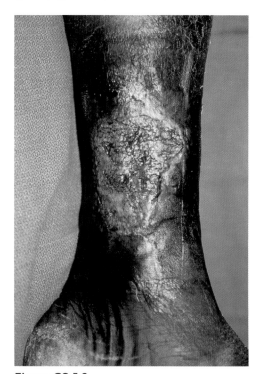

Figure CS 5.2
The leg ulcer following an autologous split thickness skin graft

Case Study 6:
A 78-year-old woman with recurrent leg ulcers

A 78-year-old woman has had recurrent ulceration on the left lateral malleolus for the last 4 years. The current ulcer has been present for 7 months. She also presents with an ulcer on the dorsum of the left foot, which has been present for 1 year. She has a past medical history of hypertension. She experiences pain in the left calf after walking more than 30 yards. She states that pain occurs with leg elevation and diminishes after lying down. She has smoked one pack of cigarettes per day for over 20 years. She does not tolerate compression bandages. She had been using topical antibiotics. Her medications include cephalexin (taken irregularly) and pentoxifylline 400 mg three times per day.

On physical examination, the skin on the leg is shiny and hairless. There is an ulcer located on the left lateral malleolus measuring 6.0 × 7.0 cm and covered with fibrinous slough and granulation tissue (Fig. CS 6.1). There is no surrounding redness or warmth. She also has an ulcer on the dorsum of the left foot of 0.9 × 3.0 cm, covered with granulation tissue. The pulses are non-palpable and almost non-audible with Doppler. There is thin, shiny, scaling on the legs with bilateral dependent rubor.

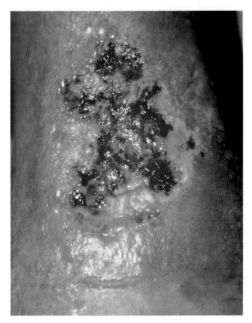

Figure CS 6.1
A leg ulcer on the left lateral malleolus

Case Study 7:
A 76-year-old man with four large oval ulcers located over a long linear scar

A 76-year-old man with non-insulin dependent diabetes mellitus for 35 years, presents with multiple punched-out ulcers on the lower extremities. The patient was referred by a vascular surgeon. The ulcers have been open for over 3 months. They developed after revascularization surgical procedures. He has a past medical history of diabetes, peripheral vascular disease, coronary artery disease and myocardial infarction. He had a pacemaker placement and coronary artery bypass graft with the use of the veins from the left lower extremity and arterial femoral–popliteal bypass on the right leg performed during the same hospitalization, a few days apart. His surgical wounds became infected with methicillin-resistant *Staphylococcus aureus* (MRSA) He received intravenous vancomycin for 1 week. The patient had smoked 1 pack of cigarettes per day for 30 years, but gave up 20 years ago. He complains of claudication and rest pain. His medications include ramipril, atorvastatin, coumadin, glypizide, insulin, and trimethoprim plus sulfamethoxazole.

On physical examination he is found to have bilateral lower extremity pitting oedema. Four large oval punched-out ulcers are noted. The ulcers are located over a long linear scar that extends from the inner thigh to the medial malleolus. The first, measuring 6.0 × 3.2 cm is located on the medial malleolus (Fig. CS 7.1). The ulcer margins are regular, and the ulcer bed has 90% fibrinous slough

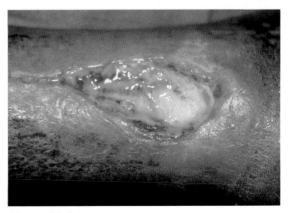

Figure CS 7.1
A leg ulcer on the medial malleolus

and 10% granulation tissue, with evidence of severe periwound maceration. The second ulcer measures 4.3 × 2.3 cm. The wound bed is covered with 60% fibrinous slough and 40% granulation tissue, with evidence of tendon exposure. The third and fourth ulcers are located on the medial leg (Fig. CS 7.2). They measure 1.8 × 0.5 cm and 4.4 × 1.0 cm, and they are covered with 80% fibrinous slough and 20% granulation tissue. The patient also has small wounds with little exudate on the right knee and left second toe. The patient has thick toenails. Pulses are not palpable and almost non-audible with Doppler. His ankle brachial pressure index on the right is 1.15 and on the left is 2.02.

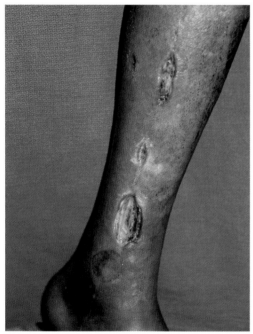

Figure CS 7.2
The lower leg showing multiple ulcers

Case study 8:
A 77-year-old man with an irregular ulcer on the right medial malleolus

A 77-year-old man presents with an ulcer on the right medial malleolus, which has been open for 4 months. The wound bed had been grafted with a split thickness skin graft but failed to heal. The ulcer had also been treated with moist-to-wet gauze. His past medical history includes hypertension, coronary artery disease, deep venous thrombosis,

peripheral vascular disease with ischaemic gangrene on the right second toe, and the fourth and fifth left toes. He has a history of percutaneous transluminal coronary angioplasty twice, and a right and left femoral posterior tibial saphenous vein bypass. His medications included aspirin, simvastatin and clopidrogel.

On physical examination, an ulcer is noted on the right medial malleolus measuring 6.0 × 8.3 cm, with flat irregular margins (Fig. CS 8.1). The wound bed is covered with mixed fibrinous and granulation tissue. A surgical staple is observed in the centre of the wound. There is a moderate amount of serous exudate and mild periwound maceration. His right lower extremity is shiny, cold and hairless, and his pulses are decreased, almost non-palpable, but audible with Doppler. His ankle brachial pressure index is 0.76. He has pitting oedema up to the knee and fine scaling of the legs. Surgical scars are observed on the inner aspect of both legs. There is no evidence of varicosities, but there is periwound woody induration.

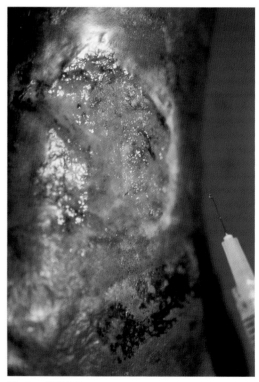

Figure CS 8.1
A leg ulcer located on the right medial malleolus with irregular margins. A staple is noticed in the centre of the wound

Case study 9:
A 65-year-old man with a diabetic foot ulcer

A 65-year-old man with non-insulin dependent diabetes mellitus for 12 years presents with a 2-month history of right plantar foot ulceration. His past medical history includes diabetic neuropathy, and amputation of the right second toe secondary to osteomyelitis. The patient has smoked two cigarettes per day for 20 years. His medications included metformin and glipizide. He uses a Darco shoe and a walking cane.

On physical examination of the plantar surface of the right foot, the patient has a full-thickness non-painful ulcer between the second and third metatarsal head, which measures 2.2 × 2.1 cm in size and is 0.5 cm deep (Fig. CS 9.1). A marked hyperkeratotic rim around the ulcer is observed but there is no undermining. A 10-g monofilament wire to test protective sensation indicates failure to feel the filament at four of the 10 sites tested (plantar aspect of the first and third digits and plantar aspect of the first and third metatarsal heads). Pulses are present and the ankle brachial pressure index is 1.0.

His glycohaemoglobin A1c is 7.6% TL Hb (normal value < 6.5), reflecting well-controlled diabetes mellitus. Blood cell count and erythrocyte sedimentation rate are within the normal range. X-ray of the right foot with three views weightbearing reveals that the second toe is absent from the metatarsophalangeal joint. The third metatarsophalangeal joint is irregular and markedly narrowed. The proximal phalanx is subluxed slightly laterally. The fourth and fifth metatarsophalangeal joints are markedly narrowed. There is no evidence of osteomyelitis.

Case study 10:
A 76-year-old woman with a large painful ulcer laterally on her right leg

A 76-year-old woman presents with a large, painful wound on the right lateral leg; this has been present for several days. The wound developed after excision of squamous cell carcinoma by Moh's surgery. She is overweight and has a history of vein stripping, multiple pregnancies, swelling of the legs that worsened at the end of the day for several years, and high cholesterol. Her medications include atorvastatin and cephalexin for the past 3 days.

On physical examination, above the right lateral malleolus, she has a full thickness ulcer measuring 15.5 × 8 cm in size and 0.9 cm deep (Fig. CS 10.1). The wound is producing a mild amount of clear exudate and mild odour. She also has a 2.5 × 2.4 cm ulcer on the dorsum of the foot. She has bilateral varicosities of the lower extremities and pitting oedema of the right leg. The pulses are palpable and strong. Her ankle brachial pressure index is 0.95.

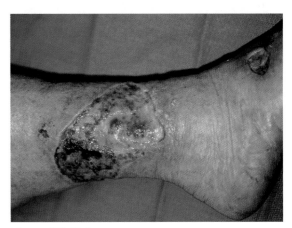

Figure CS 10.1
Ulcers located on the right lateral leg and foot. These ulcers developed after excision of a squamous cell carcinoma by Moh's surgery.

Case study 11:
A frail 80-year-old woman with extensive, sloughy leg ulcers and pressure area damage
See Box 5.1 and Figure 5.1, p 48 in Chapter 5.

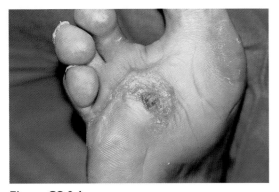

Figure CS 9.1
A diabetic foot ulcer on the plantar surface of the right foot surrounded by a hyperkeratotic rim

PART **3** | # Chronic wounds associated with malignancy

Dorothy B Doughty

Case study 12:
A 61-year-old woman with a necrotic breast wound following mastectomy

A 61-year-old woman is referred for management of a necrotic breast wound following mastectomy and placement of a tissue expander 18 days prior to referral. Significant medical and surgical history included a lumpectomy 1 year ago and recurrence of the cancer leading to the current procedure, and a coronary artery bypass graft (CABG) and placement of a coronary artery stent. She is a former smoker who gave up smoking just 18 days ago prior to the latest surgery. She is currently receiving oral chemotherapy.

Assessment reveals a wound measuring 15 × 6.2 × 2.4 cm and 75% of the wound bed is covered with soft grey eschar (Fig. CS 12.1). There is a large amount of dark yellow drainage fluid and induration of periwound tissue. The patient denies pain but reports feelings of 'tightness' in the area of the wound. She is anxious because of the wound's obvious deterioration. Baseline nutritional assessment indicates that her weight is appropriate for her height, her current intake of calories and protein are deemed sufficient to support wound healing but she is not taking any vitamin or mineral supplements.

Case study 13:
A 71-year-old man with a fungating tumour involving the right side of his face and neck

A 71-year-old man has been referred for assistance with the management of a fungating tumour involving his right face and neck (Fig. CS 13.1). He had undergone surgical resection 4 months

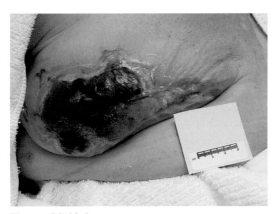

Figure CS 12.1
A necrotic breast wound following mastectomy and placement of a tissue expander

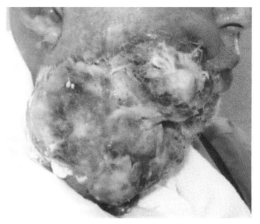

Figure CS 13.1
A fungating tumour involving the right side of the face and neck

before but the tumour recurred in a short period of time and grew rapidly, despite ongoing chemotherapy. The tumour now involves the right mandible and the entire lower right face; the carotid artery is exposed. There is a large amount of soft grey eschar on the surface of the tumour and large amounts of malodorous exudate. Additional medical problems include hypertension, diabetes mellitus and depression. He has refused hospice care and states that his goal is 'to get his skin to heal'. He is still able to eat and his pain is being managed with Roxicet and Oxycontin. However, a major difficulty is finding dressings that will stay in place, absorb the drainage and control the odour.

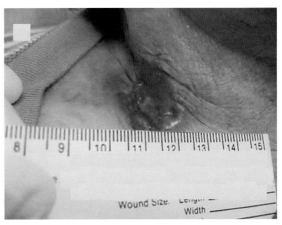

Figure CS 14.1
A radiation injury

Case study 14:
A radiation injury in a 72-year-old woman with recurrent adenocarcinoma

A 72-year old artist was referred for a non-healing wound of her right shoulder and neck secondary to a radiation injury. Her past history included a right mastectomy in 1980 for breast cancer, a prophylactic left mastectomy in 1990 and a course of radiation therapy for treatment of metastatic disease involving the sternum and right shoulder 4 months prior to the current referral. On the initial visit, the wound measured 2.5 × 1.7 × 0.4 cm; 80% of the wound bed was covered with slough and there was a moderate amount of serous exudate. The patient and her husband were trying to care for the wound at home but they explained that they were having trouble knowing what to do and the husband felt uncomfortable with changing the dressings. Topical therapy was complicated by the fact that the patient was allergic to tape. On questioning, the patient stated that her pain was well-controlled with Neurontin and Percocet.

Initial interventions included instrumental debridement of loose avascular tissue and initiation of enzymatic debridement followed by a calcium alginate dressing and transparent adhesive cover dressing. The husband was shown how to carry out the dressings and said that he was confident in his ability to provide her daily dressing changes.

One month after this initial consultation, the wound was clean and slowly granulating. There was minimal serous exudate and wound dimensions were 1.7 × 1.0 × 0.3 cm (Fig. CS 14.1).

Three months after the initial consultation, the wound was almost healed. The dimensions were 0.3 × 0.3 × 0.1 cm and the exudate remained minimal. The wound bed was clean and dark pink, with slowly progressing epithelialization. However, 2 weeks later the patient called to report that the wound was 'getting worse again'. She was brought to clinic, where assessment revealed that the wound had enlarged to 2.0 × 1.0 × 0.1 cm, the ulcer bed appeared friable, there was now a moderate amount of serosanguinous exudate, and the wound edges were described as 'rolled and closed' (Fig. CS 14.2).

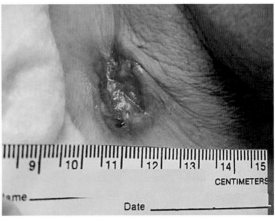

Figure CS 14.2
The same radiation injury some months later

PART **4** # Other chronic wounds

Dorothy B Doughty and Linda Russell

Case study 15:
A 21-year-old college student with a pilonidal cyst

A 21-year-old college student is referred for a non-healing wound following excision of a pilonidal cyst 5 months earlier, with a subsequent revision 1 month prior to referral. She has no other health problems and is well nourished. Her surgeon has no explanation for her failure to heal and has even performed a colonoscopy to rule out occult bowel disease. The colonoscopy was negative. Her wound, located deep in the gluteal cleft, measures 2.4 × 1.0 cm. The wound bed is viable but friable and covered with a gelatinous film (Fig. CS 15.1) Wound care

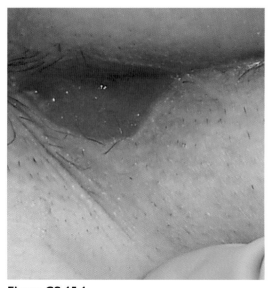

Figure CS 15.1
An excised pilonidal cyst

at the time of referral included packing with damp saline gauze. The patient complains of the gauze sticking to the wound bed and causing pain on removal. She also complains of pain while sitting, especially when sitting for prolonged periods of time.

Case study 16:
A 48-year-old woman with a dehisced surgical wound and faecal fistula

A 48-year-old woman has a dehisced surgical wound complicated by an enterocutaneous fistula. Her surgical history includes abdominal hysterectomy 8 years ago, appendectomy complicated by peritonitis 6 years ago, cholecystectomy 4 years ago and small bowel obstruction necessitating exploratory laparotomy with lysis of adhesions 2 weeks ago. The operative report notes the presence of dense adhesions and the occurrence of several enterotomies requiring repair during the procedure.

One week postoperatively, the surgical incision dehisced. Faecal drainage became apparent 10 days postoperatively and a contrast study confirmed the presence of a small bowel (ileal) fistula. Drainage is described as 'high-volume', necessitating dressing changes every 1–2 h.

Figure CS 16.1 illustrates a pectin barrier bridge and skin protection. If the fistula tract underwent epithelialization to form a 'pseudostoma' (as seen in Fig. CS 16.2), would that be predictive of probable spontaneous closure, or of probable failure to close spontaneously? Would such a development alter your care plan? How and why? (Note that Fig. CS 16.2 is of a different patient.)

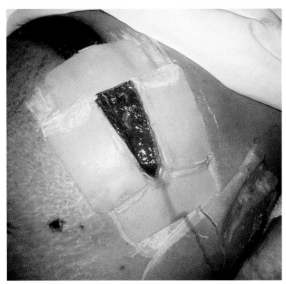

Figure CS 16.1
This illustrates a pectin barrier bridge and skin protection

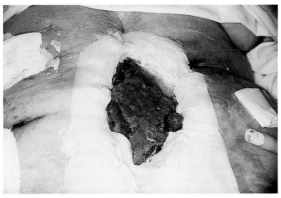

Figure CS 16.2
The fistula tract has formed a 'pseudostoma' (*note:* this is a different patient)

his right axilla has been admitted to hospital from home. He has hypertension and was diagnosed with cancer of the larynx with subsequent metastases. His medications include analgesia, sedation and a laxative for constipation. On admission he is lucid; his pain is controlled with pethidine. Prior to his admission the wound was being dressed daily with a proflavin pack prescribed by the consultant and the patient found this very uncomfortable, causing extreme pain on removal. This dressing regime had also resulted in the patient's clothes becoming wet and he was conscious of the smell. The wound is 17 × 8 cm and 10 cm in depth. Internal structures are visible and exudate levels are high (Fig. CS 17.1). The tissue is delicate following radiotherapy to his axilla.

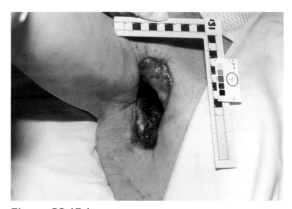

Figure CS 17.1
A non-healing wound following a excision of the right axilla

Case study 17:
A 75-year-old man with a 7-month history of a non-healing wound following excision of his right axilla
A 75-year-old man with a 7-month history of a non-healing wound following a second excision of

Case study 18:
An 18-year-old with extensive tissue necrosis following meningococcal infection
See Box 1.2 and Figs 1.2–1.4, p 9 in Chapter 1.

PART **5**

Trauma

Cathy Hess

Case study 19:
A 2½-year-old girl scalded with boiling coffee

A 2½-year-old girl is referred to the outpatient wound care team for management of scalds which resulted from boiling coffee being accidentally spilled on her. The burns are 3 days old at the time of referral. The child is initially seen by the plastic surgeon.

The base of the pectoral burn wound is 80% white with lack of sensation through most of that area (Fig. CS 19.1). The mother expresses her desire to avoid any surgical intervention, if at all possible.

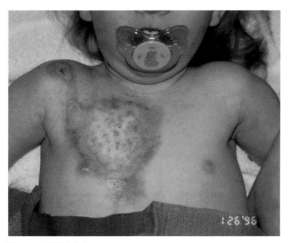

Figure CS 19.1
A scald in a young child

Case study 20:
A 53-year-old man with bilateral burns to his lower extremities

A 53-year-old male, employed as a service technician, presents to the emergency room with bilateral burns to his lower extremities. He was cleaning an engine part submerged in gasoline when the gasoline ignited. He kicked the pan of burning gas with his foot to try to remove it from the garage and, in turn, the burning gas splashed onto his legs.

Upon assessment he is found to have a non-remarkable past medical history and no known allergies. The right-leg burn is circumferential at the ankle and is well demarcated at the distal border where the shoe ceased the flame progression (Fig. CS 20.1). The hair follicles are intact in the majority of the wound. Eighty per cent of the wound is determined to be a partial thickness burn. The distal portion of the tibia, at the ankle line, has

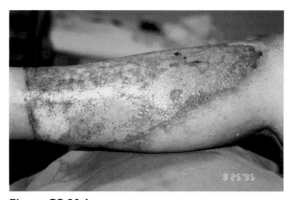

Figure CS 20.1
Burns to the lower leg

a white base with no obvious hair follicles and is insensate. The pedal pulses are intact and both feet are warm with intact sensation. A treatment programme is initiated.

Two months later the burns are completely healed and the patient is placed in compression stockings at 30–40 mmHg for scar compression. However, several months later the skin is still fragile and the patient is scratching the area and breaking through the healing tissue.

Case study 21:
A 20-year-old male who has sustained major trauma following a motor vehicle accident
A 20-year-old male arrives at the trauma unit following a motor vehicle accident. He has no significant previous medical history and no known allergies. He is unconscious and is diagnosed with a closed head injury, lacerated liver and fractures of the left arm and left leg.

After the initial treatment for his injuries, his case becomes more complicated by the development of an abscess at the site of the liver laceration. Surgical debridement and irrigation is performed and the abdominal wound is left open to heal by secondary intention. He is fitted with a PEG tube for feeding and nutritional supplementation.

He undergoes surgery for skin grafting, however the first graft fails. He is found to have a methicillin-resistant *Staphylococcus aureus* (MRSA) wound infection. After treatment for the infection a second skin graft is performed at the first failed site, using the right upper leg as the donor site. Following the stabilization of the second skin graft, the patient still has small open areas scattered throughout the site (Fig. CS 21.1). There is also a delay in the healing of the donor site, complicating this patient's return to normal activities of daily living.

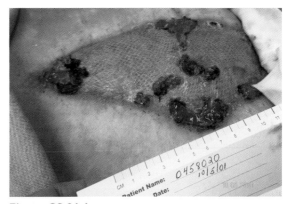

Figure CS 21.1
Skin graft

Wound management principles and resources

General principles

The physiology of wound healing

Liza G Ovington and Gregory S Schultz

CHAPTER CONTENTS

OVERVIEW OF THE PROCESS OF NORMAL WOUND HEALING

Wound healing in the skin is a highly coordinated and regulated cascade of events that can be grouped into general phases of haemostasis, inflammation, angiogenesis, matrix synthesis (granulation), epithelialization and remodelling of scar that ideally leads to functional repair of tissue injury (Fig. 6.1). The predominant cell types involved in wound repair include platelets, neutrophils, monocytes, macrophages, fibroblasts, epithelial cells and vascular endothelial cells. The healing process is highly dependent on specific communication and precise interactions between the various cell types, extracellular matrix components and soluble mediators, and there is both temporal and spatial regulation of the key events leading to repair. Growth factors, cytokines, chemokines, endocrine hormones, receptors, proteases and their inhibitors have all been shown to regulate key aspects of these processes (Bennett & Schultz 1993a, 1993b, Cherry et al 2001, Clark 1996, Kirsner & Bogensberger 2002, Mignatti et al 1996, Schultz 2000, Waldrop & Doughty 2000). In addition, key non-cellular components of the extracellular matrix, including collagen, fibrin, fibronectin and proteoglycans, also play important roles in guiding the healing process. This has led to the hypothesis that the impairment or imbalance of these key molecular regulators in wounds directly promotes the establishment and maintenance of chronic wounds (Mast & Schultz 1996, Tamuzzer & Schultz 1996). Thus, therapies that correct these imbalances and establish an

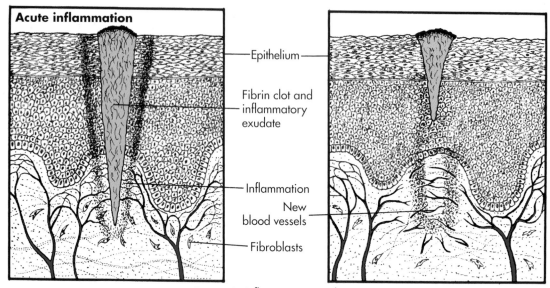

Acute inflammation

Epithelium

Fibrin clot and inflammatory exudate

Inflammation

New blood vessels

Fibroblasts

Present in inflammatory exudate:
Neutrophils
Macrophages
Bacteria and dead cells
Erythrocytes
Fibrin

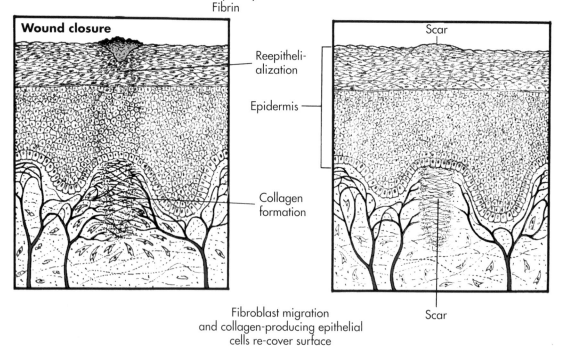

Wound closure

Scar

Reepithelialization

Epidermis

Collagen formation

Fibroblast migration and collagen-producing epithelial cells re-cover surface

Scar

Figure 6.1a
Wound healing by primary intention.

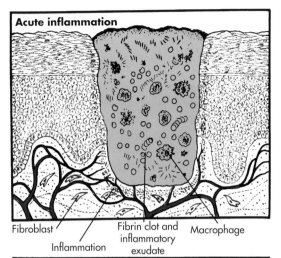

Fibroblast   Fibrin clot and   Macrophage
inflammatory
Inflammation   exudate

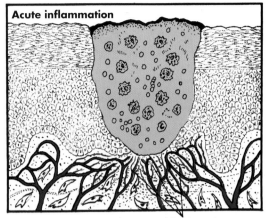

New blood vessels

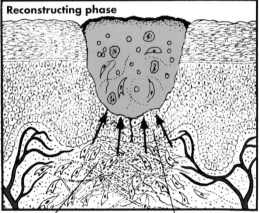

Granulation tissue

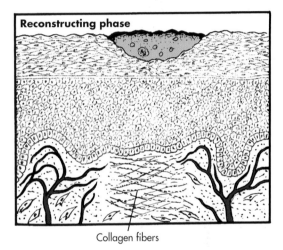

Collagen fibers

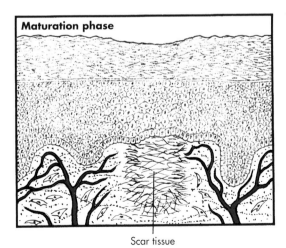

Scar tissue

Figure 6.1b
Wound healing by secondary intention.

Acute inflammation

Present in inflammatory exudate: neutrophils, macrophages, bacteria, dead cells, and erythrocytes.
Macrophages mediate the transition from the inflammatory phase to the proliferative phase of healing, releasing a wide variety of growth factors and cytokines.

Reconstructing phase

Epithelialization, formation of granulation tissue, contraction begins.

Maturation phase

This phase includes completion of contraction, differentiation, and remodeling of scar tissue.

environment in chronic wounds that permits these molecules to function normally should lead to healing of chronic wounds.

CELL–CELL COMMUNICATION

Platelets, neutrophils, monocytes, macrophages, fibroblasts, epithelial cells and endothelial cells must be able to communicate efficiently between and among themselves in order to carry out their roles in the various aspects of the healing process. Typically, one cell communicates with another cell via the intracellular synthesis and extracellular release of a molecule that conveys a specific message or signal. In order for these signalling molecules to have biological effects on target cells, they must bind physically to a receptor protein present on a target cell. The amount of mediator necessary to communicate the message is very small, frequently nanomolar quantities are effective. The more general term, soluble mediator, refers to the fact that these regulatory proteins are soluble and dynamic in achieving their effect, in other words they must be able to 'travel' in the extracellular environment from the cell of origin to a target cell.

SOLUBLE MEDIATORS – CYTOKINES, GROWTH FACTORS AND CHEMOKINES

Three major classes of soluble protein mediator are now recognized: growth factors, cytokines and chemokines. Initially, the distinction between these classes of soluble mediators arose because they appeared to target different types of cells. For example, growth factors were initially discovered for their ability to stimulate repeated cycles of mitosis of fibroblasts and epidermal cells, and they were thought to not act on immune system cells. As shown in Table 6.1, six major families of growth factors have now been identified, and whereas growth factors primarily affect non-immune cells such as fibroblasts, epithelial cells, smooth muscle cells and vascular endothelial cells, it is now know that some growth factors can stimulate inflammatory cells.

Cytokines were initially discovered based on their ability to regulate inflammation by regulating proliferation and differentiation of inflammatory cells such as monocytes, polymorphonuclear leukocytes and lymphocytes. As shown in Table 6.2, different cytokines can stimulate or inhibit inflammation and, although cytokines are synthesized by inflammatory cells, they are also synthesized by other types of cells, including keratinocytes and fibroblasts. Also, new data demonstrate that cytokines can regulate many important functions of non-inflammatory cells, such as production of matrix metalloproteinases proteases (MMPs) by fibroblasts.

The terms 'growth factors' and 'cytokines' are often used almost interchangeably now to designate proteins that regulate cell proliferation and differentiation. Both cytokines and growth factors are small-molecular-weight proteins, which are synthesized by cells and released into the extracellular environment where they can bind to specialized surface receptors on another cell. Growth factors can also be stored intracellularly (e.g. in platelet alpha granules) or by attaching to components of the extracellular matrix (such as fibronectin) where they are later activated by protease cleavage. Their regulatory actions are vital to the successful coordination of the many cellular and biochemical events in the healing cascade.

Table 6.1
Major growth factor families

Growth factor family	Cell source	Actions
Transforming growth factor beta TGFβ1, TGFβ2	Platelets Fibroblasts Macrophages	Fibroblast chemotaxis and activation ECM deposition ↑ Collagen synthesis ↑ TIMP synthesis ↓ MMP synthesis
TGFβ3		Reduces scarring ↓ Collagen ↓ Fibronectin
Platelet-derived growth factor PDGF-AA, PDGF-BB, vascular endothelial growth factor (VEGF)	Platelets Macrophages Keratinocytes Fibroblasts	Activation of immune cells and fibroblasts ECM deposition ↑ Collagen synthesis ↑ TIMP synthesis ↓ MMP synthesis Angiogenesis
Fibroblast growth factor Acidic FGF, Basic FGF, KGF	Macrophages Endothelial cells Fibroblasts	Angiogenesis Endothelial cell activation Keratinocyte proliferation and migration ECM deposition
Insulin-like growth factor IGF1, IGF2, Insulin	Liver Skeletal muscle Fibroblasts Macrophages Neutrophils	Keratinocyte proliferation Fibroblast proliferation Endothelial cell activation Angiogenesis ↑ Collagen synthesis ECM Deposition Cell metabolism
Epidermal growth factor EGF, HB-EGF, TGFα, Amphiregulin, Betacellulin	Keratinocytes Macrophages	Keratinocyte proliferation and migration ECM deposition
Connective tissue growth factor CTGF	Fibroblasts Endothelial cells Epithelial cells	Mediates action of TGFβ on collagen synthesis

The nomenclature of growth factors and cytokines can be confusing – these proteins can be named for the cell upon which they act, for the cell that was first discovered to produce them, or for the action or process that they stimulate. The name does not necessarily identify the only cell that produces the protein or the only role it plays in healing. A single type of growth factor might have more than one biological role during healing, which could depend on the time point at which it is released or the degree to which it binds. A particular type of cell can produce many types of growth factor and several different types of cell could produce a particular growth factor. For example, platelet-derived growth factor (PDGF) is produced by platelets, macrophages, fibroblasts and endothelial cells, and acts on fibroblasts and smooth muscle cells; tumour necrosis

Table 6.2
Cytokine activity in
wound healing

Cytokine	Cell source	Biological activity
Proinflammatory cytokines		
TNFα	Macrophages	PMN margination and cytotoxicity, ± collagen synthesis; provides metabolic substrate
IL1	Macrophages Keratinocytes	Fibroblast and keratinocyte chemotaxis, collagen synthesis
IL2	T lymphocytes	Increases fibroblast infiltration and metabolism
IL6	Macrophages PMNs Fibroblasts	Fibroblast proliferation, hepatic acute-phase protein synthesis
IL8	Macrophages Fibroblasts	Macrophage and PMN chemotaxis, keratinocyte maturation
IFNγ	T lymphocytes Macrophages	Macrophage and PMN activation; retards collagen synthesis and crosslinking; stimulates collagenase activity
Anti-inflammatory cytokines		
IL4	T lymphocytes Basophils Mast cells	Inhibition of TNF, IL1, IL6 production; fibroblast proliferation, collagen synthesis
IL10	T lymphocytes Macrophages Keratinocytes	Inhibition of TNF, IL1, IL6 production; inhibits macrophage and PMN activation

PMN, polymorphonuclear leukocyte cells.

factor-alpha (TNFα) is produced by macrophages and results in proliferation of fibroblasts and activation of neutrophils.

The surface binding of a growth factor or cytokine to a target cell receptor initiates intracellular changes, which ultimately result in a biological response. The response to growth factor binding could be mitogenic, chemotactic, or synthetic – in other words the target cell divides, migrates or produces something – usually a protein product such as an enzyme or collagen. Growth factors are sometimes described as having autocrine, paracrine or exocrine functions based on whether they act on the same cell that produces them, on a nearby cell or on a distant cell, respectively.

Dozens of different growth factors and cytokines are at work throughout the time course of healing. There appears to be a high level of redundancy or overlapping of their roles, which is most likely the result of an evolutionary survival strategy. An expedient healing response to tissue injury is important to avoid sepsis or blood loss. Redundancy in the regulatory pathways ensures that a potential problem in one aspect of the healing process does not have a detrimental effect on wound closure.

Chemokines, named from a contraction of chemotactic cytokines, are the newest class of soluble mediators, and were discovered for their potent chemotactic activity for inflammatory cells (Gillitzer & Goebeler 2001, Luster 1998). The structural and functional similarities among chemokines were not initially appreciated, and this has led to an idiosyncratic nomenclature consisting of many acronyms that were based on their biological functions, e.g. monocyte chemoattractant protein 1 (MCP1), macrophage inflammatory protein 1 (MIP1), their source for isolation, e.g. platelet factor 4 (PF4), their biochemical properties, e.g. interferon-inducible protein of 10 kD (IP10) or regulated upon activation normal T-cell expressed and secreted (RANTES). As their biochemical properties were established, it was recognized that the approximately 40 chemokines could be grouped into four major classes shown in Table 6.3 based on the pattern of cysteine residues located near the N-terminus (e.g. CXC, CC, C, CXXXC). In general, chemokines have two primary functions: (i) they regulate the trafficking of leukocyte populations during normal health and development; and (ii) they direct the recruitment and activation of neutrophils, lymphocytes, macrophages, eosinophils and basophils during inflammation.

Table 6.3
Chemokine families

Chemokines	Cells affected
α-Chemokines (CXC) with glutamic acid-leucine-arginine near the N-terminal Interleukin-8 (IL8)	Neutrophils
α-Chemokines (CXC) *without* glutamic acid-leucine-arginine near the N-terminal Interferon-inducible protein of 10 kD (IP-10) Monokine induced by interferon-γ (MIG) Stromal-cell-derived factor 1 (SDF1)	Activated T lymphocytes
β-Chemokines (CC) Monocyte chemoattractant proteins (MCPs): MCP1, -2, -3, -4, -5 Regulated upon activation normal T-cell expressed and secreted (RANTES) Macrophage inflammatory protein (MIP1α) Eotaxin	Eosinophils Basophils Monocytes Activated T lymphocytes
γ-Chemokines (C) Lymphotactin	Resting T lymphocytes
δ-Chemokines (CXXXC) Fractalkine	Natural killer cells

In summary, growth factors, cytokines and chemokines can be thought of as the 'words' of intercellular communication. As human beings use words and language to communicate with each other, individual cells use growth factors, cytokines and chemokines.

CELL SURFACE RECEPTORS

Growth factor receptors

To achieve the desired effect, growth factors must be produced in sufficient quantities, be released at specific time points, must survive the extracellular environment (i.e. not be degraded or permanently trapped) and must achieve physical binding with the appropriate receptors on target cells. Growth factor receptors are also proteins, and they are not uniformly distributed or even always present on cells. Receptors for growth factor are typically transmembrane proteins and consist of three segments or domains. The extracellular segment on the outside of the cell contains the site that tightly binds the soluble mediators. The transmembrane segment spans the phospholipid bilayer of the plasma membrane, and the cytoplasmic segment inside the cell typically contains a tyrosine kinase enzyme domain. Binding of a soluble mediator to the external portion of the receptor activates the tyrosine kinase enzyme domain inside the cell, which then phosphorylates tyrosine amino acids on the receptor as well as in other signal transduction proteins in the cell. Phosphorylation activates these signal transduction proteins, which usually initiates a cascade of steps that ultimately causes changes in cell functions such as altering ion channels in the membrane or initiating transcription of genes that alter the cell's function.

Cytokine receptors differ from growth factor receptors in that they typically do not contain tyrosine kinase domains that are part of the cytoplasmic segment of the receptors (Subramaniam et al 2001). Instead, the cytoplasmic segment of cytokine receptors contains binding sites that bind to other cytoplasmic proteins that are themselves kinases. It is these soluble kinases (called Jak or STAT kinases) that initiate the cascades that alter cell functions when a cytokine binds to its specific receptor protein. Chemokine receptors and their signal transduction system comprise a third type of system. All chemokines receptors are 7-transmembrane-spanning proteins, and they generate intracellular signals by interacting with trimeric G-protein-coupled systems that are functionally linked to phospholipases, which release fragments of membrane lipids that initiate signalling cascade pathways in cells.

Cell receptors are as critical to successful wound healing as the growth factors and cytokines themselves. If soluble mediators are like 'words or language' between cells, then receptors can be likened to 'ears'. Without a receptor to bind to, the soluble mediator is not 'heard' or responded to by the target cell.

Integrin receptors

Growth factor receptors are part of cell-to-cell communication. Cells must also communicate or interact with the extracellular matrix. A special family of membrane receptors, known as integrins, mediates this type of communication. Integrins are transmembrane receptors with two subunits, designated alpha and beta, that are associated in a non-covalent complex (meaning they are not chemically bound to each other). There are multiple alpha subunits and multiple beta subunits that can associate in various combinations. Over 20 alpha–beta combinations are known.

The external portion of the integrin has a globular shape and sits up above the cell membrane surface by about 20 nanometres. The internal or cytoplasmic portion of the integrin is relatively short. The specific shape of the globular external portion is determined by the particular combination of alpha and beta subunits and determines which extracellular matrix component may bind.

Specialized kinase enzymes in the cell, called focal adhesion kinases (FAKs), bind to the cytoplasmic segments of integrin receptors when they bind to a specific extracellular matrix component and initiate signalling cascades in the cell.

Aspects of wound repair that require interaction between cells and the extracellular matrix include:

- platelet interactions with fibrin and fibronectin
- leukocyte extravasation
- endothelial cell budding and capillary ingrowth
- epithelial cell migration (or any other cell's migration).

PROTEASES IN THE WOUND BED

A number of different proteolytic enzymes are produced by cells in the wound bed at different times during the healing process. Localized enzymatic breakdown of the extracellular matrix is a normal part of the repair process and is involved in wound debridement, dissolution of the basement membrane, ingrowth of capillary buds, turnover of the provisional matrix and tissue remodelling. These protease enzymes belong to different families based on their substrates and mechanism of activation, and two of the most important families are the matrix metalloproteinases (MMPs) and serine proteases. Specific MMP proteases that are necessary for wound healing are the collagenases (which degrade intact fibrillar collagen molecules), the gelatinases (which degrade damaged fibrillar collagen molecules) and the stromelysins (which very effectively degrade proteoglycans). An important serine protease is neutrophil elastase, which can degrade almost all types of protein molecules. Under normal conditions, the destructive actions of the proteolytic enzymes are tightly regulated by specific enzyme inhibitors, which are also produced by cells in the wound bed. The specific inhibitors of the MMPs are the tissue inhibitors of metalloproteinases (TIMPs) and specific inhibitors of serine protease are $\alpha1$-protease inhibitor ($\alpha1$-PI) and $\alpha2$ macroglobulin.

CELL–MATRIX INTERACTIONS

The extracellular matrix (ECM) is not merely a complex mixture of proteins, proteoglycans and glycosaminoglycans that passively supports cells. The ECM plays important active roles in regulating the proliferation, migration and differentiation of wound cells, which are key processes that help to regulate the phases of healing (Vogel 2001).

Composition of the ECM

The ECM is comprised of various classes of molecules such as proteins, glycoproteins, glycosaminoglycans (GAGs) and proteoglycans. By far the largest number of ECM molecules are proteins and glycoproteins, which are both composed of chains of amino acids. Glycoproteins also contain a few covalently attached, short, branched chains of sugars (oligosaccharides) that are often recognition signals that help provide specificity for binding. Most growth factors, cytokines, chemokines and their receptors are proteins or glycoproteins, as are the proteases and their inhibitors. Collagen and elastin molecules are also glycoproteins as are fibrin, laminin and fibronectin. The proteins and glycoproteins of the ECM provide the major tensile strength of the ECM.

Glycosaminoglycans are long, straight-chain polymers of 20 to 100 repeating disaccharide units such as hyaluronic acid (HA), dermatan sulphate, heparan sulphate and chondroitin sulphate. Usually one sugar of the disaccharide is an acid sugar (uronic acid) and the other sugar contains a sulphate group and/or a N-acetyl group (N-acetylglucosamine). The acid groups and the sulphate groups create a high density of negative charges on GAGs, which causes the GAGs to interact strongly with large numbers of water molecules. GAGs provide bulk to the ECM and enable the ECM to absorb shock forces by compressing and rebounding. Proteoglycans consist of a core protein that is chemically bound to one or more long GAG chains. In contrast to simple glycoproteins, which may contain up to a few percent carbohydrate by weight, proteoglycans may contain up to 95% or more carbohydrate. Common proteoglycans in the ECM include decorin and aggrecan. Proteoglycans such as the syndecans are also found in the plasma membranes of cells, where they help bind the ECM, interact with growth factors in the ECM, and may help in regulating the formation of collagen fibrils.

Provisional wound matrix

An injury that extends into the dermis of the skin causes disruption of the ECM and initiates the clotting cascade. Fibrin is generated at the site of injury when thrombin catalyses conversion of the plasma-derived fibrinogen to fibrin and a clot forms that stops bleeding and also forms a temporary scaffolding for the repair process. Serum-derived adhesion proteins, fibronectin and vitronectin, subsequently coat the fibrin network, forming a 'provisional wound matrix' that plays a crucial role in cellular attachment through their interactions with integrin receptors. Fibronectin facilitates the movement of cells into the wound site from the vasculature (such as leukocytes migrating from the vasculature) as well as promoting migration of fibroblasts and capillary cells through granulation tissue and epithelial cells moving over granulation tissue during resurfacing. The provisional wound matrix of fibrin/fibronectin also serves to bind and store growth factors, which are released by proteases (MMPs and serine proteases) as the provisional wound matrix is replaced by new collagen molecules in the proliferative/repair phase. Initially, type III collagen is synthesized by cells in the wound, which is slowly replaced over weeks and months by type I collagen molecules, which are found in normal skin. Furthermore, during the early phases of scar formation, the collagen molecules tend to be arranged in bundles that are oriented parallel to the edges of the wound rather than the more complex basket weave pattern of collagen bundles that is characteristic of normal dermis. As the initial scar tissue remodels over many months, the architecture and composition of the scar matrix begins to resemble non-wounded skin, but never fully regenerates non-wounded ECM.

MOLECULAR AND CELLULAR REGULATION OF THE PHASES OF WOUND HEALING

The first major event following a skin injury is haemostasis, and the platelets play key roles in this process as they undergo activation, adhesion and aggregation. These events are triggered by interactions of platelets with both soluble mediators and matrix components. Platelets become activated when exposed to extravascular collagen (such as type I collagen), which they detect via specific integrin receptors in their plasma membrane. Platelet adhesion to collagen

Haemostasis

activates them to release soluble mediators (growth factors and cyclic AMP) and adhesive glycoproteins from their alpha granules, which are in turn, signals for subsequent platelets to change their morphology, become sticky and to aggregate. The aggregated platelets become trapped in the fibrin web and provide the bulk of the clot, and their membranes act as a surface on which inactive clotting enzyme proteases are bound, activated then released to accelerate the clotting cascade. The key glycoproteins released from the platelet granules include fibrinogen, fibronectin, thrombospondin and von Willenbrand factor. Soluble mediators released from the alpha granules include platelet-derived growth factor (PDGF), transforming growth factor beta (TGFβ), transforming growth factor alpha (TGFα), basic fibroblast growth factor (bFGF), and vascular endothelial growth factor (VEGF). PDGF and TGFβ are chemotactic for neutrophils and monocytes and recruit them from the vasculature to initiate the inflammatory response. VEGF, TGFα and bFGF act on endothelial cells to initiate angiogenesis. PDGF is also chemotactic for fibroblasts, which will migrate to the area to begin the process of collagen deposition. Thus, through the interaction with the extracellular matrix and release of soluble mediators, platelets not only contribute to haemostasis but also set the stage for the subsequent events of the healing process.

Inflammatory phase

Neutrophils

Neutrophils are the first inflammatory cells to respond to the soluble mediators released by platelets and the coagulation cascade. They begin their journey from the vasculature by first adhering to the endothelial cell walls via their surface integrins and then releasing elastase and collagenase, which facilitate their migration through the basement membrane surrounding the endothelial cells and into the ECM at the wound site. Their primary role is to mount the first line of defence against infection by phagocytosing and killing bacteria, and by destroying foreign materials and devitalized tissue. They are able to interact with these extracellular targets via their integrin receptors. Neutrophils also produce and release inflammatory mediators, such as TNFα and interleukin 1 (IL1) that further recruit and activate fibroblasts and epithelial cells. Neutrophils produce and contain high levels of destructive proteases and oxygen free radicals, which they use to digest phagocytosed materials. Upon their inevitable death, neutrophils release these substances into the local wound area where they can contribute to extensive tissue damage and prolong the inflammatory phase. The persistent presence of high levels of bacteria in a wound may contribute to chronicity through continued recruitment of neutrophils and their release of proteases, cytokines and intracellular contents (Fig. 6.2).

Monocytes/macrophages

Usually, neutrophils are depleted in the wound after 2–3 days and are replaced by tissue macrophages. Macrophages begin as circulating monocytes that are attracted to the wound site, beginning about 24 h after injury by both soluble mediators and matrix degradation components such as fragments of collagen and fibronectin. Monocytes bind to the extracellular matrix via integrins and immediately differentiate into tissue macrophages. Serum factors and fibronectin mediate this differentiation. Tissue macrophages have a dual role in the healing

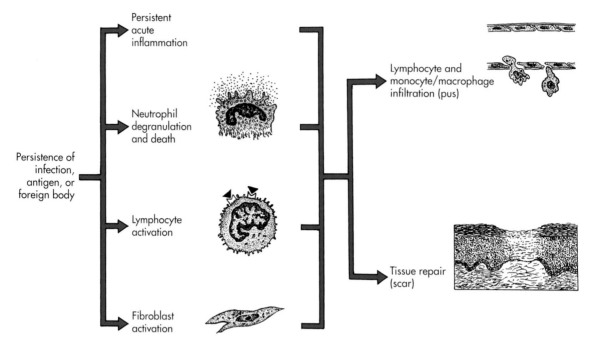

Figure 6.2
The chronic inflammatory response.

process. They are voracious phagocytes and patrol the wound area ingesting bacteria, devitalized tissue and depleted neutrophils. Macrophages also produce collagenases and elastase to assist them in breaking down devitalized tissues. They are able to regulate proteolytic destruction of tissue in the wound by producing and secreting inhibitors for these enzymes.

Soluble mediators
As well as their important phagocytic role, macrophages also mediate the transition from the inflammatory phase to the proliferative phase of healing. They release a wide variety of growth factors and cytokines including TNFα, PDGF, TGFβ, TGFα, IL1, interleukin 6 (IL6), insulin-like growth factor (IGF1) and fibroblast growth factor (FGF). Some of these soluble mediators recruit and activate fibroblasts, which will synthesize, deposit and organize the new tissue matrix, whereas others promote angiogenesis (Fig. 6.3).

Proliferative phase
Events of the proliferative, or tissue-building, phase of healing include the synthesis, deposition and organization of granulation tissue, ingrowth of new blood vessels and epithelial migration, proliferation and stratification. In this phase of healing fibroblasts, macrophages, endothelial and epithelial cells interact with matrix and with each other.

Granulation
Granulation tissue is a transitional replacement for normal dermis, which eventually matures into a scar during the remodelling phase of healing. It is charac-

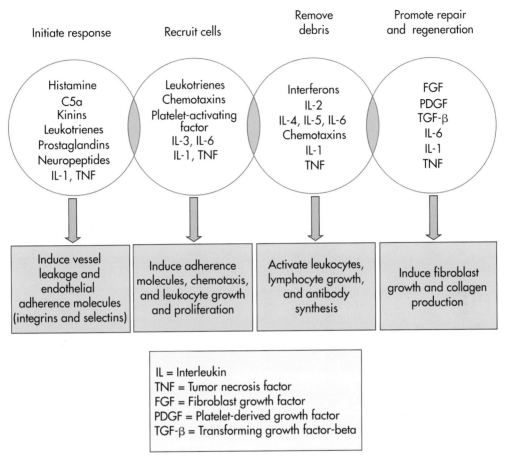

Figure 6.3
Some of the mediators and their actions.

terized from unwounded dermis by its extremely dense network of blood vessels and capillaries, elevated cellular density of fibroblasts and macrophages and randomly organized collagen fibres. It also has an elevated metabolic rate compared to normal dermis, which reflects the activity required for cellular migration and division and protein synthesis.

Fibroblasts

The collagen, proteoglycans and other components that comprise granulation tissue are synthesized and deposited primarily by fibroblasts. Fibroblasts migrate into the wound in response to multiple soluble mediators released initially by platelets and later by macrophages. Fibroblast migration in the extracellular matrix depends on precise recognition and interaction with specific components of the matrix. Fibroblasts in normal dermis are typically quiescent and sparsely distributed whereas in the provisional matrix of the wound site and in the granulation tissue, they are quite active and crowded together. Their migration and accumulation in the wound site requires them to change their morphology and to produce and secrete enzymes to clear a path for their movement from the ECM into the wound site.

Fibroblasts begin moving by first binding to matrix components such as fibronectin, vitronectin and fibrin via their integrin receptors. Integrin receptors attach to specific amino acid sequences (such as R-G-D or arginine-glycine-aspartic acid) or binding sites in these matrix components. Although one end of the fibroblast remains bound to the matrix component, the cell extends a cytoplasmic projection to find another binding site. When the next site is found the original site is released and the cell uses its cytoskeleton network of actin fibres to pull itself forward.

The direction of fibroblast movement is determined by the alignment of the fibrils in the ECM and provisional matrix and the gradient of chemotactic growth factors, cytokines and chemokines. Fibroblasts tend to migrate along these fibrils as opposed to across them. Fibroblasts secrete proteolytic enzymes locally to facilitate their forwards motion through the matrix. The enzymes secreted by the fibroblasts include three forms of the MMP family – collagenase (MMP1), gelatinases (MMP2 and MMP9, which degrade gelatin substrates) and stromelysin (MMP3, which has multiple protein substrates in the ECM).

Once the fibroblasts have migrated into the matrix they again change their morphology, settle down and begin to proliferate and to synthesize granulation tissue components, including collagen, elastin and proteoglycans.

Angiogenesis

Damaged vasculature must be replaced to maintain tissue viability. The process of angiogenesis is stimulated by local factors of the microenvironment including low oxygen tension, low pH and high lactate levels. Also, certain soluble mediators are potent angiogenic signals for endothelial cells. Many of these are produced by epidermal cells, fibroblasts, vascular endothelial cells and macrophages, and include basic fibroblast growth factor (bFGF), TGFα, and vascular endothelial growth factor (VEGF). It is now recognized that oxygen levels in tissues directly regulate angiogenesis by interacting with oxygen sensing proteins that regulate transcription of angiogenic and anti-angiogenic genes. For example, synthesis of VEGF by capillary endothelial cells is directly increased by hypoxia through the activation of the recently identified transcription factor, hypoxia-inducible factor (HIF), that binds oxygen. When oxygen levels surrounding capillary endothelial cells drop, levels of HIF increase inside the cells, HIF-1 binds to specific DNA sequences and stimulates transcription of specific genes such as VEGF that promote angiogenesis. When oxygen levels in wound tissue increase, oxygen binds to HIF, leading to the destruction of HIF molecules in cells and decreased synthesis of angiogenic factors. Regulation of angiogenesis involves both stimulatory factors like VEGF and anti-angiogenic factors like angiostatin, endostatin and pigment epithelium-derived factor (PEDF).

Binding of angiogenic factors causes endothelial cells of the capillaries adjacent to the devascularized site to begin to migrate into the matrix and then proliferate to form buds or sprouts. Once again, the migration of these cells into the matrix requires the local secretion of proteolytic enzymes, especially MMPs. As the tips of the endothelial sprouts extend and encounter another sprout, they develop a cleft that subsequently becomes the lumen of the evolving vessel and complete a new vascular loop. This process continues until the capillary system is sufficiently repaired and the tissue oxygenation and metabolic needs are met. It is these new capillary tuffs that give granulation tissue its characteristic bumpy or granular appearance.

Epithelialization

Epithelialization is a multistep process that involves epithelial cell detachment and change in their internal structure, migration, proliferation and differentiation (O'Toole 2001). The intact mature epidermis consists of five layers of differentiated epithelial cells, ranging from the cuboidal basal keratinocytes nearest the dermis up to the flattened, hexagonal, tough keratinocytes in the uppermost layer. Only the basal epithelial cells are capable of proliferation. These basal cells are normally attached to their neighbouring cells by intercellular connectors called desmosomes and to the basement membrane by hemi-desmosomes. When growth factors such as EGF, keratinocyte growth factor (KGF) and TGFα are released during the healing process, they bind to receptors on these epithelial cells and stimulate migration and proliferation. The binding of the growth factors triggers the desmosomes and hemi-desmosomes to dissolve so the cells can detach in preparation for migration. Integrin receptors are then expressed and the normally cuboidal basal epithelial cells flatten in shape and begin to migrate as a monolayer over the newly deposited granulation tissue, following along collagen fibres. Proliferation of the basal epithelial cells near the wound margin supplys new cells to the advancing monolayer apron of cells (cells that are actively migrating are incapable of proliferation). Epithelial cells in the leading edge of the monolayer produce and secrete proteolytic enzymes (MMPs), which enable the cells to penetrate scab, surface necrosis or eschar. Migration continues until the epithelial cells contact other advancing cells to form a confluent sheet. Once this contact has been made, the entire epithelial monolayer enters a proliferative mode and the stratified layers of the epidermis are re-established and begin to mature to restore barrier function. TGFβ is one growth factor that can speed up the maturation (differentiation and keratinization) of the epidermal layers. The intercellular desmosomes and the hemi-desmosome attachments to the newly formed basement membrane are also re-established. Epithelialization is the clinical hallmark of healing but it is not the final event – remodelling of the granulation tissue is yet to occur.

Remodelling

Remodelling is the final phase of the healing process in which the granulation tissue matures into scar and tissue tensile strength is increased. The maturation of granulation tissue involves a reduction in the number of capillaries via aggregation into larger vessels and a decrease in the amount of glycosaminoglycans and the water associated with the GAGs and proteoglycans. Cell density and metabolic activity in the granulation tissue drop during maturation. Changes are also made in collagen content and organization, which enhance tensile strength. The tensile strength of a newly epithelialized wound is only about 25% of normal tissue. Healed or repaired tissue is never as strong as normal tissues that have never been wounded. Tissue tensile strength is enhanced primarily by the reorganization of collagen fibers that were deposited randomly during granulation and increased covalent crosslinking of collagen molecules by the enzyme, lysyl oxidase, which is secreted into the ECM by fibroblasts. Over several months or more, changes in collagen organization in the repaired tissue will slowly increase the tensile strength to a maximum of about 80% of normal tissue.

Fibroblasts are the main cell type involved in remodelling. They synthesize new collagen, which is deposited along lines of tension. Initially, wound fibroblasts secrete type III collagen, which is then replaced by type I collagen during remodelling. Fibroblasts also secret MMPs to break down the type III collagen that was randomly deposited during the proliferative phase. A balance must be maintained between collagen removal and synthesis during remodelling and this is achieved through the action of enzyme inhibitors, which can also be produced by fibroblasts.

DIFFERENCES IN THE MOLECULAR ENVIRONMENTS OF HEALING AND CHRONIC WOUNDS

As outlined above, healing of skin wounds normally occurs in a predictable sequence of phases including haemostasis, inflammation, mitosis, angiogenesis, synthesis of extracellular matrix followed by remodelling of the scar matrix. These processes are regulated by numerous molecules including growth factors, cytokines, chemokines, receptors, proteinases and their inhibitors. It is reasonable to assume that the failure of an acute wound to progress through the phases of healing is due to conditions that interfere with the normal interactions of these molecules. Previous studies that analysed fluids collected from chronic wounds found elevated levels of inflammatory cytokines, elevated levels of proteinases and low levels of growth factor activity compared to acute, healing wounds. These observations led to the hypothesis that chronic wounds develop due to prolonged inflammation in acute wounds, which produces elevated levels of proteinases that destroy growth factors, receptors and ECM proteins that are essential for healing (Mast & Schultz 1996, Nwomeh et al 1998, Yager & Nwomeh 1999). Furthermore, analysis of fibroblasts cultured from chronic wounds indicate that they frequently have reduced capacity to proliferate in response to specific growth factors (Agren et al 2000). If this hypothesis is correct, it follows that elevated levels of inflammatory cytokines and proteinases should decrease and mitogenic activity should increase in fluids as chronic wounds begin to heal. Several studies have, indeed, reported reduced levels of inflammatory cytokines and proteases and increased mitogenic activity in wound fluids as chronic wounds begin to heal (Trengrove et al 1996, 1999, 2000). These results support the concept that treatments that shift the molecular balance in chronic wounds to a pattern that resembles the molecular profile found in acute healing wounds will promote healing (Fig. 6.4).

SUMMARY

A virtual orchestra of communication is occurring between different cell types and between cells and matrix during the healing process:

- Haemostasis and inflammation involve platelets, neutrophils and macrophages interacting with matrix components.
- Granulation tissue deposition involves fibroblasts and macrophages interacting with matrix and with each other.
- Angiogenesis requires endothelial cells to interact with matrix.
- Epithelialization requires basal epithelial cells to interact with each other and with matrix.
- Remodelling involves fibroblasts and enzymes interacting with matrix components and each other.
  Communication between cells is mediated by growth factors, and cytokines are produced and secreted and must bind to surface receptors on other cells to have an effect.

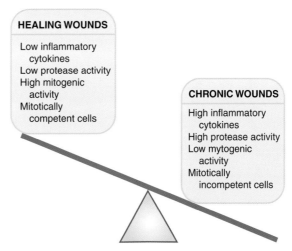

Figure 6.4
Differences in the molecular environment of healing and chronic wounds

Specific cell surface receptors called integrins enable cells to detect and interact with the extracellular matrix environment.

A variety of proteolytic enzymes is produced by cells and used intracellularly to digest phagocytosed materials and also extracellularly to assist in migration and remodelling.

The molecular environment of chronic wounds contains elevated levels of inflammatory cytokines and proteases, low levels of mitogenic activity, and cells that often respond poorly to growth factors compared to acute, healing wounds. As chronic wounds begin to heal, this molecular pattern shifts to one that resembles a healing wound.

REFERENCES

Agren M S, Eaglstein W H, Ferguson M W et al 2000 Causes and effects of the chronic inflammation in venous leg ulcers. Acta Dermato-Venereologica Supplementum (Stockholm) 210:3–17

Bennett N T, Schultz G S 1993a Growth factors and wound healing: biochemical properties of growth factors and their receptors. The American Journal of Surgery 165(June):728–737

Bennett N T, Schultz G S 1993b Growth factors and wound healing: part II. Role in normal and chronic wound healing. The American Journal of Surgery 166(July):74–81

Cherry G W, Hughes M A, Ferguson M W J, Leaper D J 2001 Wound healing. In: Morris P J, Wood W C (eds) Oxford textbook of surgery, vol 2. Oxford University Press, Oxford

Clark R A F 1996 Wound repair: overview and general considerations. In: Clark R A F (ed) The molecular and cellular biology of wound repair, vol. 2. Plenum Press, New York, p 3–50

Gillitzer R, Goebeler M 2001 Chemokines in cutaneous wound healing. Journal of Leukocyte Biology 69(4):513–521

Kirsner R S, Bogensberger G 2002 The normal process of healing. In: McCulloch J M, Kloth L C (eds) Wound healing: alternatives in management, vol 3. FA Davis, Philadelphia, p 3–34

Luster A D 1998 Chemokines – chemotactic cytokines that mediate inflammation. New England Journal of Medicine 338(7):436–445

Mast B A, Schultz G S 1996 Interactions of cytokines, growth factors, and proteases in acute and chronic wounds. Wound Repair and Regeneration 4:411–420

Mignatti P, Rifkin D B, Welgus H G, Parks W C 1996 Proteinases and tissue remodeling. In: Clark R A F (ed) The molecular and cellular biology of wound repair, vol 2. Plenum Press, New York, p 427–474

Nwomeh B C, Yager D R, Cohen I K 1998 Physiology of the chronic wound. Clinics in Plastic Surgery 25(3):341–356

O'Toole E A 2001 Extracellular matrix and keratinocyte migration. Clinical and Experimental Dermatology 26(6):525–530

Schultz G S 2000 Molecular regulation of wound healing. In: Bryant R A (ed). Acute and chronic wounds: nursing management, vol 2. Mosby; Philadelphia; p 413–429

Subramaniam P S, Torres B A, Johnson H M 2001 So many ligands, so few transcription factors: a new paradigm for signaling through the stat transcription factors. Cytokine 15(4):175–187

Tarnuzzer R W, Schultz G S 1996 Biochemical analysis of acute and chronic wound environments. Wound Repair and Regeneration 4:321–325

Tarnuzzer R W, Macauley S P, Bruce M S et al 1995 Epidermal growth factor in wound healing: a model for molecular pathogenesis of chronic wounds. In: Ziegler TR et al (eds) Growth factors and wound healing: basic science and potential clinical applications. Serono Symposia, Norwell, MA

Trengove N J, Langton S R, Stacey M C 1996 Biochemical analysis of wound fluid from nonhealing and healing chronic leg ulcers. Wound Repair and Regeneration 4:234–239

Trengove N J, Stacey M C, Macauley S et al 1999 Analysis of the acute and chronic wound environments: the role of proteases and their inhibitors. Wound Repair and Regeneration 7(6):442–452

Trengove N J, Bielefeldt-Ohmann H, Stacey M C 2000 Mitogenic activity and cytokine levels in non-healing and healing chronic leg ulcers. Wound Repair and Regeneration 8(1):13–25

Vogel W F 2001 Collagen-receptor signaling in health and disease. European Journal of Dermatology 11(6):506–514

Waldrop J, Doughty D 2000 Wound-healing physiology. In: Bryant R (ed) Acute and chronic wounds: nursing management, vol 2. Mosby, Philadelphia, p 17–39

Yager D R, Nwomeh B C 1999 The proteolytic environment of chronic wounds. Wound Repair and Regeneration 7(6):433–441

CHAPTER

7

Wound infection: Diagnosis and management

Nancy A Stotts

CHAPTER CONTENTS

INTRODUCTION

Infection is a significant problem in persons with wounds because it delays healing, increases length of hospitalization and number of physician visits, and raises the cost of care (Lalla et al 2001, Thomson & Smith 1994). Infection also has been identified as a major factor in converting acute wounds to chronic wounds (Tarnuzzer & Schultz 1996). One of the serious consequences of wound infection is osteomyelitis, in which organisms invade the bone and chronic bone infection is established (Bonham 2001). In addition, there is the possibility that bacteria that have invaded tissue will move into the bloodstream, causing bacteraemia that can lead to sepsis, multisystem organ failure and death (Singhal et al 2001, Thomson & Smith 1994).

Wound infection results when the balance between host resistance and microorganisms is disrupted and the organisms overwhelm the immune defences (Dow 2001, Robson 1997). Contamination is the presence of organisms on the surface of the wound. All wounds are contaminated and contamination opens the way to tissue colonization and infection. Colonization occurs where organisms multiply on the surface of the wound. Colonization progresses to infection when organisms invade the tissues and a systemic immune response is triggered (Stotts & Whitney 1999).

In acute wounds > 10^5 organisms per gram of tissue are associated with delayed healing and infection (Robson 1997). However, the mere presence of a few virulent organisms is also indicative of infection. For example, when beta-haemolytic streptococci are present in any concentration, the patient is treated as infected (Robson 1997, Thomson & Smith 1994).

With chronic wounds, there is some controversy about whether the number of organisms (> 10^5 organisms/gram of tissue) is diagnostic of infection (Dolynchuk 2001, Dow 2001, Falanga 2000). To understand this controversy, it is important to appreciate that, as wounds get older, they have a higher level of bioburden. Also, the specific organisms present are not those that were present when the wound was initially made (Dow 2001). More important, many chronic wounds have $> 10^5$ organisms/gram of tissue and do not have signs of infection so wound infection in chronic wounds is diagnosed based on clinical signs and symptoms rather than a specific number of organisms (Bello et al 2001).

The acute inflammatory response that is seen with inoculum of acute wounds becomes a chronic inflammatory response over time and results in injury to host tissue. Proinflammatory cytokines, including interleukin-1 (IL1) and tumour necrosis factor alpha (TNFα), rise and remain elevated. Increased levels of matrix metalloproteinases are seen, the amount of tissue inhibitors of metalloproteinases is decreased and growth factors are inhibited (Tarnuzzer & Schultz 1996).

Bacteria thus stimulate the production of local vasoactive metabolites, ischaemia, infection, and the development of chronic wounds. How the various organisms' defences, including biofilm, contribute to the development of infection is not currently understood in full (Dow 2001, Serraltra et al 2001).

Determinants of infection

The factors that determine whether infection occurs can be conceptualized as the inoculating dose of the organism, the virulence of the organism and the host resistance. In acute wounds, a small inoculating dose stimulates an immune response and activates processes that result in inflammation and lead to healing in the majority of cases and infection in a small proportion (Laato et al 1988). More frequently, a large inoculating dose is associated with infection. This often is seen with unintended contamination, as with stool into a sacral ulcer. The presence of a foreign material with a low dose of organisms can result in infection (Elek 1956). The foreign material might be something as small as a suture or as significant as an artificial joint.

Normal flora present on the skin may affect the response to the wound inoculum. The skin's normal flora has a system that controls the number of organisms present on the wound, and can prevent invasion by other organisms. Factors that disrupt the normal flora may contribute to infection (Bello et al 2001).

The virulence of the organism is evidenced by its defence system. Organisms have sophisticated defences that include the production of proteases, the release of toxins, encapsulating abilities and the formation of biofilm (Dow 2001, Serraltra et al 2001). Biofilm has recently received increased attention as it is recognized that organisms exist in an inactive form in the biofilm, a sessiling form. The organism's defence mechanisms make it difficult for the body's immune responses to kill the organism.

Host defence also determines whether infection takes place. Support for host defence is provided with adequate nutrients for production of cells and fluids for systemic circulation. Often these are considered fundamental aspects of care of any patient because they support normal defences. Recent work has explored approaches to supporting the normal immune system. For example, a study examined providing supplemental arginine to the diet of nursing home residents ($n = 32$) with pressure ulcers (Langkamp-Henken et al 2000). The purpose of the study was to determine whether arginine would increase lymphocyte proliferation and IL2 production as it did in healthy elderly with standardized wounds. Data showed that although the arginine was well tolerated, arginine supplementation at varying doses over a 4-week period did not enhance lymphocyte proliferation or IL2 production. Further work is needed in this area. Oxygen has been explored as another nutrient that supports immune function. Oxygen has been termed an 'antibiotic' because it enhances the killing effect of the normal immune system. In fact, data show that, when oxygen is given with antibiotics, the effect is synergistic (Knighton et al 1986).

Incidence of infection

The incidence of wound infection is difficult to estimate because it varies by the type of wound and there is a lack of a definitive diagnostic instrument. The incidence is well delineated in several populations, e.g. surgical wounds. About 27 million surgical procedures are performed each year in the United States and the Centers for Disease Control have set up a national surveillance system for acute hospitals. Surgical wound infection is termed surgical site infection (SSI) and its incidence varies by wound classification (Mangram et al 1999). Overall, SSI is the most frequent nosocomial infection and accounts for about 38% of all nosocomial infections. When death occurs in persons with SSI, most (77%) are related to the infection and most (93%) infections involve organs/spaces.

Determining the incidence of infection in chronic wounds presents a number of challenges. A fundamental problem is the lack of a universal definition of infection in chronic wounds. Additionally, there is no registry of chronic wounds or chronic wound infection to store data, compile it, and access it as needed.

Some data exist about infection in diabetic wounds and pressure ulcers. Infected foot wounds in diabetics are the most common reason for hospitalization of diabetics and result in the large proportion of the amputations in this population (Armstrong & Nguyen 2000). Some series suggest that infection is responsible for about 20% of hospitalizations related to diabetes (Lalla et al 2001). Pressure ulcers, recognized as heavily contaminated wounds (Bendy et al 1965), often experience associated infection. However, due to lack of studies on pressure ulcer infection reported in the literature, the extent of the problem is not known. However, the incidence of osteomyelitis in persons with chronic non-healing pressure ulcers is estimated to be 17–26% (Darouiche et al 1994).

GENERAL PRINCIPLES

Diagnosis of infection

Clinical judgement

The diagnosis of wound infection is based on clinical judgement (Bello et al 2001, Dow 2001, Mangram et al 1999). The practitioner evaluates the patient's overall condition, including whether systemic signs such as fever and malaise are present. The wound itself is evaluated and compared to its prior status. Clustering the objective and subjective signs and symptoms, both the overt and subtle, leads to the clinical diagnosis of infection.

Surgical wounds are the most common type of acute wound. Criteria to diagnose SSI by depth of infection have been established (Table 7.1). These criteria are based on statistical analyses using a large database of surgical patients (Mangram et al 1999).

There also is a universal system for identifying risk of infection in persons undergoing surgery. This classification system is based on the site of the incision

Table 7.1

The various types of surgical site infection are characterized by at least one of the following criteria (from Mangram et al 1999)

	Superficial	Deep	Organ/Space
Purulent drainage from appropriate depth site	✓	✓	✓
Culture positive	✓		✓
Signs or symptoms of infection	✓	✓	✓
Diagnosis of infection by physician	✓	✓	✓
Abscess		✓	

and level of intraoperative contamination. Each surgery is classified as clean, clean-contaminated, contaminated or dirty-infected (Mangram et al 1999). Anticipated infection rates increase as one progresses from the clean wound category to the dirty-infected wound category.

The second system classifies surgical site infection by depth: superficial, deep and organ/space. Superficial infection includes the skin or subcutaneous tissue of the incision. Deep infection involves the deep soft tissues of the incision, i.e. fascial and muscle layers. Organ/space SSI involves any part of the organs or spaces that was manipulated during surgery, other than the incision (Mangram et al 1999). All must occur within 30 days of surgery, except when an implant is utilized in which case the time extends to 1 year.

For chronic wounds, there is no uniform agreement about what signs and symptoms are associated with infection or which are diagnostic of infection (Table 7.2) (Cutting & Harding 1994, Dow 2001, Falanga 2000, Gardner et al 2001, Stotts & Whitney 1999). Inflammation, delayed healing, alterations in granulation tissue, and odour are the most frequently cited signs and symptoms. Recent work by Gardner and colleagues focused on identifying evidence-based criteria for chronic wound infection. They found that increasing pain, friable granulation tissue, foul odour, and wound breakdown were more sensitive indicators of infection in a small sample ($n = 26$) of persons with chronic wounds than the classic signs of infection (Gardner et al 2001).

Wound culture

Wound culture often is used to confirm the clinical diagnosis of wound infection and identify the sensitivity of the organism(s) to various antibiotics. It is important to recognize that the interpretation of the findings of the number and type of organism may differ based on whether the wound is acute or chronic and whether the clinician views the number $> 10^5$ per gram of tissue as diagnostic of infection.

Several commonly used wound culture techniques include biopsy, swab and aspiration. Important to the accuracy of the culture are the selection of the culture site, preparation of the tissue, its transport to the laboratory and the preparation of the accompanying laboratory requisition. These do not differ based on the type of culture technique utilized and are summarized in Box 7.1.

Tissue biopsy is the standard against which other methods are compared (Table 7.3). The procedure involves removing a piece of tissue using a punch biopsy or a scalpel. The tissue is placed in a sterile container and transported to

Table 7.2
Comparison of signs and symptoms of infection in chronic wounds

	Cutting & Harding (1994)	Stotts & Whitney (1999)	Falanga (2000)	Gardner et al (2001)	Dow (2001)
Inflammation	✓*	✓	✓		✓
Altered granulation tissue**	✓	✓	✓	✓	✓
Odour	✓	✓		✓	✓
Wound breakdown	✓			✓	
Pocketing at the base of the wound	✓				
Delayed healing	✓	✓	✓	✓	✓
Pain		✓	✓	✓	
Increased exudate		✓			✓
Elevated glucose		✓			
Necrotic tissue			✓		
Systemic signs and symptoms			✓		✓
Translucent film over base of wound			✓		
Cellulitis			✓		✓

*With serous drainage.
**Friable (Cutting & Harding 1994, Dow 2001, Gardner et al 2001); exuberant (Falanga 2000); boggy and oedematous, grey or deep maroon in colour, prone to bleeding (Dow 2001).

Box 7.1
Practices that maximize the accuracy of culture data

The culture site
Culture clean tissue
Do not culture eschar
Do not culture pus on the surface of the wound

Preparation of the tissue
Remove loose debris
Do not use abrasion to remove debris because it damages tissue
Irrigate the wound with a physiological solution (normal saline)
Do not use antiseptics prior to culture (if used cleanse well prior to culture)

Management of the specimen
Use a container that is appropriate to the purpose of the culture

continued

Box 7.1
continued

All containers should be sterile
Handle the specimen using sterile technique

Transport to the laboratory
Transport the specimen to the laboratory as quickly as possible (delay
    can result in death of organisms and overgrowth of others)
If transport will be delayed, consider use of a different transport medium

Preparation of the laboratory requisition
Identify the site of the culture accurately
Describe the wound history
Provide data about use of antibiotics

Table 7.3
Major types of culture
techniques

	Biopsy	Swab	Aspiration
How is it performed?	Tissue from the wound is removed with a punch biopsy or scalpel. A suture may be used to close the wound	The tip of an applicator is moved back and forth in a small-circumscribed area until the tip of the applicator is moistened with tissue fluid	A 23 needle with a 10-cc syringe is inserted into intact skin next to the wound and moved back and forth while applying negative pressure to the syringe. The negative pressure is maintained until the needle is removed from the tissue
What are the advantages of using it?	Considered the standard in practice	Easy to use, requires minimal training, accessible in most settings	Provides information about tissue involvement without additional damage to the wound
What are the disadvantages of using it?	Causes pain (no anaesthesia used as it would dilute the findings). May delay healing. Requires skill in performing the technique. Appropriate for use only in the office or hospital	Surface contamination results in overestimation of bacterial count when compared with biopsy	Underestimates number of organisms when compared with biopsy

the laboratory, where the tissue is flamed, ground and plated in progressive dilutions. It is used in many facilities, especially in surgical patients during the intraoperative period, in which case removal of tissue is performed under anaesthesia. Its strength is that it provides an accurate view of the organisms in the tissue (Robson 1997). Tissue biopsy may not be used due to lack of equipment, technical expertise to perform the procedure, or cost. It is also often not used because the procedure is painful, often requires a suture to close the biopsy site and because it might delay healing.

Alternative approaches are used to culture wounds including swab and aspiration. For the *swab culture*, an area is identified and the tissue swabbed until the tip of the swab is saturated with tissue fluid. The size of the area to be swabbed is not well established. Because infection is in the tissue and not on the wound's surface, utilizing a small area probably will result in culturing fewer surface contaminants. Thus, the work of Levine (Levine et al 1976) is attractive to some people who recommend that the swabbing is performed in a 1-cm^2 area. When compared with biopsy, the swab technique overestimates the number of organisms present because it includes those on the surface as well as those in the tissue (Herruzo-Cabrera et al 1992, Levine et al 1976).

Wound culture using *aspiration technique* involves inserting a needle attached to a syringe through the intact skin next to the wound. Negative pressure is applied and the needle shaft inserted in several different directions to obtain wound fluid. The negative pressure is maintained while the needle is withdrawn from the tissue. Air is then removed from the syringe and the syringe transported to the laboratory for culture of its contents. When compared with biopsy, aspiration underestimates the number of organisms present (Rudensky et al 1992), probably because the specific organism(s) cultured depend on the site where the aspiration is performed.

Diagnosis of osteomyelitis

Osteomyelitis is a special case of wound infection where the infection invades the bone. The most accurate clinical diagnosis is made by probing the bone (Grayson et al 1995). While the bone biopsy is considered the community standard for diagnosing infection by some authors (Bonham 2001, Lewis et al 1988, Sugarman 1987), how often it is used in clinical practice is not known. Bone biopsy can be performed on hospitalized patients at the bedside or in an outpatient setting using a rongeur. One concern is the need to obtain the biopsy through a non-contaminated area to avoid contamination. In a non-surgical situation, this can be a challenging requirement (Bonham 2001).

Authors have sought a non-invasive diagnostic test for osteomyelitis and so have studied a variety of techniques including magnetic resonance imaging, X-ray, bone scans (three-phase), Tc 99m-labelled antigranulocyte antibody scintillography, and ^{111}In leukocyte scans. A series of small studies has shown MRI to be effective (Bonham 2001); however, the high cost often is described as the reason the test is not routinely undertaken. Of significance is the fact that there is no gold standard or community standard that is the reference standard for diagnosing osteomyelitis. While multicentre, randomized clinical trials are recommended to address the diagnosis and treatment issues, until a reference standard is developed, drawing implications from studies performed will remain a challenge.

Prevention of wound infection

Cleansing, debridement, topical antiseptics and prophylactic antibiotics are approaches used to prevent wound infection. Cleansing is the removal of loose debris and metabolic wastes from the surface of the wound; debridement is removal of dead tissue from a wound. Topical agents are antiseptics that are applied to the surface of the wound to reduce the bacteria load. The prophylactic use of antibiotics occurs when patients are prescribed antibiotics without evidence of an infection in the hope that they will not become infected.

Controlled studies supporting these preventive activities exist in the area of debridement (Steed et al 1996) and the use of prophylactic antibiotics in specific types of surgery (Mangram et al 1999). Rodeheaver, an authority in the area of control of bioburden, identifies the current lack of evidence to support both cleansing and the use of topical antiseptics (Rodeheaver 2001). Best practices support the use of cleansing. The use of topical antiseptics is controversial (Falanga 2000, Rodeheaver 2001).

Cleansing

Cleansing is usually done at each dressing change, utilizing a physiological solution under pressures of 4–15 pounds per square inch (PSI). Cleansing may be done utilizing a 35-cc syringe and a 19 angiocath or a commercially available spray bottle that provides the fluid with the appropriate amount of force. A physiological solution is recommended. Commercially available solutions often have surfactants in them to help reduce the surface tension and remove more debris and metabolic wastes than would be possible with a solution alone (Rodeheaver 2001). Antiseptic solutions may increase the toxicity to surface cells and are not recommended. There are no data about the volume of fluid that is to be used, although the rule in practice is to use enough to remove visible debris.

Debridement

Prevention and treatment of infection require debridement whenever dead tissue is present as it is a nidus for infection. By definition, debridement is the removal of dead material from a wound. It can be accomplished by several different methods: sharp, chemical, mechanical and autolytic; less frequent is the use of biodebridement.

Sharp debridement is removal of tissue with a scalpel or scissors. When done with a scalpel in the operating room with anaesthesia it is called surgical debridement. Surgical debridement provides the most rapid approach to removal of dead tissue and is the treatment of choice when the wound is infected. It is contraindicated in an ischaemic limb (Dolynchuk 2001). Unfortunately, healthy tissue may be sacrificed with sharp debridement because it is not a precise technique. Additionally, it is possible that organisms are showered into the bloodstream during the debridement process, resulting in bacteraemia and its sequellae. This method requires special training and should be performed only by physicians and others who have been properly educated and whose licensing boards and facility policies permit this activity (Singhal et al 2001). Data show that in diabetics with foot ulcers, surgical debridement augments healing as it reactivates the acute healing processes (Steed et al 1996).

Chemical debridment involves the use of an enzymatic debriding agent to remove dead tissue. This approach does not remove necrotic tissue as rapidly as surgical debridement but it does not sacrifice healthy tissue. It may be used in conjunction with surgical debridement and is often used for moderately sized areas of necrotic tissue. It is an appropriate choice for patients who are unable to tolerate surgery. In using chemical debridement when the wound is filled with eschar, it is important that the eschar be cross-hatched so the medication can penetrate into the dead tissue. Box 7.2 compares several common products available for chemical debridement. Important considerations include selectivity of the agent, the pH at which it functions and the side-effects experienced by the patient.

| **Box 7.2** *Commonly used enzymatic debriding agents* | **Accuzyme (Healthpoint)** |

Accuzyme (Healthpoint)

This ointment contains papain and urea and is active at a pH of 3–12. It digests non-viable protein, including necrotic tissue and slough, but does not damage viable tissue. Papain may be inactivated by hydrogen peroxide and heavy metals, including lead, silver and mercury.

Use*: Manufacturer recommends the wound be cleansed with wound cleanser or saline. Accuzyme is applied daily or twice daily to the cleansed wound bed. If needed, irrigation may be used to remove the liquefied materials prior to redressing the wound. Transient 'burning' has been reported by a small proportion of people. The liquefied material that is in contact with intact skin may cause irritation.

Collagenase Santyl Ointment (Smith & Nephew)

This product contains collagenase derived from *Clostridium histolyticum*. It digests collagen but is not harmful to healthy tissue. It is most effective at pH 6–8. Detergents and heavy metals (lead, mercury) inactivate it. Cleansing agents such as hydrogen peroxide and Dakin's solution are compatible with it.

Use*: Manufacturer recommends debris and digested material be removed by gentle rubbing with a gauze saturated in normal saline or other agent that is compatible with the Collagenase Santyl. When infection is present, an antibiotic powder is applied to the wound prior to the Santyl. The Collagenase Santyl is applied daily directly to the wound or on a gauze pad that is applied to the wound. The ointment should be stopped when debridement of necrotic tissue is complete and granulation tissue well established. Skin irritation is reported, especially when the exudate gets on healthy skin.

Panafil (Healthpoint)

This is a proteolytic enzyme derived from papayne. It digests non-viable protein matter but is not harmful to healthy tissue. It contains chlorophyllin copper complex sodium that supports healing. It works best in a pH of 3–12.

Use*: Cleanse the wound with normal saline or wound cleanser. Avoid cleaning with hydrogen peroxide because it can inactivate the ingredients. It also is inactivated by heavy metals (lead, silver, mercury). Apply directly to the wound. It is applied daily or twice daily; it can be redressed at 2–3 day intervals as the wound progresses. A small percentage of persons report 'burning' on application.

*Data from package inserts.

Mechanical debridement is removal of dead tissue using either removal of dressings that were inserted moist and allowed to dry or irrigation. With removal of the dry dressing, desiccated exudates, adherent slough and necrotic material are removed. Most people consider removal of dead tissue with wet-to-dry dressings (put in moist and removed after they dry) as less desirable than other, more modern approaches. It is non-selective and so may disrupt healthy tissue and in this way delay healing. It is also reportedly quite painful.

Irrigation is old terminology for what today is called cleansing, i.e. removal of debris and metabolic wastes by flushing with solution. Irrigation, however, usually carries with it the connotation of large quantities of fluid, such as are used in the emergency department to cleanse wounds that are highly contaminated with 'road rash' (gravel imbedded into tissues after sliding on the pavement in a motor vehicle accident).

Irrigation can be done using a continuous stream of fluid, e.g. intravenous fluid is raised above the bed and the stream controlled by the size of angiocath (ideally a 19) used to deliver the fluid. Similarly, taking a shower and removing the dressing so the shower flow is directly on the wound is recommended for many patients. Irrigation may also be delivered in a pulsatile form and, when it is, it is called pulsed lavage. Using a special machine, the irrigation pressure is adjusted to meet patient needs.

Autolytic debridement is the breakdown of dead tissue by the person's own immune system that takes place beneath a dressing. This type of debridement is the slowest, intended for non-infected wounds, and is useful for small areas of necrosis. Hydrogel and hydrocolloids promote autolysis by hyperhydration (Singhal et al 2001).

Biodebridement is the use of sterile maggots for debridement. Sterile maggots are inserted into the wound and a dressing applied so they are contained within the wound. After 48–72 h, they are flushed from the wound and disposed of as biological waste (Thomas et al 1998). If the wound needs further debridement, additional maggots are applied and the process is repeated. Some patients have difficulty accepting this therapy. Currently, there are no studies comparing this form of debridement with other approaches.

Topical agents

Topical agents are a two-edged sword: they reduce bacterial burden in wounds but they also impair the function of some cells necessary for healing (Rodeheaver 2001). Iodine products are frequently cited as the offending products, although a host of other agents fall into this category, including Dakin's solution, hydrogen peroxide, acetic acid and triple antibiotic.

While many authors oppose their use under any circumstances (Rodeheaver 2001), others believe that topical antiseptics have a place in clinical care (Falanga 2000). Those who support their use would suggest that topical antiseptics should be used only when needed, therefore topical agents should never be used *routinely* in wounds. They suggest that using topical antiseptics reduces bacterial load. Some newer products, such as cadexomer iodine and dressings impregnated with silver, are being used by some practitioners (Bello et al 2001, Falanga 2000). There is agreement, however, that one group in whom topical agents should be limited is those with venous disease, as they have a higher incidence of skin sensitivity (Falanga 2000).

Prophylactic antibiotics

Prophylactic antibiotics are used in surgical patients prior to surgery so that the antibiotic can be at the site when the incision is made. They are also used in high-risk patients (those who are neutropenic or who have an artificial joint) when the skin or mucous membranes may be damaged (Lehne 2001).

With the surgical population, antibiotics are given prior to surgery to reduce the bacterial load at the site where the incision is made. There is usually a preoperative dose and several postoperative doses, varying somewhat by body system and surgeon experience. The critical part of this process for nursing is the timely administration of the doses of the antibiotic. The initial dose is started as the patient goes to the operation room, within 1 h of the surgical incision (Mangram et al 1999). After surgery, blood levels need to be maintained so timely administration again becomes paramount to prevent wound infection.

With the neutropenic population, prophylactic antibiotics have been shown to decrease bacterial infection. However, there is a trade-off when the bacterial flora is reduced because the risk of fungal infection increases when it is not kept under control by the bacterial population (Lehne 2001).

Treatment of wound infection

Infected wounds involve invasion of the tissues by organisms and so treatment is aimed at removal of the organisms from the tissue. Pivotal to treatment is addressing the underlying cause, identifying the causative organism(s), treating the organisms that have invaded the tissues, removing dead tissue and providing systemic support for immune function.

Treating the underlying cause

The cause of the infection needs to be identified through history taking, physical examination and laboratory techniques. The history may be a key item to identifying the source of infection so it can be treated. For example, in a patient with a chronic leg wound infection, treatment of faecal incontinence may be key to control of the source of the infection. Alternatively, identifying and treating the cause of the infection may require more extensive work. For example, a staphylococcal outbreak in the cardiac surgery population might require the infection control department to do an extensive evaluation of all the operating room staff.

Treating the organism(s) causing the infection

The primary treatment of infection is antibiotics. There are two phases to treatment. The first focuses on obtaining a wound culture, performing a Gram stain and providing empirical treatment. Although the culture will take 48 h for results to be completed, the Gram stain is a more rapid (15–20-min) approach that will confirm that infection is present and whether the organisms are Gram-positive, Gram-negative, or a combination. Empirical antibiotic therapy is then selected based on all available data, including knowledge of the usual organisms in the specific institution. Current treatment regimes are outlined in recent publications (Dow 2001, O'Meara et al 2001).

The second phase of treatment is based on the culture results. Preliminary culture results are available at 24 h and final results are completed usually about 48 h after the culture. At that time, the antibiotic regime will be modified as necessary, taking into account sensitivity of the various organisms to specific antibiotics, the availability of the products and the cost of the various alternative regimes.

Identification of the organism and its susceptibility to various antibiotics is pivotal to appropriate therapy. Narrow-spectrum antibiotics are usually preferred to broad-spectrum antibiotics because they reduce the number of organisms for whom resistance may develop. Susceptibility of organisms to various anti-microbials is identified by either the disk-diffusion method, also known as the Kirby–Bauer test, or the broth dilution technique. The disk-diffusion method indicates the antibiotics to which the organism is sensitive. The broth dilution technique provides more precise information in that it is used to define both the minimal inhibitory concentration (MIC), i.e. the lowest concentration of anti-biotic that completely inhibits bacterial growth, and the minimal bactericidal concentration (MBC), i.e. the lowest concentration of drug that produces a 99.9% decrease in bacterial colonies (Lehne 2001).

Antibiotics must get to the site of the wound infection in appropriate concen-trations. This means that management of collateral issues, such as whether the patient has oedema at the wound site or decreased perfusion, need to be consid-ered in the therapeutic plan. The importance of administration of antibiotics on an appropriate timeline and with or without food and fluids seems funda-mental but often requires sophisticated juggling, especially when patients are on multiple medications or have dietary and fluid restrictions.

When patients are to take medication at home, education of the patient and family is critical to the success of the treatment. Understanding when the drug is to be taken, whether it is to be administered with food/fluids, appreciating the side-effects, having an understanding of the interaction of the antimicrobial with their other drugs and appreciating the importance of taking the entire regime (i.e. not stopping when the side-effects abate) are pieces of information that are basic to safe care (Lehne 2001).

Removing dead tissue

See the section 'Debridement' (p. 108).

Providing support for immune function

Oxygenation and perfusion are fundamental to the success of the immune system in fighting infection (Hunt & Hopf 1997). Early studies explored the effects of innoculum of organisms on wounds of animals housed in a hypoxic (12%), normoxic (21%), and hyperoxic (45%) environment (Hunt et al 1975). Infection rates were highest in the hypoxic group and lowest in the hyperoxic group. The authors speculated that increased levels of oxygen support the oxidative production of hydrogen peroxide. Subsequent work has confirmed their speculation and extended our knowledge of the importance of oxygen and perfusion in supporting healing and mitigating infection (Knighton et al 1986).

Recent work has explored the importance of provision of oxygen as a strategy to reduce surgical wound infection rates (Greif et al 2000). Patients ($n = 500$) undergoing colorectal surgery were randomized to receive 30% or 80% inspired oxygen during surgery. Anaesthesia was standardized and patients were managed routinely throughout the surgical period by their surgeon, who was blind to group assignment. There was a 6% lower infection rate (5.2% versus 11.2%) in those who received the higher concentration of oxygen, indicating that normal immune function can be augmented with the use of supplemental oxygen in the intraoperative period.

A number of additional factors that support perfusion has been explored as possible factors to mitigate infection and promote healing in persons with wounds. The relationship between temperature modulation at the time of surgery has been explored as a factor to reduce infection (Kurtz et al 1996). Using an experimental design, colorectal surgical patients ($n = 200$) were randomly assigned to usual operating room temperature or to a normothermia environment. Data showed that those in the warmer environment had significantly fewer infections ($p = 0.009$).

Similarly, temperature modulation in the preoperative period has been shown to reduce the infection rate in persons undergoing a clean surgical procedure (Melling et al 2001). A sample of subjects ($n = 416$) were randomly assigned to routine preoperative care and treatment with either systemic heating or local incision area heating. Data showed that the heating groups, individually and together, had lower infection rates and received fewer antibiotics than those who received routine care. These data suggest that maintaining a normothermic environment decreases the incidence of infection in acute surgical wounds.

Several factors that support oxygenation and perfusion probably also affect the development of infection, although controlled studies have not examined the direct link to infection. Pain management is important in maximizing blood flow. Data show that blood flow measured with subcutaneous oxygen is greater in persons with good pain control than in those with poor pain control (Acka et al 1999). If blood flow is greater, the opportunity to clear the tissues of organisms will be enhanced.

Similarly, provision of fluids to patients with wounds should help maximize local availability of the immune response. Chang et al (1983) showed that there is a group of patients who are subclinically hypovolaemic. Subsequent randomized clinical trials showed that when fluids were provided based on subcutaneous oxygen levels, more fluids were administered than when fluids were based on traditional formulas (Hartman et al 1992, Jonsson et al 1987). However, the samples for these studies were small and so precluded evaluation of the effect on infection.

Recent work by Armstrong & Nguyen (2000) examined the effect of reducing oedema in diabetics with foot infection on the rate of healing. They randomized patients ($n = 115$) to treatment and found foot compression resulted in a significantly greater proportion of patients healing. Thus, adding oedema reduction to traditional antibiotic treatment resulted in greater healing, probably because the medication was able to reach the affected tissues when the oedema was reduced.

CONCLUSIONS

Infection is a serious problem in people with wounds. The diagnosis of infection is based on clinical signs and symptoms. In acute wounds there is agreement as to the criteria for diagnosis but in chronic wounds there is only moderate agreement as to the criteria for diagnosis of wound infection. There is agreement that a wound culture of $> 10^5$ organisms/gram of tissue is diagnostic of infection in acute wounds, or a lower number with very virulent organisms. Controversy remains as to whether this same number is diagnostic of wound infection in chronic wounds.

Prevention of infection and its treatment focus on reducing the bacterial load and supporting immune defences. Bacterial load is reduced by cleansing, debriding, application of topical agents and administration of systemic anti-biotics. Immune defences are supported with oxygenation-perfusion, including supplemental oxygen, management of temperature, provision of fluids and optimizing pain levels.

REFERENCES

Akca O, Melischek M, Scheck T et al 1999 Postoperative pain and subcutaneous oxygen tension [letter]. Lancet 354(9172):41–42

Armstrong D G, Nguyen H C 2000 Improvement in healing with aggressive edema reduction after debridement of foot infection in persons with diabetes. Archives of Surgery 135:1405–1409

Bello Y M, Falabella A F, De Carbalho H et al 2001 Infection and wound healing. Wounds 13(4):127–135

Bendy R H, Nuccio P A, Wolfe E et al 1965 Relationship of quantitative wound bacterial counts to healing of decubiti: effect of topical gentamicin. Antimicrobial Agents and Chemotherapy 4:147–155

Bonham P 2001 A critical review of the literature: part 1. Diagnosing osteomyelitis in patients with diabetes and foot ulcers. Journal of Wound Ostomy and Continence Nursing 28:73–88

Chang N, Goodson W H III, Gottrup F, Hunt T K 1983 Direct measurement of wound and tissue oxygen tension in postoperative patients. Annals of Surgery 197(4):470–478

Cutting K F, Harding K G 1994 Criteria for identifying wound infection. Journal of Wound Care 3:198–201

Darouiche R O, Landon G C, Klima M, et al 1994 Osteomyelitis associated with pressure sores. Archives of Internal Medicine 154(7):753–758

Dolynchuk K N 2001 Debridement. In: Krasner D L, Rodeheaver G T, Sibbald RG (eds) Chronic wound care: a clinical source book for healthcare professionals, 3rd edn. HMP Communications, Wayne, PA, p 385–390

Dow G 2001 Infection in chronic wounds. In: Krasner D L, Rodeheaver G T, Sibbald R G (eds) Chronic wound care: a clinical source book for healthcare professionals, 3rd edn. HMP Communications, Wayne, PA, p 343–356

Elek S 1956 Experimental staphylococcal infections in the skin of man. Annals of the New York Academy of Science 65:85–90

Falanga V 2000 Wounds and infection. In: Falanga V (ed) Text atlas of wound management. Martin Dunitz, London, p 61–96

Gardner S E, Frantz R A, Doebbeling B N 2001 The validity of the clinical signs and symptoms used to identify localized chronic wound infection. Wound Repair and Regeneration 9:178–186

Grayson M, Gibbons G, Balogh K et al 1995 Probing to bone in infected pedal ulcers: a clinical sign of underlying osteomyelitis in diabetic patients. Journal of the American Medical Association 273:721–723

Grief R, Akca O, Horn E P et al 2000 Supplemental perioperative oxygen to reduce the incidence of surgical-wound infection. Study by the Outcomes Research Group. New England Journal of Medicine 342(3):161–167

Hartman M, Jonsson K, Zederfeldt B 1992 Effect of tissue perfusion and oxygenation on accumulation of collagen in healing wounds: randomized study in patients after major abdominal operations. European Journal of Surgery 158:521–526

Herruzo-Cabrera R, Vizcaino-Alcaide M J, Pindeso-Castillo C, Rey-Calero J 1992 Diagnosis of local infection of a burn by semiquantitative culture of the eschar surface. Journal of Burn Care & Rehabilitation 13:639–641

Hunt T K, Hopf H W 1997 Wound healing and wound infection. What surgeons and anesthesiologists can do. Surgical Clinics of North America 77:587–606

Hunt T K, Linsey M, Grislis G 1975 The effect of differing ambient oxygen tensions on wound infection. Annals of Surgery 181(1):35–39

Jonsson K, Jensen J A, Goodson W H et al 1987 Assessment of perfusion in postoperative patients using tissue oxygen measures. British Journal of Surgery 74:263–267

Knighton D R, Halliday B, Hunt T K 1986 Oxygen as an antibiotic. A comparison of the effects of inspired oxygen concentration and antibiotic administration on in vivo bacterial clearance. Archives of Surgery 121(2):191–195

Kurz A, Sessler D I, Lenhardt R 1996 Perioperative normothermia to reduce the incidence of surgical-wound infection and shorten hospitalization. Study by the Wound Infection and Temperature Group. New England Journal of Medicine 334(19):1209–1215

Laato M, Niiikoski J, Lunberg C, Gerdin B 1988 Inflammatory reaction and blood flow in experimental wounds inoculated with *Staphylococcus aureus*. European Surgical Research 10(1):33–38

Lalla F, Pellizzer G, Strazzabosco M 2001 Randomized prospective controlled trial of recombinant granulocyte colony-stimulating factor as adjunctive therapy for limb-threatening diabetic foot infection. Antimicrobial Agents and Chemotherapy 45(4):1094–1098

Langkamp-Henken B, Herrlinger-Garcia K A, Stechmiller J K 2000 Arginine supplementation is well tolerated but does not enhance mitogen-induced lymphocyte proliferation in elderly nursing home residents with pressure ulcers. Journal of Parenteral and Enteral Nutrition 24(5):280–287

Lehne R E 2001 Pharmacology for nursing care, 4th edn. W B Saunders, Philadelphia, p 1071–1075

Levine N S, Lindberg R B, Mason R B, Pruitt A D 1976 The quantitative swab culture and smear: a quick simple method for determining the number of viable aerobic bacteria on open wounds. Journal of Trauma 16:L89–L94

Lewis V L Jr, Bailey M H, Pulawski G et al 1988 The diagnosis of osteomyelitis in patients with pressure sores. Plastic and Reconstructive Surgery 2:229–232

Mangram A J, Horan T C, Pearson M L et al 1999 Guidelines for prevention of surgical site infection, 1999. Infection Control and Hospital Epidemiology 20(4):247–278

Melling A C, Ali B, Scott E M, Leaper D J 2001 Effects of preoperative warming on the incidence of wound infection after clean surgery: a randomized controlled trial. Lancet 358:876–880

O'Meara S M, Cullum N A, Majid M, Sheldon T A 2001 Systemic review of antimicrobial agents used for chronic wounds. British Journal of Surgery 88:4–21

Robson M C 1997 Wound infection: a failure of wound healing caused by an imbalance of bacteria. Surgical Clinics of North America 77(3):637–650

Rodeheaver G T 2001 Wound cleansing, wound irrigation, wound disinfection. In: Krasner D L, Rodeheaver G T, Sibbald R G (eds) Chronic wound care: a clinical source book for healthcare professionals, 3rd edn. HMP Communications, Wayne, PA, p 369–383

Rudensky R, Lipschits M, Isaacsohn M, Sonnenblick M 1992 Infected pressure sores: comparison of methods for bacterial identification. Southern Medical Journal 85:901–903

Serralta V W, Harrison-Balestra C, Cazzaniga A L et al 2001 Lifestyles of bacteria in wounds: presence of biofilms? Wounds 13(1):29–34

Singhal A, Reis E A, Kerstein M D 2001 Option for nonsurgical debridement of necrotic wounds. Advances in Wound Care 14:96–103

Steed D L, Donohoe D, Webster M W, Lindsley L 1996 Effect of extensive debridement and treatment of diabetic foot ulcers. Journal of the American College of Surgeons 183:61–64

Stotts N A, Whitney J D 1999 Identifying and evaluating wound infection. Home Healthcare Nurse 17(3):159–164

Sugarman B 1987 Pressure sores and underlying bone infection. Archives of Internal Medicine 147:553–555

Tarnuzzer R W, Schultz G S 1996 Biochemical analysis of acute and chronic wound environments. Wound Repair and Regeneration 4:321–325

Thomas S, Andrews A, Jones M 1998 The use of larval therapy in wound management. Journal of Wound Care 7:521–524

Thomson P D, Smith D J Jr 1994 What is infection? American Journal of Surgery 167 (1A Suppl):7S–11S

FURTHER READING

Bennett L L, Rosenblum R S, Perlov C et al 2001 An in vivo comparison of topical agents on wound repair. Plastic and Reconstructive Surgery 108(3):686–687

Bowler P G, Duerden B I, Armstrong D G 2001 Wound microbiology and associated approaches to wound management. Clinical Microbiology Reviews 14(2):244–269

Gross P A, Pujat D 2001 Implementing practice guidelines for appropriate antimicrobial usage: a systematic review. Medical Care 39(8 Suppl 2):II55–II69

Heggers J P, Robson M C 1991 Quantitative bacteriology: its role in the armamentarium of the surgeon. CRC Press, Boca Raton, FL

Kirsner R S, Federman D G 1998 The ethical dilemma of population-based medical decision making. American Journal of Managed Care 4(11):1571–1576

Mangram A J, Horan T C, Pearson M L 1999 Guidelines for prevention of surgical site infection, 1999. Infection Control and Hospital Epidemiology 20(4):247–278

Robson M C 1999 Award recipient address: lessons gleaned from the sport of wound watching. Wound Repair and Regeneration 7(1):2–6

Robson M C, Mannari R J, Smith P D, Payne W G 1999 Maintenance of wound bacterial balance. American Journal of Surgery 178(5):399–402

Dressings and cleansing agents

Liza G Ovington and David Eisenbud

INTRODUCTION

Wound healing is the result of a complex and highly ordered series of biochemical and cellular processes that involve the coordinated action of multiple cell types in response to humoral peptide mediators and to aspects of the cellular environment such as oxygen tension, temperature and pH. Under normal physiological conditions, when the various cells are healthy and efficient and their environment is within normal homeostatic parameters, the healing process proceeds predictably and without incident. When those cells and the wound environment are compromised by alterations in local or systemic conditions, repair is hindered and the wound does not close in an orderly or timely fashion.

Optimal management of the non-healing wound involves understanding both the local and systemic wound environment. The patient must be approached in a holistic manner (Krasner & Sibbald 1999). Socioeconomic factors (such as the setting where the patient is to be treated, his or her social support systems and the requirements of the payer), systemic factors affecting the patient's whole-body physiology, the function of the extremity or body part that is wounded, and the actual tissue contained within the physical boundaries of the wound, must all be considered. The healthcare system in general, as well as the specific setting in which care is rendered, may affect what treatments and therapies are available for use by the medical community. The availability or absence of support in the home from a spouse or family member can influence certain product selections or regimens for elderly and debilitated patients. Systemic conditions including nutritional status, blood glucose levels, immune function, and a variety of disease processes and oral medications may have significant impact on wound healing and must be considered in the overall plan for management. Finally, the local environment of the wound itself plays a critical role in determining certain aspects of wound treatment. Status of the exposed tissues and structures, condition of the surrounding skin, level and nature of exudate, and microbial status influence decisions related to topical management.

LOCAL WOUND MANAGEMENT

This chapter will focus on local wound management, specifically the use and selection of cleansing agents and dressings. However, it is important to keep in mind that local management is a necessary but not sufficient part of caring for a wounded patient. Patients with chronic wounds who present to the wound-care expert have often been treated by one or more providers using inappropriate cleansing and dressing techniques that can hinder or prevent healing; sometimes merely instituting more optimal cleansing and dressing techniques can restore healing progress. Frequently, however, a non-healing wound is but the visible manifestation of underlying pathology. In these cases, changes in cleansing and dressing techniques will generally not result in improved healing. Medical and/or surgical management of this underlying pathology and elimination or minimization of complicating factors is often the most critical aspect of care; these issues are addressed in other chapters in this text. In addition, education of the patient and family regarding both the care and the cause of the wound is vital not only for optimal healing but also for health maintenance and prevention of wound recurrence.

REMOVAL OF IMPEDIMENTS TO HEALING

The time-honoured approach to wound care can be viewed as 'passive': impediments to healing – infection, ischaemia, diabetes, etc. – are identified and controlled, thereby allowing endogenous repair processes to resume at a normal pace. The majority of topical wound treatment options, including wound cleansing and dressings, aim to reduce bacterial burden, reduce necrotic tissue, restore physiological levels of pH, temperature and moisture and improve the microcirculation in the wound bed. 'Active' approaches to wound healing attempt to accelerate natural healing processes beyond their natural speed. These include the topical application of bioengineered tissues and growth factors, which are discussed elsewhere in this text.

Products and processes for wound cleansing, which aim to reduce bacterial colonization and minimize necrosis, will be addressed first. It is logical to begin local wound management with attention to these two factors because they are among the most common impediments to healing, and can culminate in infection. Without preliminary attention to these problems, attempts to address others will likely be unsuccessful.

Microbial states of tissue

Before discussing specific cleansing products, it is of value to first examine the target to be cleansed – the wound. No open wound is devoid of any bacteria. There are three microbiological states that are encountered in a wound – contamination, colonization and infection (Gilchrist 1997). Contamination is characterized as the simple presence of microorganisms in the wound but without proliferation. It is generally accepted that all wounds, regardless of aetiology are contaminated. Human skin, respiratory passages and the gastrointestinal tract harbour at least 10^{14} microorganisms (Williams & Leaper 1998) and such endogenous bacteria are the most common source of wound colonization (see Chapter 7 for a more detailed discussion of bacterial colonization and infection).

The germ is nothing; it is the terrain in which it grows that is everything (attributed to Pasteur circa 1880)

Wound cleansing and debridement

Pasteur's caveat about 'terrain' is relevant to a discussion of bacterial levels and wound infection. The wound terrain comprises the environmental conditions that will enable or discourage the 'germ' or microorganism to successfully colonize the wound surface or to invade viable tissue. Acute and chronic wounds offer distinctly different environments for colonization. Chronic wounds are often characterized by an impaired vascular supply and devitalized tissues that offer a nutritional supply to microorganisms, as well as by a varied topography of crevices, undermining and tunnels that can represent 'safe harbour' for proliferation. Acute wounds by comparison are in general relatively free of debris and are well vascularized. For these reasons, wound cleansing and debridement are important processes related to preventing infection in chronic wound management. Cleansing is the first line of defence in the removal of microorganisms and foreign materials and devitalized tissue from the wound. Debridement can be considered a 'special type of cleansing' that is indicated when devitalized tissue is present in large amounts.

Cleansing materials and methods

The aforementioned semantics are important because in the realm of wound management, the three processes – cleansing, disinfection and antisepsis – have been misused interchangeably in discussing products used and developed for wound cleansing. The primary objective of cleansing a wound is to remove foreign materials and reduce the bioburden, in the hope of treating or preventing wound infection, preparing the wound bed for grafting and reducing odour and exudate (Eaglstein & Falanga 1997). Topical products commonly used in wound cleansing include antiseptics, antibiotics, detergents, surfactants and saline and water.

Intact skin is a formidable barrier, primarily because of the tough, keratinized (non-living) stratum corneum layer and secretions from sebaceous and sweat glands. When this barrier is breached, viable tissues are exposed and vulnerable. The use of many solutions considered safe on intact skin may be damaging in an open wound. Although cleansing has been defined as a physical process of removal, many clinicians feel the need to use an antiseptic solution as a cleansing agent in an effort to kill potential pathogens in the wound and thereby stave off infection. Interestingly, it has been shown that even the surface of intact skin cannot be rendered bacteria-free by any antiseptic. Bacteria exist deep in adnexal structures and are brought to the skin surface by secretions of sweat and sebum. Even if one's hands are scrubbed with 70% ethanol to achieve a 99.7% reduction of surface bacteria, subsequent washing with soap and water results in a significant increase in surface bacteria (Laufman 1989). This effect is thought to be due to the friction-induced shedding of epithelial squames that harbour viable bacteria.

Tissue toxicity issues

The potential for deleterious effects of cleansing solutions on open wounds has long been recognized:

> It is necessary in the estimation of the value of an antiseptic to study its effect on the tissues more than its effect on the bacteria (Fleming 1919)

It is not logical that antiseptics developed for use on intact skin would be compatible with internal tissues and, in fact, they may have cytotoxic effects that could delay wound healing (Bennett 2001). Most antiseptics work by destroying bacterial cell walls and do not spare non-bacterial cells such as wound fibroblasts and macrophages (Hellewell et al 1997). Some antiseptics such as iodine and various alcohols also evaporate rapidly and are drying to tissues, causing desiccation necrosis. A large variety of antiseptics have demonstrated adverse effects on many of the cellular events in wound healing. Specific inhibition of key steps includes prolonging inflammation, inhibiting fibroblast and endothelial cell proliferation, interfering with wound contraction and toxicity to keratinocytes (Cho 1998).

It should be recognized that the pendulum, having pointed in favour of antiseptic use in wounds for so many years, then having swung greatly against its use, is moving back towards the centre again (Eaglstein & Falanga 1997). A large body of evidence has emerged to clarify lower concentrations and dose exposures to povidone–iodine, hydrogen peroxide and chlorhexidine that may not be detrimental to wound repair. In an extensive test of five common antiseptics, Bennett was unable to demonstrate any consistent ill effect on fibroblast proliferation, angiogenesis or reepithelialization (Bennett et al 2001).

At present, the general consensus among wound-care practitioners is that normal saline is the safest cleansing agent for chronic wounds that do not have significant amounts of devitalized tissue or signs of clinical infection. There have even been arguments for the use of regular tap water as a cleansing solution (Moscati et al 1998, Riyat & Quinton 1997). In one randomized controlled study of 705 consecutive accident and emergency patients, the infection rate in wounds irrigated with sterile saline was 10.3%, compared with 5.4% in wounds irrigated with tap water (Angeras et al 1992).

Cleansing technique

As important as the choice of the specific cleansing solution are the temperature of the solution and the method of its delivery to the wound surface. Cleansing solutions that are refrigerated or even at room temperature can reduce the surface temperature of the wound, resulting in local hypothermia. It is known from surgical experience that tissue hypothermia can result in decreased mitogenesis and decreased phagocyte activity. It can take as long as 40 min for a wound to regain its original temperature after cleansing, and several hours for cellular activities to normalize (Flannagan 1997).

Cleansing solutions must be delivered with sufficient volume and force to loosen and wash away microorganisms and debris, although excessive force may drive the loosened material into viable tissue rather than out (Rodeheaver et al 1975). A safe range of effective irrigation pressures has been established as 4 to 15 pounds per square inch (psi). A 35-ml syringe fitted with a 19-gauge angiocatheter tip delivers a stream of liquid at a pressure of 8 psi. Increasing the bore of the angiocatheter or decreasing the size of the syringe result in higher-pressure streams, whereas decreasing the bore or increasing the size of the syringe result in lower pressures.

In summary, a wound is not a static entity or an inanimate surface, but a complex, fragile and dynamic milieu of viable endogenous cells and structures, exogenous microorganisms, labile chemicals and chemical reactions, devitalized cells and microorganisms, and potential foreign particulate matter from the external environment. The differential impact of cleansing solutions and methods on all of these components of the wound must be weighed in terms of overall benefit to the healing process.

Topical antibiotics

Despite their widespread use, the exact role of topical antibiotics in treating chronic wounds is controversial (O'Meara et al 2001). Topical application has a potential advantage over systemic administration in its ability to deliver higher concentrations of antibiotic directly to the wound tissues. This is particularly pertinent when the wound has impaired arterial or venous circulation. Indications for prophylactic use of topical antibiotics in wounds that are not clinically infected, and their ability to reduce bacterial count better than antiseptics, irrigation and debridement, are unclear. Many studies have supported the concept of enhanced wound healing using topical antibiotics (Cho 1998); others have failed to show a benefit over controls and a few reports have claimed a negative effect on wound repair.

The most common topical antibiotics in use include bacitracin zinc (alone or in combination with polymyxin B sulfate and/or neomycin sulfate), mupirocin, silver sulfadiazine, gentamicin and erythromycin. Because no one agent covers the full range of organisms found in chronic wounds, combination therapy is typical. It is important to note that mupirocin, cadexomer iodine and elemental silver preparations are effective against antibiotic-resistant species.

In addition to the potential to promote resistant bacterial strains, indiscriminate use of topical antibiotics can also result in skin irritation or allergic reactions. Contact dermatitis to bacitracin occurs in up to 13% of patients, and to neomycin in 34%, with prolonged use.

Debridement versus cleansing

If significant amounts of devitalized tissues are present in the wound, they will delay healing and predispose the wound to colonization and infection by providing a site of attachment and source of nutrients for bacteria. Therefore the expedient removal of devitalized tissue or debridement is advisable for optimal healing. Devitalized or necrotic tissue may have a variety of appearances from loosely adherent yellow slough to tightly adherent, leathery black eschar. Removal or debridement can be achieved by multiple methods, depending on the amount and nature of the necrotic tissue and the patient's overall status.

In general, there is no single 'best' method of debridement; each technique is appropriate for certain clinical scenarios. Furthermore, the methods can be used to great effect in combination. For example, a surgically debrided wound can be treated with high-pressure irrigation and a proteolytic enzyme ointment to control further build-up of protein and cellular debris on the wound surface.

In other cases, tightly adherent eschar might be treated with enzymatic agents to make future surgical debridement easier and less painful.

Promotion of tissue viability and proliferation

Once the wound environment has been optimized in terms of removing impediments to healing by cleansing and/or debridement, attention should be turned towards maintaining the viability of the healthy tissue and establishing conditions that facilitate the proliferation of new tissues to close the wound. Important systemic factors that promote healing include adequate blood supply and nutrition; however, the focus in this chapter is on local factors, specifically those that are impacted by wound dressing materials.

Maintenance of appropriate tissue hydration

Perhaps the single most pertinent parameter of the local wound environment relative to tissue viability and proliferation is that of tissue hydration. Cells and tissues are only viable within a narrow range of hydration. One of the critical functions of intact skin is to maintain functional hydration levels in the underlying tissues by acting as a barrier to moisture loss to the atmosphere. The stratum corneum is the key to this barrier function. Moisture loss from intact skin can be measured as the moisture vapour transmission rate (or MVTR) and varies with anatomical location. The mean value for the MVTR of intact skin is around 200 g of moisture vapour per square metre per day ($g/m^2/d$) (Lamke 1977). The MVTR of skin without the stratum corneum (a wound) is almost 40 times as high or $7874 \, g/m^2/day$ (Rovee et al 1972).

The impact that wound dressing materials could have on replacing this moisture barrier function of the stratum corneum was not fully recognized and reduced to practice until the latter half of the twentieth century. In the early 1960s, studies in both animal and human models documented increased healing rates for wounds maintained in a physiologically moist local environment relative to wounds exposed to air and allowed to desiccate (Hinnman & Maibach 1963, Winter 1962). Since that time, research data have suggested that a physiologically moist local wound environment also contributes to diminution of pain and enhancement of cosmesis relative to a dry desiccated wound environment (Hedman 1988, Nemeth et al 1991).

Multiple mechanisms have been suggested for the effects of a moist local environment on healing. Histological studies of wounds healing in a moist environment versus wounds healing in a dry environment have revealed that the dry environment results in further tissue death or 'dehydration necrosis' (Rovee et al 1972, Winter 1972). It has been shown that resurfacing epithelial cells move further and faster in a moist environment, whereas a dry environment retards their progress (Winter 1972). Further studies of wounds healing in a moist environment have shown that the fluid that is retained at the wound surface by a semiocclusive dressing contains proteolytic enzymes and functional growth factors (polypeptides that promote cellular movement or proliferation) that enhance the healing process (Chen et al 1992). In dry wounds, these enzymes and proteins are present only deeper in the tissues, and in lesser concentrations. Another proposed mechanism for the reduced healing times associated with moist wound healing involves the 'current of injury' that flows because of the natural electrical potential that exists between the layers of the skin after an injury. This current 'flows' in a moist wound but is turned 'off' when the wound is allowed to dry out (Jaffe & Vanable 1984). This endogenous electrical current may play a role in enhancing healing by promoting cell migration and by influencing cells to express more receptors for growth factors (Falanga et al 1987). Finally, maintenance of stable wound temperature may play a role in the benefit of semiocclusive dressings. When moisture vapour escapes freely from tissue, the evaporative process results in local cooling, with the previously discussed effects on cellular mitosis and phagocyte efficiency. A dressing that slows the evaporative process may therefore reduce tissue temperature loss. Certain dressings, such as foams and hydrocolloids, have been demonstrated to have an insulating effect on wound tissues relative to air exposure or gauze (Thomas 1990).

The concept of maintaining or establishing a physiologically moist wound environment is inherently logical. Cells and tissues subsist and function in a moist milieu beneath an intact stratum corneum. Yet in the case of a wound, the conventional wisdom of both the housewife and the surgeon is to allow or even encourage the exposed tissues to desiccate. There is an underlying fear of promoting infection with moisture. A number of retrospective and prospective studies of wounds managed topically by materials that sustain a moist environment or by conventional materials (gauze and saline) have documented that this fear is not, in fact, borne out. Observed rates of infection have actually been lower for wounds dressed with semiocclusive dressings relative to gauze. Another common misconception among patients who are concerned about covering wounds is the concept that wounds should be left open to 'breathe'. This of course, is patently false; the ability of wounds to absorb oxygen from the environment is minimal, and limited to the uppermost 2 mm of tissue.

The development of materials that sustain a moist wound environment for optimal healing has become a thriving industry. Such materials are largely synthetic polymers that are fashioned into fibres, mats, wafers or membranes that are semipermeable to gases such as oxygen, carbon dioxide and moisture, yet often impermeable to liquids. This characteristic earns them the general term 'semiocclusive'. These different types of semiocclusive dressings create or maintain a moist local environment by capturing transpired moisture vapour or liquid drainage from the wound and holding it at the surface. It is possible to use gauze and saline to establish and maintain a continuously moist wound environment, however, it has been shown to require substantially more dressing changes, labour and overall cost than the polymeric (semiocclusive) materials.

THE ROLES OF DRESSINGS: FORM VERSUS FUNCTION

Science is nothing but trained and organized common sense. (attributed to Huxley circa 1860)

Choosing among the vast and expanding array of dressing products for a specific patient can seem a daunting task. Novices may deal with this problem by adopting a 'one size fits all' approach, in which they identify a dressing with certain attractive characteristics and use it indiscriminately for a wide variety of cases. However, this approach does not make optimal use of the technology. A basic understanding of the categories and functions of dressings, and the use of common sense, will generally point to one or more acceptable choices in each case. Fortunately, there is often more than one right answer!

Semiocclusive wound dressings are commonly categorized, discussed and reviewed from the standpoint of their composition. Descriptions of what a wound dressing consists of from a materials point of view is informative and it has been done well by many authors (Ovington 1998, Thomas 1990, Turner 1989). However, such discussions are not always instructive in terms of selecting a wound dressing for clinical use. What the product is made of or what it contains is only a part of the selection equation. Additional information needed relates to the function or performance of the dressing. So, rather than launch into another description of physical form and characteristics of generic dressing categories such as transparent films, foams, alginate fibres, hydrocolloid wafers, hydrogel wafers, amorphous hydrogels, collagen sheets and newer specialty materials, we will attempt to weave this information into the broader context of dressing functions and performance parameters.

A performance-based approach to dressing utilization

Performance is the way in which something functions, or the action for which a thing is especially fit or employed. In general, the dressing products that survive the regulatory process and are commercialized have acceptable safety profiles. However, some products are more suited than others for a specific phase of wound healing or wound condition. In spite of this, many dressings are often promoted as being a uniform solution for any wound. As a dressing almost never addresses or corrects the underlying pathology of a wound, it should not be selected based on wound aetiology but on local wound needs determined by a thorough assessment of the wound and periwound skin. The requirements of an individual wound provide criteria for dressing performance, which then become the basis of product selection.

This type of performance-based approach to product selection is a familiar concept in prescribing drugs. First the desired performance is identified, then the available products with that function are examined. Drugs can be classified based on their chemical structures but clinical selection usually begins with their classification by function. With respect to wound dressings, the focus has been more on their composition rather than their functions. Recent discussions have surfaced in the literature that take note of this situation. Krasner calls for a paradigm shift in decision making about dressing (Krasner 1997). The shift is described as the interactive and active utilization of dressing materials in the same way as drugs; with specific actions, interactions, contraindications, indications and side-effects. Van Rijswijk presents arguments for the classification of dressings based on clinically valid functions as opposed to product components in order to increase clinical utility (Van Rijswijk & Beitz 1998).

Some manufacturers have realized that their products would be better utilized if they were viewed in terms of their functions and have attempted to convey functions of their products in their advertising. Others have devised charts that categorize their products based on the absorbent capacity of each. What is needed is more than a guide to a particular line of products, but an approach to thinking differently about all available dressing products.

A more general, performance-based approach to utilizing wound dressings might be guided by six basic questions:

1. What does the wound need?
2. What does the product do?

3. How well does it do it?
4. What does the patient need?
5. What is available?
6. What is practical?

Answers to what the wound needs are found by thorough local assessment of the wound in terms of its three dimensions, the type or types of tissue present in the wound bed (granulation, epithelial, slough, eschar), the quality and quantity of drainage and the condition of the periwound skin and its microbial status.

This assessment must be performed not only initially but also at each dressing change. Wounds are not static entities; their needs change as they progress or deteriorate. A dressing that was appropriate in the early, exudative inflammatory phase of wound healing becomes inappropriate for optimal healing during the later, less exudative phase of re-epithelialization. As the wound evolves in either direction, dressing choices must similarly evolve to meet local needs.

Answers to what the product does should be sought in multiple places, including marketing materials, data from controlled clinical trials and data from in vitro evaluations. Other sources of information are the product package insert and labelling. Product material safety datasheets (MSDS) are available on request from manufacturers and contain detailed information regarding composition. If there are concerns about components of a dressing related to allergic reactions, this is a valuable document to have on file.

Answers to how well a product performs relative to other products in the same material category or of similar function are ideally found in randomized controlled clinical trials that make head-to-head comparisons. Unfortunately, such trials are few in number. In the absence of controlled clinical data, comparative laboratory data may be of value in gauging relative product performance. Such laboratory studies of different commercial brands of transparent films, hydrocolloids and hydrogels have suggested that there is indeed variable performance between different brands of a particular category of dressing (Thomas & Lovelace 1988, 1997, Sprung et al 1998). A few important caveats concerning laboratory testing of dressing products are worth mentioning. The testing conditions should model as closely as possible clinically relevant parameters. For example, one particular in vitro study examined the absorptive capacity of 23 different amorphous hydrogels and used three different test fluids – water, normal saline and actual wound fluid. A wide variation in absorptive capacity was observed for many products, depending on what test fluid was used. It was found that water absorption was significantly higher and not predictive of wound fluid absorption. However, normal saline absorption correlated quite well with wound fluid absorption. This difference is probably due to the fact that both saline and wound fluid are ionic solutions whereas water is not. The same study examined the effects of fluid temperature on absorption by 17 different hydrocolloid wafers. Saline or water at room temperature and at body temperature was differentially absorbed by all products tested. Some products absorbed more when the test fluid was at room temperature and others when the test fluid was at body temperature.

Returning to the six questions that can guide performance-based dressing selection; the question of what the patient needs is answered by comprehensive medical and psychosocial evaluation. As mentioned earlier, a dressing cannot address underlying causes or systemic factors that contribute to impaired healing. The question of what is available pertains to the patient's healthcare plan or the broader healthcare environment in terms of availability, payment and cost effectiveness of the product. Finally, the question of what is practical relates to the overall care plan and goals of treatment, as well as to how complicated the product is to use and whether it will be changed by a healthcare professional, a family member or the patient.

Dressing performance parameters

Performance parameters or functions may be either general or wound specific and not every dressing can be expected to do everything well or even at all. The

Table 8.1
Performance parameters of dressings and categories that meet them

Dressing performance parameters	Appropriate dressing material categories
Optimize local environment	Any material *if* used appropriately
Adherent to skin	Many dressings with adhesive borders or surface coatings
Non-adherent	Tubular products Contact layers
Conformable to topography	Extra-thin versions of hydrocolloids Extra-thin versions of foams Transparent films
Conformable to depth	Amorphous gels Rope versions of alginates Pastes, powders
Absorb excess exudate	Foams Alginates Superabsorbents Textile fibres
Promote tissue hydration	Films Hydrocolloids
Promote autolytic debridement	Gel wafers Amorphous gels
Promote phases/attract cells of the healing process	Collagen Acemannan Beta glucan Hyaluronic acid
Assist in bacterial control	Materials that provide impermeable mechanical barrier Silver-releasing products Iodine-releasing products
Assist in odour control	Absorptive products in general Products containing activated charcoal
Easy to use	Products used in appropriate situations and according to instructions
Range of use	Varies by situation and product

need for variable performance based on the needs of different wounds, or even the same wound throughout its healing course, has played a part in the current proliferation of wound dressing products. By adopting a performance-based approach, the clinician attempts to match available dressings and their functions to wound needs. General areas of dressing function and the categories of dressing materials that meet them are summarized in Table 8.1.

Important functional considerations include: the degree of adherence to the periwound skin, conformability to challenging anatomical topography; the ability to absorb wound exudate or, alternatively, to promote tissue hydration; promotion of autolytic debridement; the ability to support the healing process or to recruit or activate critical cells involved in the healing process; infection control; odour management; ease of application and range of use. The latter two areas depend primarily on the care setting and the training of the end user. It is important to recognize that it may not be possible to find a dressing that optimally fulfils all of these criteria; priorities may need to be selected and compromises made.

Caveat emptor – product price versus treatment costs

As a final caveat, almost all types of semiocclusive dressing that create or maintain a physiologically moist wound environment have a unit price higher that that of gauze. Taking a global view of the patient and considering all the resources that are expended to evaluate and manage the wound, the cost of dressings used may be minor in comparison with other costs. Examples of other expenses include ancillary supplies (cleansers, tapes, gloves, pain medications, etc.), labour costs associated with caregiver time (windshield time, dressing change time, etc.), costs associated with length of stay, and even the cost to the patient in terms of lost work days. It is possible for a product to be inexpensive to acquire but expensive to use because it results in delayed wound healing (relative to another treatment) or increased complications. Conversely, a product that is more expensive to acquire may actually be less expensive to use if it facilitates more rapid healing with fewer complications.

REFERENCES

Angeras M H, Brandberg A, Falk A, Seeman T 1992 Comparison between sterile saline and tap water for the cleaning of acute traumatic soft tissue wounds. European Journal of Surgery 158(6–7):347–350

Bennett L L, Rosenblum R S, Perlov C et al 2001 An in vivo comparison of topical agents on wound repair. Plastic and Reconstructive Surgery 108:675–683

Chen W Y, Rogers A A, Lydon M J 1992 Characterization of biologic properties of wound fluid collected during the early stages of wound healing. Journal of Investigative Dermatology 99(5):559–564

Cho C Y, Lo J S 1998 Dressing the part. Dermatology Clinics 16:25–36

Eaglstein W H, Falanga V 1997 Chronic wounds. Surgical Clinics of North America 77:689–700

Falanga V, Bourguignon G J, Bourguignon L Y 1987 Electrical stimulation increases the expression of fibroblast receptors for transforming growth factor beta. Journal of Investigative Dermatology 88:488

Flanagan M 1997 Wound cleansing. In: Morison M et al, (eds) Nursing management of chronic wounds. Mosby, London, p 87–101

Fleming A (1919) The action of chemical and physiological antiseptics in a septic wound. British Journal of Surgery 7:99–129

Gilchrist B 1997 Infection and culturing. In: Krasner D, Kane D (eds) Chronic wound care, 2nd edn. Health Management Publications Inc, Wayne, PA, p 109–114

Hedman L A 1988 Effect of a hydrocolloid dressing on the pain level from abrasions on the feet during intensive marching. Military Medicine 153:188–190

Hellewell T B, Major D A, Foresman P A, Rodeheaver G T 1997 A cytotoxicity evaluation of antimicrobial and non-antimicrobial wound cleansers. Wounds 9(1):15–20

Hinnman C D, Maibach H I 1963 Effect of air exposure and occlusion on experimental human skin wounds. Nature 200:377–378

Jaffe L F, Vanable J W 1984 Electrical fields and wound healing. Clinics in Dermatology 2(3):34–44

Krasner D 1997 Dressing decisions for the twenty-first century: on the cusp of a paradigm shift. In: Krasner D, Kane D (eds) Chronic wound care, 2nd edn. Health Management Publications Inc, Wayne, PA, p 139–151

Krasner D L, Sibbald R G 1999 Nursing management of chronic wounds: best practices across the continuum of care. Nursing Clinics of North America 34:933–945

Lamke L O 1977 The evaporative water loss from burns and water vapor permeability of grafts and artificial membranes used in the treatment of burns. Burns 3:159–165

Laufman H 1989 Current use of skin and wound cleanser and antiseptics. American Journal of Surgery 157:359–365

Moscati R M, Reardon R F, Lerner E B, Mayrose J 1998 Wound irrigation with tap water. Acad Emerg Med 5(11):1076–1080

Nemeth A J, Eaglstein W H, Taylor J R et al 1991 Faster healing and less pain in skin biopsy sites treated with an occlusive dressing. Archives of Dermatology 127:1679–1683

O'Meara S M, Cullum N A, Majid M et al 2001 Systematic review of antimicrobial agents used for chronic wounds. British Journal of Surgery 88:4–21

Ovington L G 1998 The well-dressed wound: an overview of dressing types. Wounds 10 (Suppl A):1A–11A

Riyat M S, Quinton D N 1997 Tap water as a wound cleansing agent in accident and emergency. Journal of Accident and Emergency Medicine 14(3):165–166

Rodeheaver G T, Pettry D, Thacker J G et al 1975 Wound cleansing by high pressure irrigation. Surgery in Gynecology and Obstetrics 141(3):357–362

Rovee D T, Kurowsky C A, Labun J, Downes A M 1972 Effect of local wound environment. In: Rovee D T, Maibach H I (eds) Epidermal wound healing. Year Book Medical Publishers, Chicago, p 159–181

Sprung P, Hou Z, Ladin D A 1998 Hydrogels and hydrocolloids: an objective product comparison. Ostomy/Wound Management 44(1):36–53

Thomas S 1990 Functions of a wound dressing. In: Thomas S (ed) Wound management and dressings. Pharmaceutical Press, London, p 9–19

Thomas S, Loveless P 1988 Comparative review of the properties of six semipermeable film dressings. The Pharmaceutical Journal, June 18:785–788

Thomas S, Loveless P 1997 A comparative study of the properties of twelve hydrocolloid dressings. World Wide Wounds, July 1997. Online. Available: www.smtl.co.uk/World-Wide-Wounds

Turner T D 1989 The development of wound management products. Wounds 1(3):155–171

Van Rijswijk L, Beitz J 1998 The traditions and terminology of wound dressings: food for thought. Journal of Wound Ostomy and Continence Nursing 25:116–122

Williams N A, Leaper D J 1998 Infection. In: Leaper D J, Harding K G (eds) Wounds: biology and management. Oxford Medical Publications, Oxford, p 71–87

Winter G D 1962 Formation of scab and the rate of epithelialization of superficial wounds in the skin of the young domestic pig. Nature 193:293–294

Winter G D 1972 Epidermal regeneration studied in the domestic pig. In Rovee D T, Maibach H I (eds) Epidermal wound healing. Year Book Medical Publishers, Chicago, p 71–112

CHAPTER 9

Adjuvant therapies: ultrasound, laser therapy, electrical stimulation, hyperbaric oxygen and negative pressure therapy

Mary Dyson

CHAPTER CONTENTS

INTRODUCTION

The adjuvant therapies currently available for the stimulation of wound healing and improvement of scar tissue quality include the physical modalities of ultrasound, laser therapy and other forms of photobiomodulation, electrical stimulation, hyperbaric oxygen and negative pressure therapy. Used in addition to best clinical practice in wound management, these can help in the healing of wounds. These modalities are described in this chapter, the emphasis being on how they work, so that the practitioner has sufficient knowledge to decide which to use, on what types of wound and how to monitor their effectiveness. Selection of the appropriate adjuvant therapy should be based on an understanding of the healing process and on the properties and mode of action of the different therapies.

ULTRASOUND

Ultrasound (US) has been used in wound care for over 50 years. Originally only megahertz (MHz) US was available, but in the 1990s kilohertz (kHz) devices were tested successfully. In this section the physical properties and biological effects of MHz and kHz US are described, together with how they can be used in wound care. Sufficient information is provided for the user to select the most appropriate method of treatment for wounds of different types and in different locations.

What is ultrasound?

Ultrasound is a mechanical vibration transmitted at a frequency above the upper limit of human hearing (i.e. above 20 kHz, where 1 hertz [Hz] = 1 cycle per second and 1 kHz = 1000 cycles per second). It causes the molecules of media that can transmit it (e.g. biological tissues) to oscillate or vibrate, and can be used therapeutically to accelerate wound healing (Dyson 1995). Megahertz US, typically between 0.5 and 3 MHz (i.e. 0.5 and 3 million cycles per second) has been used for more than 50 years to stimulate healing. During the 1990s, 30 kHz and 50 kHz US were also demonstrated to have therapeutic effects (Peschen et al 1997); this new form of therapeutic US is growing rapidly in use.

Frequency
Many of the clinically relevant properties of US are related to its *frequency*, i.e. number of times per second that a molecule displaced by the US completes a cycle of movement and returns to its original position. Frequencies (*f*) are expressed in hertz (i.e. cycles per second) (Fig. 9.1). The time taken to complete a cycle is termed a *period* (*T*). Frequency and wavelength are inversely related; the lower the frequency the longer the wavelength. This is why kilohertz US is also known as long-wave US.

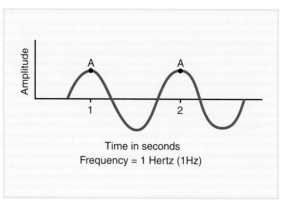

Figure 9.1
Frequency

Attenuation

Attenuation is the reduction of the power of the US wave as it is *absorbed, scattered* or *reflected* by the tissues. Lower frequencies penetrate deeper than higher frequencies because they are less readily attenuated. At higher frequencies, more of the energy is absorbed superficially than penetrates into deeper structures. Both kHz and MHz US are absorbed by proteins but are transmitted readily through water and fat; kHz ultrasound can also pass through metal and bone. If a wound is superficial, then 3 MHz US is effective, whereas if it is several centimeters deep, then 1 MHz will be a more suitable choice. If bone is involved, e.g. in type IV pressure ulcers, or if a metal implant is present, then kHz may be more effective. US is reflected from interfaces between substances differing acoustically, e.g. skin and air, collagen and tissue fluid, soft tissues and bone. A coupling medium acoustically similar to skin therefore has to be used between the head of the probe and the surface of either the skin or the wound so that US can be transmitted into them. Some film and hydrocolloid dressings are good coupling agents, as is saline.

Half-value Thickness

When US is transmitted through tissue, its intensity gradually decreases as a result of absorption, scattering, and reflection. The thickness of tissue necessary for the intensity (measured in W/cm^2) to be reduced to one-half of the level applied to its surface is termed the half-value thickness (Fig 9.2). The intensity available at any depth within the tissue is inversely proportional to the depth of penetration (i.e. the greater the depth, the less the remaining available intensity). For example, if 1 W/cm^2 of 1 MHz US is applied to the skin, at a

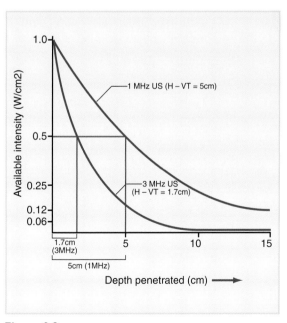

Figure 9.2
Half-value thickness

depth of 5 cm, only 0.25 W/cm^2 would be available. Absorption, which is a major cause of attenuation (e.g. loss of intensity), is frequency dependent. The greater the frequency, the shorter the wavelength; the shorter the wavelength, the greater the absorption. For a US beam of 3 MHz, the wavelength is shorter than that at 1 MHz, and therefore absorption occurs more readily than at 1 MHz, reducing the half-value thickness by 3. Thus, in the example above, the half-value thickness would be 5/3 = 1.7 cm. A frequency of 3 MHz is an efficient one to use to treat superficial regions, such as injured skin, but lower frequencies are indicated for deeper targets, such as injured muscle or bone; kHz US is even more penetrative, i.e. has a greater half-value thickness (Sussman & Dyson 1998). Applied to intact skin on the lateral aspect of a limb, kHz US can reach a wound on the medial aspect, so there is no need for the probe to be in contact with the wound, even through a dressing; this is clinically important if the wound is infected or if it is painful when pressure is applied to it.

The amount of absorption varies with the composition of the tissues as well as with the wavelength, which, as described above, is inversely related to frequency. Bone is more absorptive than highly proteinaceous tissues (e.g. dermis and muscle); protein is more absorptive than fat (e.g. adipose tissue); and fat is more absorptive than water-rich materials (e.g. oedematous tissues). Because of this, the half-value thickness of bone is less than that of muscle, which is less than that of fat, which is less than that of oedematous soft connective tissue. US can therefore penetrate skin, fat and oedematous tissues to reach a sinus extending beyond the wound surface.

Wavelength

The *wavelength* (γ) is the shortest distance, measured parallel to the direction of wave propagation, between molecules that are at equivalent points of vibration in the repeated cycle of movement, which constitutes a wave. It is related to the *frequency* and *velocity* (c) of the wave by the following equation:

$$\gamma = c/f.$$

The velocity of US in water, blood, interstitial fluid and soft tissues is approximately 1500 m/s. The higher the frequency, the shorter the wavelength. This is important diagnostically, because the shorter the wavelength, the greater the degree of resolution. The frequency of 20 MHz that is used by some high-resolution diagnostic US devices to examine skin and wounds non-invasively produces a wavelength that is sufficiently short to allow the stratum corneum and stratum Malpighii of the epidermis, the papillary and reticular layers of the dermis, the adipose hypodermis, collagen fibre bundles, necrotic tissue, oedematous tissue, granulation tissue and scar tissue to be distinguished and measured (Dyson et al 2003).

High frequencies are more readily absorbed by tissues than low frequencies and produce a greater thermal effect in them but they are more easily attenuated and therefore are less penetrative. Lower frequencies produce cavitation and the microstreaming associated with it more readily than do higher frequencies; there is evidence that many of the biological effects produced by therapeutic US are caused by stable cavitation and microstreaming (Dyson 1995).

Therapeutic ultrasound equipment

The equipment used to produce therapeutic levels of megahertz US typically consists of a microcomputer-controlled high-frequency generator linked by a coaxial cable to an applicator or treatment head. The treatment head contains a disc of a piezoelectric material, such as lead zirconate titanate (PZT), which acts as a transducer changing one form of energy into another, in this case into *ultrasound*. When an alternating voltage is applied across such a disc, it expands and contracts at the same frequency as the oscillation, transducing electrical energy into US. A similar system is made use of for kilohertz US, but the frequency of vibration is much lower, and the transducers have a different composition and mode of operation. Examples of equipment for generating MHz US, kHZ US and for kHz and MHz US are shown in Figs 9.3, 9.4 and 9.5, respectively. There is evidence that both MHz and kHz US can stimulate the healing of chronic wounds, as described below.

CLINICAL POINTS

- Use whatever therapeutic device is available, because whatever the frequency some of the energy will be absorbed into the injured tissue and can produce clinically relevant biological effects.
- If you have a choice of frequencies, use a higher frequency for superficial injuries and a lower frequency for deeper injuries.
- kHz US is recommended for painful and/or infected wounds.

The ultrasonic field

The ultrasonic pressure field generated by the transducer depends on the size and shape of the transducer and on how it is mounted in the applicator. The pressure varies across the surface of the applicator and also with the distance from it. The pressure changes experienced by the tissues being treated, therefore, depend in part on their position relative to the applicator. Ultrasound is emitted from a disc-shaped transducer of the type used with megahertz therapeutic US as a beam, which is at first cylindrical; this region is termed the *near field* or *Fresnel zone*, and the energy distribution in it is extremely variable. Beyond this, the beam starts to diverge and the energy distribution within it becomes more regular; this region is termed the *far field* or *Fraunhofer zone*. The distance

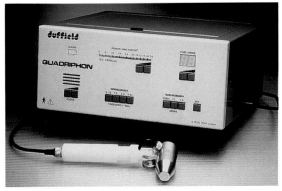

Figure 9.3
Ultrasound therapy device producing MHz ultrasound

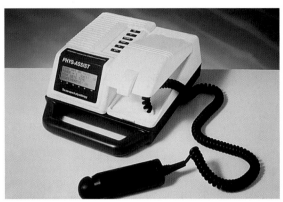

Figure 9.4
Ultrasound therapy device producing kHz ultrasound

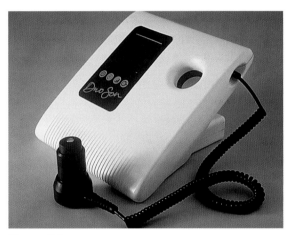

Figure 9.5
Ultrasound therapy device producing kHz and MHz
ultrasound either separately or simultaneously

(*d*) from the transducer to the beginning of the far field is related to the radius
(*a*) of the transducer and the wavelength (γ) of the ultrasound:

$$d = a^2/\gamma$$

Unless the part to be treated is immersed in a water bath large enough for the
target tissues to be in the far field, US therapy usually involves treatment of
tissue in the non-uniform near field. The *beam non-uniformity ratio* (BNR) is a
measure of this non-uniformity, and is the ratio of the spatial peak intensity
(I[SP]) to the spatial average intensity (I[SA]). These terms are defined below.
Applicators with low BNRs give more *predictable* results and are *safer* than those
with higher BNRs, since the higher spatial peak intensities of the latter are
potentially damaging (Ziskin & Michlovitz 1990).

Intensity

Intensity (I) is the amount of energy (in watts) per unit area per unit time. Applicators typically have an *effective radiating area* (ERA) of a few square centimetres. The I can be averaged in space over the face of the applicator (termed *spatial average* [SA]) or in time (termed *temporal average* [TA]). When pulsed US is used, pulse average (PA) intensity (i.e. the temporal average during the period of the pulse) should be noted, as should the temporal average during the full pulse repetition cycle. The type of intensity should be specified as either I(SATA) if continuous or both I(SATA) and I(SAPA) if pulsed.

Application of ultrasound to a wound

US is reflected from the interfaces between air and skin, and between air and soft tissues, so it has to be transmitted into the tissues through a suitable coupling medium such as a gel with a high water content, a film dressing, water or saline. Wounds should be filled with warm sterile saline and covered with either a film dressing such as Opsite (Smith & Nephew) or a hydrocolloid dressing such as Granuflex (ConvaTec), all of which transmit US from the applicator into the tissues to be treated. Putting a coupling medium such as Aquasonic 100 Gel (Parker Laboratories Inc.) onto the US-emitting face of the applicator facilitates moving it over the skin or over the dressing covering the wound.

Treatment parameters

The following parameters should be recorded when using US to treat a wound:

- frequency (in Hz)
- duration of treatment (in minutes)
- continuous or pulsed application
- if pulsed, pulse duration (in ms) and space duration (also in ms)
- intensity (in W/cm^2):
  — as I(SATA) for both continuous and pulsed applications and
  — either I(SAPA) or I(SATP) if pulsed.

A typical treatment of a wound is as follows:

- frequency = 3 MHz
- duration of treatment = 5 min
- pulsed
- pulse duration = 2 ms; space duration = 8 ms (duty cycle = 20%)
- I(SATA) = 0.2 W/cm^2
- I(SAPA) = I(SATP) = 1.0 W/cm^2.

Ultrasound bioeffects

The safe and effective use of US depends on an understanding of the effects it has on intact and injured living tissues. These bioeffects can be classified into:

- thermal
- predominantly non-thermal.

Thermal effects

US applied to vascularized tissue in the I(SATP) range of 1.0–2.0 W/cm^2 for between 5 and 10 min increases its temperature to between 40°C and 45°C, which is the therapeutically beneficial level (Ziskin & Michlovitz 1990). This is acceptable only in adequately vascularized tissues. Temperatures above this cause *thermal necrosis* and must be avoided. Clinically beneficial thermal effects occur with both 1 MHz and 3 MHz continuous US but at different tissue depths. At a frequency of 3 MHz, energy absorption occurs mainly in superficial tissues (up to 2 cm beneath the surface). At a frequency of 1 MHz, less energy is absorbed by the superficial tissues. This frequency also penetrates into deeper tissues, with effective energy levels being available up to 5 cm below the surface. Because pulsing the wave reduces the temporal average intensity, it reduces the thermal effects. Whenever US is absorbed, heat is produced, but if the temperature increases less than 1°C this is not considered to be physiologically relevant; the therapeutic effects are then due predominantly to non-thermal mechanisms.

CLINICAL POINTS

- **Because many wounds are inadequately vascularized, care must be taken when applying thermal levels of US. In these situations there is reduced ability to dissipate heat and burns can result. Continuous MHz therapeutic US is contraindicated in the presence of arterial occlusion.**
- **Pulsed therapeutic MHz US and continuous kHz US, which produce their effects by predominantly non-thermal mechanisms, are safe and clinically effective over areas of impaired circulation.**

Predominantly non-thermal effects
Non-thermal effects of MHz US occur at low spatial average intensities, which can be achieved by pulsing at, for example, a 20% duty cycle. They are attributed to *cavitation*, *standing wave formation* and *acoustic streaming*.

Cavitation involves the production and vibration of micron-sized bubbles within fluids including tissue fluid. The US beam affects small, gaseous bubbles that move within the fluids. These bubbles oscillate in the US field, alternately expanding and contracting during each cycle of the US wave. The movement and compression of the bubbles can cause changes in the cellular activities of tissues subjected to US.

- *Stable cavitation* occurs at intensities low enough for the bubbles to change little in size during each cycle. The effect of stable cavitation can result in diffusional changes across the membranes of cells located close to these bubbles. They can also distort the cell membranes causing, for example, reversible increase in membrane permeability to calcium ions, thus affecting cell activity. Stable cavitation is potentially beneficial and can stimulate healing.
- *Unstable or transient cavitation* refers to collapse of the bubbles mentioned above. Transient bubbles implode, causing local mechanical damage and free-radical formation. This is potentially very hazardous. It occurs at high intensities, particularly when the sound head is not moved during treatment and standing waves develop (Sussman & Dyson 2001).

Standing waves occur if the applicator is kept still during treatment. The US is then reflected backwards and forwards between the applicator and any reflective surface, for example that between soft tissue and bone, producing a standing wave in which energy can accumulate to damaging levels. There is evidence that the intravascular flow of blood cells can be stopped temporarily and that endothelial cells can be damaged (Dyson & Pond 1973). Moving the transducer disrupts the standing waves.

Acoustic streaming is the unidirectional movement of fluids along acoustic boundaries (e.g. bubbles or cell membranes) as a result of the mechanical pressure wave associated with the US beam (Ziskin & Michelovitz 1990). Outcomes attributable to this effect include a reversible increase in cell membrane permeability and increased protein synthesis.

It has been proposed that stable cavitation and microstreaming are responsible for the stimulatory effects of low intensity US (Dyson 1995).

CLINICAL POINTS

- **Low-intensity therapeutic US stimulates wound healing by acting as a non-thermal stimulus, which reversibly increases cell membrane permeability and thus modulates the activity of cells active in the healing process.**
- **Transient cavitation and standing wave formation are potentially damaging but are readily avoided by using low intensities and keeping the applicator moving during treatment.**

How ultrasound stimulates wound healing

Mechanism

Wound healing can occur only if the cells involved in the process are activated. The entry of calcium ions into cells can activate them. Increase in the permeability of the plasma membranes of cells to calcium ions follows exposure to non-thermal levels of ultrasound (Dyson 1995). The physical mechanisms producing this are stable cavitation and acoustic streaming of the fluid around the cells.

Cells in the path of the beam of ultrasound migrate, divide, differentiate, grow, phagocytose and synthesize growth factors and matrix materials such as collagen according to their capabilities. Collectively, these activities heal the wound, providing they occur in an organized fashion. Therapeutic US acts as a stimulus that the cells transduce. An amplified response occurs in each affected cell, the type of which depends upon the type of cell involved, for example polymorphs phagocytose debris, fibroblasts synthesize collagen and other matrix materials, endothelial cells migrate and divide forming new capillaries.

Effect of US on acute wounds

When wounds begin to heal they enter a phase of temporary acute inflammation. Treatment with therapeutic US during acute inflammation can shorten this. The wound consequently progresses into the subsequent proliferative phase more rapidly (Dyson 1995). US should therefore be applied as soon as possible after an injury. During acute inflammation the growth factors necessary to progress healing are produced and secreted; this is stimulated by therapeutic US. What US therapy does is to assist the body to heal itself. It is of value if healing is suboptimal, as is generally the situation. In such circumstances healing can be accelerated. There is also evidence that acute skin injuries treated with US in the acute inflammatory phase develop stronger reparative tissue than do control wounds (Hart 1993).

CLINICAL POINT

- **Begin treatment of acute wounds as soon as possible after injury, so that they progress as rapidly as possible into the proliferative phase of repair and develop stronger reparative tissue.**

Effect of US on chronic wounds

To assist the healing of chronic wounds, the wounds must first be activated so that at least part of each wound is in the acute inflammatory phase of repair. This can be achieved by debriding the wound. Treatment with:

- kHz ultrasound via a water bath or
- one application of MHz US at an intensity high enough to produce thermal effects

can also activate chronic wounds. When acute inflammation has commenced, the application of lower-intensity, predominantly non-thermal, US has been shown to accelerate healing of venous leg ulcers (Dyson et al 1976). The following treatment regime has been shown to be effective:

- frequency = 3 MHz
- duration of treatment = 5–10 min, three times each week
- pulsed
- pulse duration = 2 ms; space duration = 8 ms
- $I(SATA) = 0.2$ W/cm^2
- $I(SAPA) = I(SATP) = 1.0$ W/cm^2.

The treatment was applied to the periwound area following the initiation of acute inflammation.

An alternative method utilizing long-wave (i.e. kHz) US has also been shown to be effective as an adjunctive treatment for venous leg ulcers (Peschen et al 1997). Here the treatment is applied via a water bath similar to the podiatry bath shown in Fig. 9.6. The acoustic streaming produced in the bath removes superficial necrotic tissue and occasionally produces a tingling sensation and pinhead-sized points of bleeding. Further treatments with kHz US were shown by Peschen et al (1997) to accelerate healing in comparison with a control group. The following treatment regime was used:

- frequency = 30 kHz
- duration of treatment = 10 min, three times per week
- continuous
- $I(SATA) = 0.1$ W/cm^2.

Both the US-treated and the control wounds were covered with hydrocolloid dressings and compression therapy was applied. After 12 weeks, the US-treated group of wounds showed an average decrease in surface area of 55.4% compared with only 16.5% in the control wounds ($P < 0.007$; $n = 24$).

MHz US has also been shown to accelerate the healing of pressure ulcers (Sussman & Dyson 1998). The following treatment regime was used:

- frequency = 1 MHz
- duration of treatment = 5 min daily
- pulsed
- pulse duration = 2 ms; space duration = 8 ms
- $I(SATA) = 0.1$ W/cm^2
- $I(SAPA) = I(SATP) = 0.5$ W/cm^2.

The treatment was applied to the periwound area following the initiation of acute inflammation. The effects of kHz US on pressure ulcer healing remain to be examined.

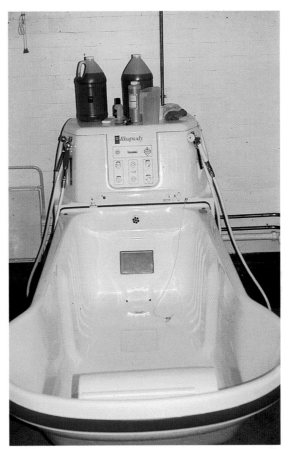

Figure 9.6
Podiatry bath incorporating a rectangular kHz ultrasound therapy transducer.

Expected outcomes

Ultrasound is most effective when treating in the acute inflammatory phase of healing. During this phase, expect an acceleration of inflammation and early progression to the proliferative phase of healing. In chronic wounds the first outcomes to treatment will be increased perfusion, observed as warmth, oedema, and darkening of tissue colour compared with adjacent skin colour tones. In necrotic wounds, expect to see autolysis of the necrotic tissue; the outcome will be a clean wound bed. Wounds in two clinical trials of MHz US progressed to closure in a mean time of 4 to 6 weeks (McDiarmid et al 1985, Nussbaum et al 1994). However, these times could be longer for patients with intrinsic and extrinsic factors that limit healing. Published research is a valuable guide in prediction of outcomes (Sussman & Bates-Jensen 2001) and the progress of repair should be compared with this. It is therefore necessary, as with any therapy, for the progress of repair of each wound to be monitored throughout the course of treatment.

If the wound does not change phase and/or become reduced in size (surface area and depth) within 2 to 4 weeks, the clinical status of the patient should be reassessed. If this has deteriorated, it may, for example, be necessary for clinical or surgical intervention. If it has not deteriorated, then the treatment regimen should be reviewed and, if necessary, revised. It may, for example, be necessary to reinitiate acute inflammation.

The use of high-resolution ultrasound imaging to monitor wound healing

In addition to its therapeutic role, US is also of value in wound care as a diagnostic technique (Dyson et al 2003). In these days of evidence-based clinical practice it is essential that the effectiveness of treatment is monitored objectively. US imaging permits this to be done non-invasively, rapidly and painlessly. Unlike surface photography, it allows tissue changes within, throughout and around the wound to be visualized in the manner of a biopsy, but without any damage to the patient. Magnified, high-resolution images of living tissue akin to low power micrographs are produced by using 20 MHz US; the technique is therefore often referred to as *ultrasound biomicroscopy*. The images obtained are digital, can be archived, and can be e-mailed to remote sites for analysis if this is required, an example of telemedicine in action.

Portable, user- and patient-friendly high-resolution scanners such as that shown in Fig. 9.7 are now commercially available. It is recommended that the surface appearance of the wound be recorded with a digital camera and the tissue changes within and around the wound with a high-resolution US scanner every time the wound is treated. Taking these scans can be done by the nurse or other clinician treating and/or dressing the wound and adds only a few minutes to the time spent with each patient. The scanner shown in Fig. 9.7 (see www.longportinc.com for further information), which operates at a frequency of 20 MHz, provides a vertical resolution of the order of 65 µm and clear

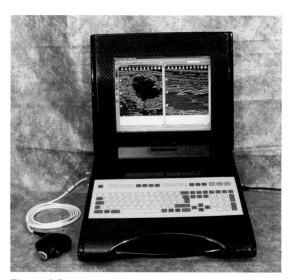

Figure 9.7
Portable high-resolution diagnostic ultrasound scanner
(Longport Inc.)

discrimination between acoustically different materials such as tissue fluid, debris, granulation tissue, scar tissue and the various layers of the epidermis, dermis and hypodermis. The software incorporated into the scanner allows linear and area measurements to be made from the scans. These are then stored, together with the scans, digital photographs and the patient's notes, in a secure, retrievable fashion. Examples of scans of intact skin and of healing skin 7 and 14 days after taking a punch biopsy are illustrated in Figs 9.8, 9.9 and 9.10, respectively.

Digital photographs and high-resolution US scans should be taken before treatment is commenced and throughout the course of any treatment so that its effectiveness can be monitored and changes made if the response of the patient indicates this.

LOW INTENSITY LASER THERAPY (LILT)

Electromagnetic radiation in the form of photons, delivered in either laser or non-laser form, has been applied to wounds as a means of stimulating healing for over 30 years. The technique is now often referred to as *photobiomodulation*, the use of photons to modulate biological activity (Dyson et al 2002). Light consists of those wavelengths of the electromagnetic spectrum that are visible

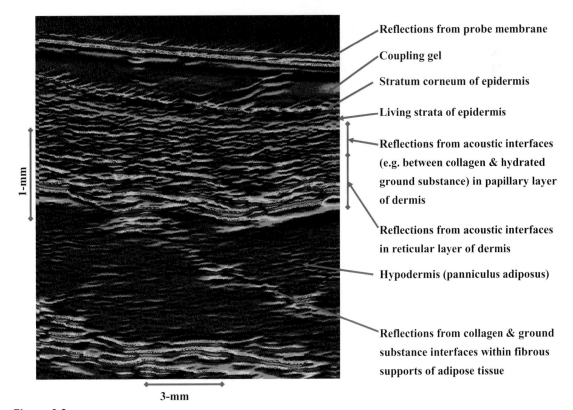

Intact Skin

Reflections from probe membrane

Coupling gel

Stratum corneum of epidermis

Living strata of epidermis

Reflections from acoustic interfaces (e.g. between collagen & hydrated ground substance) in papillary layer of dermis

Reflections from acoustic interfaces in reticular layer of dermis

Hypodermis (panniculus adiposus)

Reflections from collagen & ground substance interfaces within fibrous supports of adipose tissue

1-mm

3-mm

Figure 9.8
High-resolution ultrasound scan of intact skin on the inner aspect of the forearm

Wound Day 7

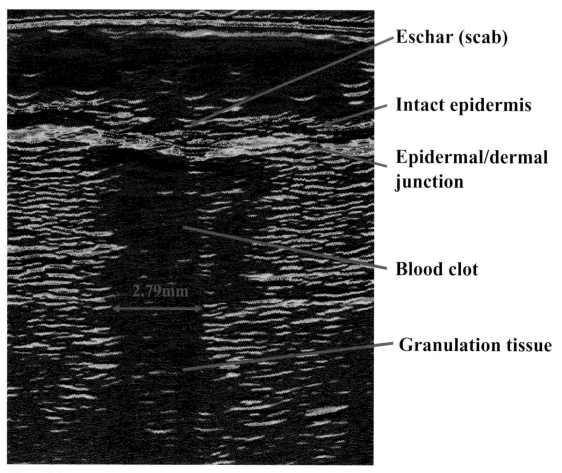

Eschar (scab)

Intact epidermis

Epidermal/dermal junction

Blood clot

Granulation tissue

2.79mm

Figure 9.9
High-resolution ultrasound scan of healing skin 7 days after a full-thickness punch biopsy

to the human eye. This part of the spectrum extends from violet (the shortest visible wavelength) to red (the longest visible wavelength). Infrared (IR) is just beyond the visible range. The perceived colour depends on the wavelength. White light is a mixture of all the visible wavelengths. For photons to reach a wound all that is required is that the wound be either exposed to air or sterile saline, or be covered by a transparent dressing. Exposure to red light and/or infrared radiation can stimulate the healing of both chronic wounds (Mester et al 1985) and acute wounds (Dyson & Young 1986).

Laser is an acronym for **l**ight **a**mplification by the **s**timulated **e**mission of **r**adiation. The stimulated emission of radiation occurs when a photon interacts with an energized atom. When an atom is energized, for example by electricity, one of its electrons is excited, that is, raised to a higher energy orbit than its orbit when in the resting state. If the energy of the incident photon is equal to

Wound Day 14

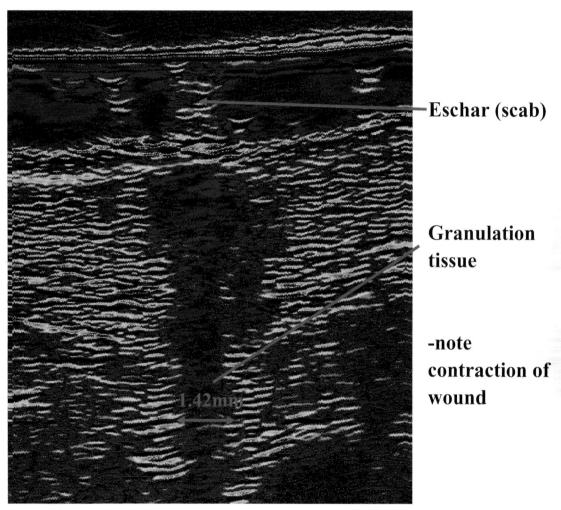

Figure 9.10
High-resolution ultrasound scan of healing skin 14 days after a full-thickness punch biopsy

the energy difference between the electron's excited and resting states, the stimulated emission of a photon occurs and the excited electron returns to its resting state. This photon has the same properties as the incident photon, which it also emitted. This process is repeated in the adjacent energized atoms, producing a laser beam. Unlike light from non-laser sources, this light is:

- monochromatic, i.e. of a single wavelength
- collimated, i.e. its light rays are non-divergent
- coherent, i.e. in phase, the troughs and peaks of the waves coinciding in time and space.

With regard to laser therapy, monochromaticity is its most important characteristic. To produce an effect, the light must be absorbed, and absorption is wavelength-specific. Different substances absorb light of different wavelengths. Mitochondria, present in all cells, contain cytochromes that absorb red light. Some cells absorb some wavelengths of infrared radiation, while other cell types absorb other IR wavelengths.

LILT is an acronym for low-intensity laser therapy (Baxter 1994). Unlike the high-intensity medical lasers used to thermally cut and coagulate tissues, LILT involves the use of medical lasers that operate at intensities too low to damage living tissues. Their action is photobiomodulation; they can stimulate inactivated tissue components and inhibit activated components (Agaiby et al 1998).

LILT equipment   This has three essential components:

1. a *lasing medium*, which is capable of being energized sufficiently for lasing to occur
2. a *resonating cavity* containing the lasing medium
3. a *power source* that transmits energy into the lasing medium.

The lasing medium.   The type of lasing medium used determines the wavelength, and therefore the colour, of the laser beam. For example, an HeNe laser, in which the lasing medium is a mixture of helium and neon gases, produces red light with a wavelength of 632.8 nm. Gallium, aluminium and arsenide, the lasing medium of GaAlAs semiconductor diodes, also produces monochromatic radiation, but the wavelength of this depends on the ratio of these three materials and is in the red–infrared range of the electromagnetic spectrum, typically 630–950 nm.

The resonating cavity.   The resonating cavity containing the lasing medium has two parallel surfaces, one being totally reflecting, the other being partially reflecting. Photons emitted from the lasing medium are reflected between these surfaces, some of them leaving through the partially reflecting surface as the laser beam. The cavity of an HeNe laser is many centimetres long, whereas that of a GaAlAs semiconductor diode is tiny, the diode being the lasing medium and its polished ends the reflecting surfaces. Most LILT devices are currently of the GaAlAs type. Their treatment heads may contain either one or several diodes. Those with one diode resemble laser pointers and are designed to treat acupuncture and trigger points; they can also be used to treat points in and around wounds. Those with many diodes are generally called cluster probes and allow large areas to be treated rapidly. The diodes may be housed in a rigid head (Fig. 9.11) or in a flexible material. The latter can be applied around curved surfaces such as the shoulder. Cluster probes housing up to 50 diodes are available, groups of these diodes emit different wavelengths in the red and infrared range. The red light targets all cells, while different wavelengths in the infrared range appear to target specific cell types. In cluster probes usually only some of the diodes produce coherent radiation but all produce monochromatic radiation. *Power source.*   The power source for a LILT device may be either a battery or mains electricity. Many LILT devices are portable. The main function of the power source is to energize the lasing medium.

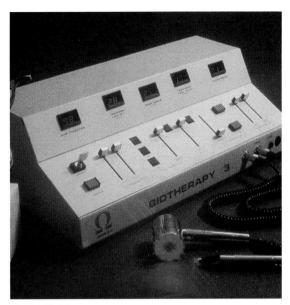

Figure 9.11
A LILT device showing a single diode probe and a
multidiode cluster probe

**Application of LILT
to a wound**

When treating an open wound, LILT is usually applied through a transparent dressing via a cluster probe. This can either be placed in contact with the dressing or held a few centimetres above it if the wound is painful. Mester et al (1985) recommended the use of an energy density of 4 J/cm², joules being calculated by multiplying the power density (in W/cm²) by the irradiation time in seconds. In addition to treating the wound bed, Baxter (1996) recommends treating the intact skin around the wound with a single diode probe at points about 1–2 cm from the wound margin and about 2–3 cm apart. The probe should be pressed firmly onto the intact skin. This reduces attenuation by temporarily displacing erythrocytes that would absorb some of the incident energy. It is usually recom-mended that the energy density applied be no more that 10 J/cm².

When LILT is used to treat a patient the following treatment parameters should be recorded:

- wavelength (in nm)
- treatment duration (in min)
- power output (in mW)
- power density (in mW/cm²) calculated by dividing the power output by the irradiating area (or spot size) of the laser. The spot of a semiconductor diode is typically 0.1–0.125 cm². This is multiplied by the number of diodes when a cluster probe is used
- energy density (in J/cm²) calculated by multiplying the power density by the irradiation time in seconds
- if LILT is used in pulsed mode then the pulse repetition rate in Hz (i.e. number of pulses per second) should also be recorded.

LILT bioeffects

For LILT to be effective, photons must be absorbed by the tissue targeted. Absorption is wavelength dependent. Red light is absorbed by cytochromes in the mitochondria of all living cells, whereas certain wavelengths of infrared are absorbed by specific proteins of the cell membrane, these proteins varying according to the type of cell. Provided that appropriate wavelengths and energy densities are used, cell activity can be stimulated if it is suboptimal. Cells in which this has been investigated include mammalian keratinocytes, lymphocytes, macrophages, fibroblasts and endothelial cells, all cells of significance in tissue repair. Much of this work has been reviewed by Baxter (1994). Cells affected by LILT show a temporary increase in permeability of their cell membranes to calcium ions (Young et al 1990). This may be the mechanism by which LILT modulates cell activity, as has been shown to occur following US treatment. Other electrotherapeutic modalities may act in a similar fashion.

How lilt stimulates wound healing

Mechanism

The triggering of cell activity by reversible changes in membrane permeability when photons are absorbed could be responsible for the stimulation of tissue repair (Young & Dyson 1993). Increase in calcium uptake by macrophages exposed to red light and infrared in vitro has been shown to be wavelength- and energy-density-dependent. Of the wavelengths tested, 660, 820 and 870 nm were effective; 880 nm was ineffective. These same wavelengths also affected growth factor production by the macrophages, 660, 820 and 870 nm being stimulatory whereas 880 nm was not. Energy densities of 4 and 8 J/cm^2 were found to be effective; 2 and 19 J/cm^2 were not (Young et al 1990). Red light of 660 nm wavelength is absorbed by the cytochromes of mitochondria, where it stimulates adenosine triphosphate (ATP) production and increases cytoplasmic H$^+$ concentration, which can affect cell membrane permeability (Karu 1988). Infrared radiation of 820 and 870 nm may be absorbed by components of the cell membrane. Some of these components vary in different cell types, which may be why the infrared wavelengths absorbed by cells differ according to the cell type. For example, 870 nm affects macrophages (Young et al 1990) but not mast cells (El Sayed & Dyson 1990). It may be possible to selectively stimulate macrophages, but not mast cells, in vivo by exposure to an 870-nm probe; this remains to be investigated.

Following a reversible change in membrane permeability to calcium ions, the cell responds by doing what it is designed to do. In the case of macrophages, this is to produce growth factors and to phagocytose debris; mast cells degranulate, releasing histamine and other substances.

The molecular mechanisms by which LILT affects cell activity begin with photoreception, when the photons are absorbed. This is followed by signal transduction, amplification and a photoresponse, for example cell proliferation, protein synthesis and growth factor production, all of which may assist in tissue repair. Membrane structure differs according to the cell type, which, if infrared is absorbed by parts of the membrane, may explain why different cell types absorb different wavelengths of infrared. Theoretically, it should be possible by the judicious selection of infrared wavelengths to affect some cell types while leaving others unaffected. Red light lacks this sensitivity, being absorbed by the mitochondrial cytochromes present in all living cells.

The cellular effects of LILT relevant to tissue repair include the stimulation of:

- ATP production
- mast cell recruitment and degranulation
- growth factor release by macrophages
- keratinocyte proliferation
- collagen synthesis
- angiogenesis.

At the tissue level there is an acceleration of the resolution of acute inflammation, resulting in the more rapid formation of granulation tissue and re-epithelialization than in sham-irradiated control tissue. Any or all of these effects could help to explain why wound healing can be stimulated by LILT.

CLINICAL POINTS

- Red light will affect all the cells involved in the healing process.
- To stimulate macrophages while leaving mast cells unaffected, use 870 nm infrared radiation.

Effect of LILT on acute wounds
As with any other technique, the healing of acute wounds can only be stimulated by LILT if they are healing suboptimally, for example if they are in a dry environment. In such wounds, granulation tissue production can be stimulated as can wound contraction (Dyson & Young 1986). The most effective energy density reported is 4 J/cm^2.

Effect of LILT on chronic wounds
In 1985, Mester et al surveyed the LILT treatment of over 1000 patients with chronic ulcers; using an energy density of 4 J/cm^2, they showed 50–100% healing, variation being related to the type of lesion and the clinical condition of the patient. It has been suggested that the induction of acute inflammation in the chronic wounds by, for example, debridement, should precede treatment with LILT, since growth factors released during acute inflammation stimulate healing, and it has been shown that LILT can accelerate this phase of healing (Young & Dyson 1993).

ELECTRICAL STIMULATION

Electrical stimulation, often referred to as E-stim, has been used since the 1960s to promote wound healing (Assimacopoulos 1968). More recent investigations include those of Gault & Gatens (1976), Akers & Gabrielson (1984) and Feedar et al (1992).

What is E-stim?

According to Sussman & Byl (2001), E-stim is 'the use of a capacitive coupled electric current to transfer energy to a wound'. Although there are other methods of transferring electricity to tissues, capacitive coupling is the most widely available and is non-invasive. It involves the transference of electric current through an electrode pad applied to moistened skin or to the wound bed, both of which act as a wet conductive medium. At least two electrodes are needed to complete the circuit. The electrodes can be placed either within the wound bed or on the intact skin near the wound. The polarity of the electrodes can be varied to alter their effects on the wound. Polarity determines the direction of current flow; electrons move from the negative pole (the cathode) to the positive pole (the anode). Current flow can be either unidirectional or bidirectional.

E-stim can be delivered in a variety of waveforms:

- continous unidirectional direct current, also known as galvanic current
- monophasic pulsed direct current, the pulses or phases being either square wave, or containing two peaks
- continuous alternating current, also know as biphasic or bipolar. This can be either:
    - o balanced or unbalanced
    - o symmetrical or asymmetrical.

These wave forms are illustrated in Fig. 9.12.

E-stim equipment

Electrical stimulators consist of a *power source*, an *oscillator circuit*, an *output amplifier* and *electrodes*. Portable stimulators are battery powered; the larger devices have a mains supply. Many incorporate *microprocessors* that provide the user with a choice of waveforms and treatment protocols.

The electrodes complete the circuit between the stimulator and the patient. Sussman & Byl (2001) recommend using aluminium foil as electrodes because it is non-toxic, inexpensive, disposable, conformable, a good conductor and can be cut to the size required. The surface area of the electrode affects current density – the smaller the surface area, the greater the current density, the deeper the penetration of the current and the greater its effect. Increasing the distance between the electrodes increases the penetration depth, as does increasing the amplitude of the voltage. One electrode is usually smaller than the other. The smaller electrode is referred to as the active electrode, the larger as the disper-sive electrode.

Direct current devices of both low voltage (typically 60–100 V) and high voltage (typically 100–500 V) are available commercially, as are alternating current devices, which resemble the transcutaneous neural stimulators (TENS) used to reduce pain but have a different waveform.

Application of E-stim to a wound

The dressing covering the wound and on which one of the electrodes is often placed must be a good conductor and keep the wound moist so that the current can be transmitted into the wound bed. According to Bourguignon et al (1991), occlusive film dressings are poor conductors. By contrast, fully hydrated hydrocolloid dressings and hydrogels are good conductors and promote heal-ing by:

- maintaining a moist environment
- promoting an injury current through this moisture
- retaining growth factors which stimulate healing.

Treatment parameters
Selection of treatment. The biological requirements of the wound vary as it progresses through the healing process. The biological effects of polarity,

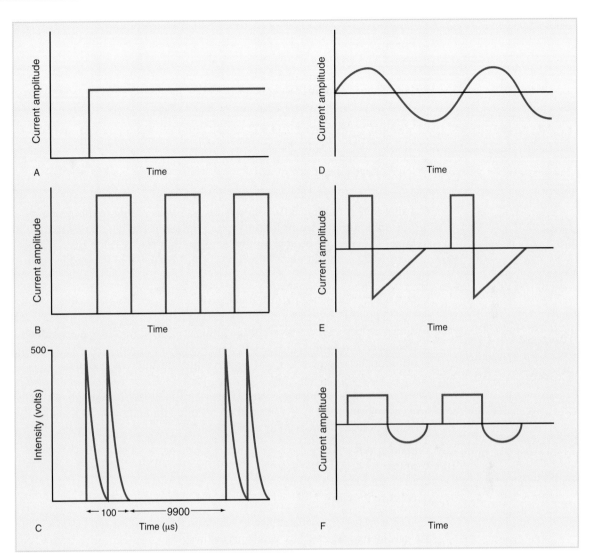

Figure 9.12
Waveforms used in electrical stimulation. (A) Unidirectional direct current; (B) monophasic pulsed current; (C) high-voltage pulsed current showing twin-peaked monophasic waveform; (D) balanced symmetrical alternating (biphasic) current; (E) balanced asymmetrical alternating (biphasic) current; (F) unbalanced asymmetrical alternating (biphasic) current. (Modified from Sussman & Byl 1998.)

biphasic currents, frequency and voltage amplitude should all be considered before deciding on an appropriate treatment (Dyson & Lyder 2001):

- *Polarity.* The negative pole is generally used as the active pole during acute inflammation or when the wound is infected. Once this has been resolved the polarity is varied with the aim of matching polarity with changes in the polarity of the injury potential (Kloth & Feedar 1988).

- *Biphasic current.* Baker et al (1996) in their investigations into the effect of biphasic current on pressure ulcers in patients with spinal cord injuries found that the best results were obtained with an asymmetrical waveform biased toward the negative pole.
- *Pulsing frequency.* Varying this for high-voltage pulsed currents affects blood flow, with lower-pulsing frequencies producing higher bloodflow velocities (Mohr et al 1987).
- *Amplitude.* This is usually kept constant throughout treatment and is reported as either voltage for high-voltage pulsed currents or as milliamperes (mA) for low-voltage direct current.

The response of the wound to treatment should be monitored non-invasively and subsequent treatments modified if necessary according to this response.

The optimum pattern of treatments using E-stim is not yet known and the treatments used have been arrived at empirically. Polarity is the main variable to have been tested. Sussman & Byl (2001) recommend that the smaller, active, electrode:

- be negative during the acute inflammatory phase and when treating oedematous regions
- alternate between positive and negative every 3 days during granulation tissue development
- alternate between positive and negative daily during remodelling.

Direct current. *High-voltage pulsed current* usually has a monophasic twin-peak waveform (see Fig. 9.10C). When used to stimulate wound healing, the parameters selected are usually as follows:

- voltage = 80–200 V
- pulse rate = 50–120 Hz
- peak duration = 5–20 μs
- polarity, variable.

Monophasic low-voltage microcurrent. When used to stimulate soft tissue healing the parameters selected are usually as follows:

- Voltage < 100 V
- Amperage = 200–300 μA.

Alternating current. This is used without pulsing. It appears to be most effective as a wound-healing stimulator when its waveform is unbalanced and asymmetrical, in contrast to the balanced, symmetrical waveform used in TENS devices to reduce pain (Sussman & Byl 2001).

E-stim bioeffects

Living cells interact creating a bioelectrical environment that is modified by injury. The aim of E-stim is to help normalize this environment and, in doing so, accelerate healing. The intact epidermis has an electrical potential across it and acts as a battery that maintains this potential. Positively charged sodium ions are moved by the sodium pump to the deep aspect of the epidermis, leaving an excess of negatively charged chloride ions on its outer surface, which develops an electronegative charge of about −23 mV. When the epidermis is injured, current can flow as ions are transmitted through the tissue fluid linking the damaged regions of the epidermis. This unidirectional flow attracts reparative cells to the wound bed by a process termed *galvanotaxis*. When healing is either completed or arrested this current, referred to as the *injury current*, disappears. Debriding a chronic wound restores the injury current.

How electricity stimulates wound healing

Mechanism

This is unknown, but it has been suggested that E-stim mimics the injury current and thus initiates healing in a chronic wound. This change in the bioelectric environment of a chronic wound may be sufficient to jump-start the healing process (Gentzkow et al 1991). Varying the treatment parameters may act as stimuli that accelerate the healing process.

Effect of E-stim on acute wounds

When used correctly, E-stim accelerates the resolution of acute inflammation with the result that the proliferative phase begins more rapidly.

Effect of E-stim on chronic wounds

The restoration of an injury current by E-stim may initiate acute inflammation and thus trigger the healing process. Further treatments can accelerate healing. If healing decelerates or stops then the treatment parameters should be changed. In such cases, Kloth (1995) recommends using a high-voltage pulsed current stimulator with daily reversal of the polarity. Regular non-invasive monitoring of the healing process is essential if E-stim is to be used effectively.

CLINICAL POINT

- Using E-stim with dressings that keep the wound moist increases its effectiveness.

HYPERBARIC OXYGEN

Hyperbaric oxygen (HBO), i.e. oxygen at a pressure greater that 1 atmosphere, has been used extensively in medicine as a therapeutic modality since the nineteenth century, when it was used to treat bacterial infections (Irvin & Smith 1968). Among the medical uses of HBO relevant to wound healing and approved by the Undersea and Hyperbaric Medical Society (Thom 1992) are:

- crush injury, the compartment syndrome, and other acute traumatic ischaemias
- enhancement of healing in selected problem wounds
- necrotizing soft tissue infections
- thermal burns.

What is HBO therapy?

HBO therapy is the administration of oxygen at pressures greater than 1 atmosphere. It has properties more akin to a drug than to a physical therapy (Kindwall 1993). Its actions include:

- reducing oedema by about 50% in postischaemic muscle by preserving ATP (Nylander et al 1984)
- reducing fluid requirements in acute burns by 35% in the first 24 h, thus reducing oedema (Ciani et al 1989)
- stimulating angiogenesis in ischaemic wounds (Heng 1993).

It can be administered either systemically or topically. The advantages of the topical approach include low cost and lack of systemic oxygen toxicity.

HBO equipment

Systemic

HBO chambers used for systemic HBO therapy are effectively small rooms in which the patient spends several hours breathing oxygen at 2–3 atmospheres pressure. This increases the amount of dissolved oxygen in the blood and enhances oxygen delivery to hypoxic tissues, provided that the tissues have an adequate blood supply. The chambers can be *monoplace*, accommodating one patient, or *multiplace*, accommodating several patients.

Topical

Hyperbaric oxygen chambers used topically are generally engineered to fit around an injured limb, although disposable polyethylene bags in which oxygen is kept at 1.04 atmospheres have also been used (Heng et al 1983). They enclose the injury and adjacent intact skin. The chamber is sealed onto the intact skin to stop oxygen loss from the chamber. The HBO is applied directly to the open wound where it dissolves in tissue fluid, improving the oxygen content of the fluid bathing the cells without necessarily entering the blood capillaries. This extravascular route for oxygenation is of particular importance in ischaemic wounds 'where some prior oxygenation of the ischaemic tissue is necessary before endothelial proliferation and neovascularisation can take place' (Heng 1993). With topical HBO delivery, the oxygen is only a few microns from the cells. Since diffusion kinetics of gases such as oxygen depend largely on diffusion distances, and with topical administration to an open wound these are minute, the topical HBO devices are very efficient and require lower pressures to stimulate angiogenesis than the 2–3 atmospheres necessary with systemic HBO chambers. There is a reduced risk of systemic oxygen toxicity with topical HBO chambers because there is little increase in systemic absorption of oxygen. Ways in which systemic oxygen toxicity can manifest itself include grand mal seizures and pulmonary haemorrhage (Morgan et al 1963). However, local oxygen toxicity can occur and particular care must be taken with diabetic ulcers, which are prone to develop oxygen toxicity, probably due to increased levels of glutathione peroxidase induced by HBO (Morykwas & Argenta 1997).

Application of HBO to a wound

If the wound is open, then topical HBO is recommended. All dressings should be removed so that the oxygen can reach the tissue fluid bathing the wound unimpeded. Topical HBO is unsuitable for treating closed injuries, where the only effective method of delivering HBO is systemic. Necrotizing soft tissue infections, myonecrosis, crush injuries, compartment syndrome, refractory osteomyelitis, osteoradionecrosis and compromised skin grafts and flaps all respond well to HBO delivered systemically (Kindwall 1993).

Treatment parameters

Systemic HBO   The usual regime consists of:

- duration = 90–120 min
- pressure = 2.0–2.5 atmospheres
- treatment spacing = 1 per day or 2 per day
- number of treatments = 10–60, depending on the condition being treated.

Topical HBO

- Duration: this is variable, for example: 20 min twice daily, or 4–6 h daily.
- Pressure = 1.04–2 atmospheres.
- Treatment spacing = one per day or two per day, with a rest period of 2–3 days per week to decrease local endothelia cell toxicity.
- Number of treatments: variable.

The above treatment schedules are cited by Morykwas & Argenta (1997); they are empirical. With open wounds there should be frequent monitoring of response and modification of the treatment regime when indicated by this response.

HBO bioeffects Soft tissue oxygen levels are in normal conditions approximately 40 mmHg. If the levels drop to less than 30 mmHg, metabolic activity is significantly impaired (Grim et al 1990). Local oxygen levels are frequently less than 30 mmHg in injured or infected tissue. Bacterial infection reduces local tissue perfusion and therefore oxygenation. Neutrophils use a significant amount of oxygen when they phagocytose bacteria. Oxygen has been described as an antibiotic (Knighton et al 1984). If the level of oxygen can be increased, this assists in healing and in the fight against infection. HBO is a means of achieving this objective.

Mechanism

The use of HBO in treating open wounds is based on the increased solubility of oxygen in blood and tissue fluids under hyperbaric conditions (Illingworth et al 1961). The extra dissolved oxygen carried in the blood of a patient breathing oxygen at an elevated pressure of 2–3 atmospheres enhances delivery to hypoxic tissues, provided that these tissues are adequately vascularized. However, the problem in wound healing is not so much the level of oxygenation of the blood but rather the inadequate vascularization of the wound. When HBO is supplied topically it reaches the tissue fluid bathing the cells of the wound bed directly, bypassing the blood vessels supplying the wound. The cells involved in the healing process are therefore better oxygenated for the period that the oxygen is supplied. This temporary oxygenation of the wound bed is necessary for many of the processes involved in wound healing, including:

- phagocytosis of bacteria by neutrophils
- endothelial cell proliferation, and thus for vascularization of the wound bed
- collagen synthesis.

It should be appreciated that, even with topical HBO, there is a risk of oxygen toxicity, although this is purely local. It includes the destruction of newly formed blood vessels but can be avoided by allowing several days of rest from HBO therapy each week (Heng 1993). Furthermore, the relative hypoxia occurring during the rest periods is a stimulus to the release of growth factor and to capillary formation. When cells are hypoxic they are unable to generate reduced glutathione or glutathione stimulating hormone (GSH), which protects them against free radical attack (Andreoli et al 1986), When oxygen is reintroduced into ischaemic tissues during reperfusion, lipid peroxidation and damage of the cell membranes can occur from an excess of free radicals. However, HBO inhibits lipid peroxidation, thus protecting cell membranes from damage (Raskin et al 1971). It is important to realize that the effects on injured tissues of the presence and absence of oxygen are complex. The beneficial aspects of hyperbaric oxygen on wound healing may be negated by failure to identify and react to signs of oxygen toxicity. Tissue responses should therefore be monitored non-invasively throughout the healing process and treatments amended where appropriate.

Effect of HBO on acute wounds

Minor burns and scalds show accelerated healing when treated with topical HBO. Reported effects cited by Heng (1993) include:

- oedema reduction
- increased collagen sythesis
- increased angiogenesis
- accelerated re-epithelialization.

Effect of HBO on chronic wounds

Chronic ischaemic wounds benefit from HBO. It can initiate healing and within about 3 weeks the wound bed is usually well vascularized. Healing generally continues after the HBO therapy has been discontinued (Heng et al 1984).

CLINICAL POINTS

- **Topical HBO is more effective than systemic HBO in treating open wounds with a compromised blood supply.**
- **Remember that oxygen can be toxic as well as being a stimulator of healing, so monitor tissue changes and change your treatment of the wound if necessary.**

NEGATIVE PRESSURE THERAPY

Also known as vacuum-assisted closure (VAC), this is a non-invasive technique entailing exposure of a wound to subatmospheric pressure (Morykwas & Argenta 1997). The effects of this include:

- dilation of the arterioles, improving the blood supply to the wound
- removal of excess fluid, thus reducing oedema
- reduction in bacterial colonization of a wound by drawing off many of the bacteria with this fluid
- improved granulation tissue formation, resulting in progressive wound closure.

What is negative pressure therapy?

Negative pressure therapy is the application of subatmospheric pressure, either continuously or intermittently, to an open wound. A VAC device to do this has been manufactured for clinical use in wound healing by Kinetic Concepts Inc (KCI). It delivers negative pressure (vacuum) uniformly to the wound bed and to the tissue adjacent to it. Case studies have documented its effectiveness (Morykwas & Argenta 1997) in the treatment of acute and chronic cavity wounds.

VAC equipment

The VAC negative pressure equipment consists of:

- VAC negative pressure unit (Fig. 9.13)
- VAC PAC dressing pack, containing sterile foam dressing, suction tubing, occlusive transparent drapes
- Canister to collect the exudate and tubing for connection between the VAC unit and the foam dressing.

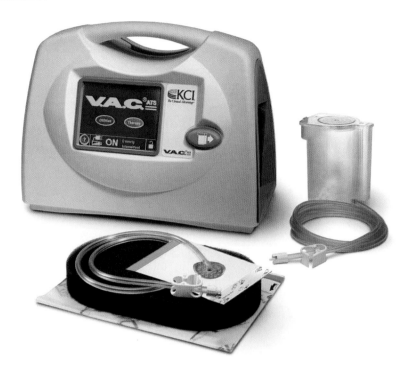

Figure 9.13
The VAC negative pressure unit (KCI)

Application of VAC to a wound

- The foam dressing is cut to the shape of the wound and applied to the wound, which has been irrigated with normal saline.
- The foam dressing and at least 3.5 cm of surrounding intact skin is covered with the occlusive transparent drapes to ensure an occlusive seal and convert the open wound into a controlled closed wound. The drape is also sealed to the tube leaving the dressing.
- The free end of the tubing from the foam dressing is connected to the tubing on the unit.
- The unit is set to deliver type of negative pressure required, continuous or intermittent, and the device is switched on.

Treatment parameters (supplied by KCI)
These vary according to the type of wound being treated. The following example is for pressure ulcers:

- cycle: continuous for first 48 h to evacuate excess fluid from the wound; intermittent thereafter (standard: 5 min on, 2 min off) to promote granulation tissue formation
- duration: ideally 24 h a day
- target pressure: 125 mmHg
- dressing change: every 48 h or every 12 h if the wound is infected.

VAC bioeffects

The continuous negative pressure used at the commencement of treatment draws fluid from the wound bed and surrounding tissue, decreasing local interstitial pressure and allowing vessels previously compressed or collapsed to dilate, restoring blood flow. The intermittent negative pressure applied later assists the proliferative phase of repair when granulation tissue forms.

Mechanism

The use of negative pressure therapy to remove tissue fluid from the wound bed and its oedematous surroundings is based on the supposition that the removal of this fluid will enhance the healing process. Certainly, reduction in oedema and therefore of pressure on the microcirculatory system is advantageous in that the reduced pressure allows the vessels to dilate, with the result that perfusion of the wound is improved. Also the fluid from chronic wounds contains factors that, when applied to cells in vitro, suppress cell division and protein synthesis. However, later in the healing process the fluid contains beneficial growth factors secreted by macrophages and other cells, factors that can enhance the development of granulation tissue. Analysis of the fluid withdrawn from chronic and healing wounds has demonstrated this change (Morykwas & Argenta 1997).

Another mechanism of action of the VAC is the mechanical stimulation of cells by tensile forces placed on the surrounding tissue when the applied vacuum collapses the foam dressing. This results in deformation of the cells anchored in the tissues. Integrins act as transmembrane bridges between the applied extra-cellular forces and the cytoskeleton. Perturbation of the integrin bridges distorts the cell membrane and results in the release of second messengers that trigger changes in gene expression with subsequent increases in cell proliferation and protein synthesis.

Effect of negative pressure therapy on acute wounds

When the same treatment parameters as for pressure ulcers are used, there is a rapid reduction in oedema followed by an acceleration of granulation tissue formation.

Effect of negative pressure on chronic wounds

The VAC has been used successfully to treat venous ulcers, arterial insufficiency and neuropathic (diabetic) ulcers. The recommended treatment parameters are continuous treatment for the duration of the therapy, with a target pressure of 50–75 mmHg and a dressing change every 48 h, or every 12 h if infected.

CLINICAL POINTS

- The removal of fluid from a chronic wound removes bacteria and other suppressors of healing.
- The reduced pressure allows the vessels of the microcirculation to dilate.
- Deformation of cell membranes activates cells.

CONCLUSIONS

All the adjunctive therapies described can assist in wound healing if used in an appropriate manner. Most act by assisting in the resolution of inflammation so that the proliferative phase of healing begins earlier, leading to speedier wound closure. Cell activity is jump-started by changes in membrane permeability;

with the result that healing is accelerated. The clinician responsible for treating an injured patient is better equipped to select the most beneficial treatment for the patient if armed with an understanding of each therapy and of its mode of action.

The ultimate test of any treatment is the way in which the patient responds to it. Systemic changes in patients should be documented and their wounds should be imaged non-invasively throughout healing by, for example, digital photography and high-resolution diagnostic ultrasound. Changes in wound structure and physiology should be quantified where possible so that valid comparisons can be made. The sharing of findings via peer-reviewed journals and conference presentations will add to our understanding of these therapies and improve the lot of injured patients.

REFERENCES

Agaiby A, Ghali L, Dyson M 1998 Laser modulation of T-lymphocyte proliferation in vitro. Laser Therapy 10:153–158

Akers T K, Gabrielson A L 1984 The effect of high voltage galvanic stimulation on the rate of healing of decubitus ulcers. Biomedical Sciences Instrumentation 20:99–100

Andreoli S P, Mallet C P, Bergstein J M 1986 Role of glutathione in protecting cells against hydrogen peroxide oxidant injury. Journal of Laboratory and Clinical Medicine 108:190–198

Assimacopoulos D 1968 Wound healing promotion by the use of negative electric current. The American Surgeon 34:423–442

Baker L L, Rubayi S, Villar R 1996 Effect of electrical stimulation on healing of ulcers in human beings with spinal cord injury. Wound Repair and Regeneration 4:21–28

Baxter D 1994 Therapeutic lasers: theory and practice. Churchill Livingstone, Edinburgh

Baxter D 1996 Low intensity laser therapy. In: Kitchen S, Bazin S (eds) Clayton's electrotherapy, 10th edn. W B Saunders, London, p 197–217

Bourguignon G L et al 1991 Occlusive dressings unsuitable for use with eletrical stimulation. Wounds 3(3):127

Ciani P, Lueders H M et al 1989 Adjunctive hyperbaric oxygen therapy reduced length of hospitalization in thermal burns. Journal of Burn Care and Rehabilitation 19: 432–435

Dyson M 1995 Role of ultrasound in wound healing. In: McCulloch J M, Kloth L C, Fudar J A (eds) Wound healing: alternatives in management, 2nd edn. F.A. Davis, Philadelphia, p 318–346

Dyson M, Lyder C 2001 Wound management: physical modalities. In: Morison M J (ed) The prevention and treatment of presure ulcers. Mosby, Edinburgh, p 177–193

Dyson M, Pond J 1973 The effects of ultrasound on circulation. Physiotherapy 59:284–287

Dyson M, Young S R 1986 The effects of laser therapy on wound contraction and cellularity. Lasers in Medical Science 1:125–130

Dyson M, Franks C, Suckling J 1976 Stimulation of healing of varicose ulcers by ultrasound. Ultrasonics 14:232–236

Dyson M, Agaiby A, Ghali L 2002 Photobiomodulation of human T-lymphocyte proliferation in vitro. Lasers in Medical Science 17(4):A22

Dyson M, Moodley S, Verjee L et al 2003 Wound healing assessment using 20 MHz ultrasound and macrophotography. Skin Research and Techonology 9:116–121

El Sayed S, Dyson M 1990 A comparison of the effect of multi-wavelength light produced by a cluster of semiconductor diodes and each individual diode on mast cell number and degranulation in intact and injured skin. Lasers and Surgical Medicine 10:559–568

Feedar J F, Kloth L C, Gentzkow G D 1992 Chronic dermal ulcer healing enhances with monophasic pulsed electrical stimulation. Physical Therapy 72:539

Gault W R, Gatens P F Jr 1976 Use of low intensity direct current in management of ischemic skin ulcers. Physical Therapy 56:265–269

Gentzkow G D, Miller K H 1991 Improved healing of pressure ulcers using Dermapulse, a new electrical stimulation device. Wounds 3:158–160

Grim O, Gottlieb L, Boddie A 1990 Hyperbaric oxygen therapy. Journal of the American Medical Association 263:2216–2220

Hart J 1993 The effect of therapeutic ultrasound on dermal repair with emphasis on fibroblast activity. University of London, London UK (PhD Thesis)

Heng M C Y 1993 Topical hyperbaric therapy for problem skin wounds. Journal of Dermatologic Surgery and Oncology 19:784–793

Heng M C Y, Pilgrim J P, Beck F W J 1984 A simplified hyperbaric oxygen technique for leg ulcers. Archives of Dermatology 120:640–645

Illingworth C F, Smith G, Lawson D D et al 1961 Surgical and physiological observations in experimental pressure chambers. British Journal of Surgery 49:111–117

Irvin T, Smith G 1968 Treatment of bacterial infections with hyperbaric oxygen. Surgery 63: 362–376

Karu T I 1988 Molecular mechanisms of the therapeutic effect of low-intensity laser irradiation. Lasers in Medical Science 2:53–74

Kindwall E P 1993 Hyperbaric oxygen. More indications than many doctors realize. British Medical Journal 307:515–516

Kloth L C 1995 Electrical stimulation in tissue repair. In: McCulloch J M, Kloth L C, Feedar J A (eds) Wound healing: alternatives in management, 2nd edn. F. A. Davis, Philadelphia, p 275–310

Kloth L C, Feedar J 1988 Acceleration of wound healing with high voltage, monophasic, pulsed current. Physical Therapy 68:503–508

Knighton D, Halliday B, Hunt T K 1984 Oxygen as an antibiotic. Archives of Surgery 119:199–204

McDiarmid T, Burns P N, Lewith G T, Machin D 1985 Ultrasound and the treatment of pressure sores. Physiotherapy 71:66–70

Mester E, Mester A F, Mester A 1985 The biomedical effects of laser application. Lasers in Surgery and Medicine 5:31–39

Mohr T, Akers T, Wessman H C 1987 Effect of high voltage stimulation on blood flow in the rat hind leg. Physical Therapy 67:526–533

Morgan T E Jr et al 1963 Effects on man of prolonged exposure at a total pressure of 190 mmHg. Aerospace Medicine 34:589–592

Morykwas M J, Argenta L C 1997 Nonsurgical modalities to enhance healing and care of soft tissue injuries. Journal of the Southern Orthopaedic Association 6:279–288

Nussbaum E L, Biemann I, Mustard B 1994 Comparison of ultrasound, ultraviolet C and laser for treatment of pressure ulcers in patients with spinal cord injury. Physical Therapy 74:812–825

Nylander G, Norstrom H, Eriksson E 1984 Effects of hyperbaric oxygen on oedema formation after a scald burn. Burns 10:193–196

Peschen M, Weichenthal M, Schopf E, Vanscheidt W 1997 Low-frequency ultrasound treatment of chronic venous ulcers in an outpatient therapy. Acta Dermato-venereologica 77:311–314

Raskin P, Lipman R L, Oloff C M 1971 Effect of hyperbaric oxygen on lipid peroxidation in the lung. Aerospace Medicine 42:28–30

Sussman C, Bates-Jensen B M (eds) 2001 Wound care: a collaborative manual for physical therapists and nurses, 2nd edn. Aspen Publishers, Gaithersburg, MD

Sussman C, Byl N 1998 Electrical stimulation for wound healing. In: Sussman C, Bates-Jensen B M (eds). Wound care: a collaborative manual for physical therapists and nurses. Aspen Publishers, Gaithersburg, MD, p 357–388

Sussman C, Byl N 2001 Electrical stimulation for wound healing. In: Sussman C, Bates-Jensen M (eds). Wound care: a collaborative practice manual for physical therapists and nurses, 2nd edn. Aspen Publishers Inc, Gaithersburg, MD, p 497–545

Sussman C, Dyson M 1998 Therapeutic and diagnostic ultrasound. In: Sussman C, Bates-Jensen B M (eds). Wound care: a collaborative manual for physical therapists and nurses. Aspen Publishers, Gaithersburg, MD, p 427–445

Sussman C, Dyson M 2001 Therapeutic and diagnostic ultrasound. In: Sussman C, Bates-Jensen M (eds). Wound care: a collaborative practice manual for physical therapists and nurses, 2nd edn. Aspen Publishers Inc, Gaithersburg, MD p 596–620

Thom S R 1992 Hyperbaric oxygen therapy: a committee report. Undersea and Hyperbaric Medical Society, Bethesda, MD

Young Sr, Dyson M 1993 The effect of ultrasound and light therapy on tissue repair. In: Macleod D A D, Maughan C, Williams C R, Sharo J C M, Nutton R (eds) Intermittent high intensity exercise. Chapman and Hall, London, p 321–328

Young S R, Dyson M, Bolton P 1990 Effect of light on calcium uptake by macrophages. Laser Therapy 2:53–57

Ziskin M C, Michlovitz S L 1990 Therapeutic ultrasound. In: Michlovitz S L (ed) Thermal agents in rehabilitation. F.A. Davis, Philadelphia, p 141–176

CHAPTER

10

Dermatological aspects of wound healing

Janice Cameron and Heather Newton

INTRODUCTION

The management of the skin around wounds is often complex and challenging for both professional and lay carers. This chapter focuses on factors associated with skin assessment and maintaining skin integrity around wounds, and discusses the management of a number of skin problems that may be encountered.

THE SKIN

The skin is the largest organ in the body and forms a barrier between the internal organs and the external environment. Its primary functions include protection against bacteria, thermoregulation, excretion, prevention of moisture loss, vitamin D synthesis and sensory perception.

As illustrated in Fig. 10.1, the skin is made up of two main layers: the epidermis and the dermis. The epidermis is itself composed of several layers. The outermost layer of the epidermis is called the stratum corneum (the horny or cornified layer), which consists of keratin and lipids. Keratin provides a waterproof layer, prevents fluid evaporation from underlying tissue and gives protection from bacteria. Skin scale is dry keratin. The skin continually repairs and regenerates itself with new epithelial cells that migrate upwards from the deeper basal cells of the epidermis to replace the dead cells in the stratum corneum, a process that takes approximately 28 days. The thickness of the epidermis varies according to its function, being thick on the palms of the hands and soles of the feet and thin over the eyelids. The epidermis is supported by the dermis, which is thicker than the epidermis and composed of collagen,

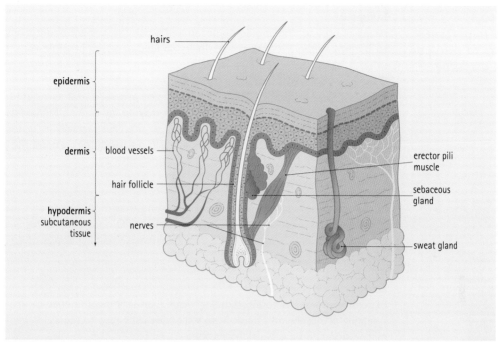

Figure 10.1
Structure of the skin. (From Cameron 1997)

reticulum and elastin fibres, which form a framework for the nerve endings, blood vessels, lymphatic capillaries, sweat glands, sebaceous glands and hair follicles. A layer of subcutaneous fatty tissue (the hypodermis) merges with the deepest layer of the dermis providing thermal insulation (Ebbling 1992, Ebbling et al 1992).

ASSESSMENT OF THE SKIN

The aim of the skin assessment is to identify any risk factors associated with the maintenance of skin integrity. A detailed clinical history should be taken, together with examination of the skin itself. An individualized plan of care can then be implemented. By continuous assessment of the skin, potential problems can be identified and early implementation of appropriate interventions may prevent skin deterioration. Some important factors to consider are summarized in Box 10.1.

All assessment findings should be documented in the patient's case notes as a baseline for measuring the effectiveness of implemented interventions. Where possible, a photograph of the wound and surrounding skin should be taken. If it is not possible to take a photograph, a grid transparency may be used to trace the wound. Any areas of concern in the surrounding skin can be traced and marked on the transparency and should be accompanied by a description of the skin condition.

Box 10.1
Some important factors to consider when assessing skin

Integrity
Areas of broken skin should be noted and a risk assessment undertaken to determine the patient's susceptibility to further tissue breakdown.

Colour and temperature
Erythema may be a consequence of unrelieved pressure or, if associated with a localized increase in temperature, it may be indicative of inflammation. Pallor or bluish tones and skin that is cold to the touch usually indicates poor vascularization. Brown staining (haemosiderin pigmentation) around the gaiter area of the lower leg is an indication of venous disease.

Texture
In old age skin becomes thinner and dryer and thus more prone to trauma (Davies 1992). Thick, dry skin scale (hyperkeratosis) on the lower leg is a chronic condition associated with venous disease. Weeping skin is often associated with an acute condition.

Exposure to moisture
Patients who have a heavily exuding wound, urinary incontinence or are sweating profusely are at risk from excessive exposure to moisture, leading to maceration and possible skin erosion.

MANAGEMENT OF SKIN PROBLEMS COMMONLY ASSOCIATED WITH WOUNDS

A number of commonly presenting problems are now described.

Blisters or bullae

Blisters can form within the epidermis or at the dermal–epidermal junction. They may be a result of thermal injury, acute inflammatory reaction, friction, eczema, oedema or a blistering disorder such as bullous pemphigoid. When assessing the risk factors associated with leaving a blister intact or removing the fluid it is important to consider the cause and the position of any blisters. In a review of research evidence on the management of burn blisters Flannagan (2001) found conflicting views, with some authors supporting aspiration and others suggesting it was more beneficial to leave the blister intact. Blisters may occur from external damage such as friction or tight bandaging pinching the skin. Protection of the skin, especially over the shin and around bony prominences in the ankle and foot, with a wadding bandage layer, either made of synthetic or natural fibres, is essential before applying a compression bandage. The condition of bullous pemphigoid is an autoimmune disease that affects mainly the elderly population. The eruption presents as large, tense blisters on an urticarial base; they are often very itchy (Fry & Cornell 1985). Treatment is with systemic or topical corticosteroids. Locally, the fluid is released by lightly using a scalpel blade to split the blister. Dressings should be non-adherent.

Maceration

Maceration is a result of excessive amounts of moisture remaining in contact with the skin for extended periods. Whereas wound exudate has a beneficial role in wound repair, prolonged exposure can irritate the skin and lead to maceration and loss of epithelium (Fig. 10.2). A barrier preparation, such as zinc oxide paste, applied to the skin around the wound will protect the skin from wound exudate. A small amount of a mixture of 50% white soft paraffin and 50% liquid paraffin (50/50) added to the zinc oxide paste will facilitate easier application and removal (Cameron 1998). Alternatively, skin barriers that leave a protective film on the skin surface may be used around the periulcer area. They are particularly useful under adhesive dressings and around ostomies to form a good seal and prevent skin trauma when the dressing or appliance is removed. Many types of dressing are available for the management of wound exudate. However, the performance of absorbent dressings may be compromised by external pressure from compression bandages or positioning of the patient (Thomas 1997).

Eczema/dermatitis

This inflammatory disorder of the skin is characterized in the acute stage by erythema, exudation, vesiculation and irritation. In the chronic phase there is little or no exudate, more skin scale and also irritation.

Dry eczematous skin. This is managed with regular use of an emollient. Immersing the leg in warm tap water for 10–20 min prior to application of the emollient, will soften and loosen skin scales. Emollients come in the form of creams and ointments. Creams are an emulsion of oil in water in semisolid form. When applied to the skin, most of the cream evaporates because of the high water content. However, creams contain emulsifiers and preservatives that can cause sensitivity problems in patients with a leg ulcer and, where possible, should be avoided and an ointment used as an alternative. Ointments have little or no water, are occlusive and rehydrate the skin. A simple, cost-effective emollient that is unlikely to sensitize is a mixture of 50% white soft paraffin in 50% liquid paraffin (50/50) (Cameron 1997).

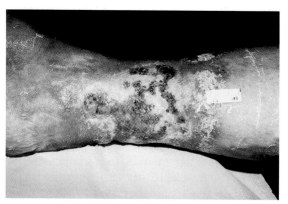

Figure 10.2
Failure to manage wound exudate resulting in maceration

Acute weeping eczema. This can be treated with a dilute solution of potassium permanganate (using only enough potassium permanganate for the solution to be pale pink in colour). The leg should be immersed in the solution daily for 10–15 min, followed by application of a topical corticosteroid ointment (Hunter & Savin 1983). The potency of the corticosteroid required will depend on the degree of eczema present on the limb. A potent steroid (betamethasone 0.1% or beclomethasone dipropionate 0.025%) should be applied daily for a few days then the amount reduced over several days by gradually replacing the steroid ointment with a simple emollient such as 50/50 white soft paraffin mixture (Cameron 1995).

Irritant contact dermatitis

Irritant contact dermatitis is described as a non-immunological inflammatory reaction of the skin to an external agent. Irritants can affect the skin in different ways with the clinical spectrum ranging from slight scaling and redness to marked eczema (Frosch 1992). The severity of the reaction will vary according to the skin area exposed, the method of exposure, the substance used and the concentration (Lahti 1992). Patients most at risk to an irritant contact dermatitis are those where the skin barrier function has been disturbed by an endogenous condition, such as venous stasis eczema. The patient may complain of pain, burning, stinging and itching. Antiseptics have been shown to cause irritant skin reactions when applied to broken skin (Patti et al 1990). Regular skin contact with a mild irritant can result in 'hardening' of the skin, where the skin becomes hyperkeratotic (McOsker & Beck 1967).

Allergic contact dermatitis

Allergic contact dermatitis, also referred to as contact sensitivity, is common in patients with venous leg ulcers. It has long been considered that the occlusive nature of leg ulcer treatments on skin where the barrier function has been disturbed by maceration and eczema can create the perfect environment for sensitization to occur (Stolze 1966). Sensitization may occur after a short period of exposure to an allergen or following a long period of use. Allergic contact dermatitis is a delayed type IV hypersensitivity induced by the reaction between an antigen and sensitized T lymphocytes (Baer 1986). An allergen sensitizes through skin contact and, on renewed contact with the allergen, the skin produces a reaction that is seen clinically as eczema (Scheper & Blomberg 1992). Allergic contact dermatitis usually presents in the area of direct contact with the allergen. However, this is not always the case and it is possible for the sensitivity to be expressed as poor ulcer healing or persistent irritation (Fisher et al 1971). Failure to recognize sensitivity was reported by Cameron (1990) who found 23% of 52 patients with chronic venous leg ulcers were sensitized to their current treatment. Patients suspected of having contact dermatitis should be referred to a dermatologist for patch testing to identify the responsible allergens. Common leg ulcer allergens can be found in a wide range of topical treatments, including emollients, medicaments, dressings, bandages and hosiery. A number of important leg ulcer allergens are described in Box 10.2. Although the allergens mentioned in Box 10.2 are considered to be the main sensitizers in leg ulcer patients, other preparations used in the management of the skin have been reported as causing sensitivity and much will depend on local prescribing habits. Some potential sources of leg ulcer allergens are summarized in Table 10.1.

Box 10.2
Leg ulcer allergens

Rubber

Mercapto mix, thiuram mix and carba mix belong to a group of chemicals used in the rubber industry. The rubber in bandages is usually covered in cotton to help prevent contact with the skin, although this may not be enough to prevent a skin reaction in a sensitized patient (Fig. 10.3). Another potential source of rubber coming into contact with the skin is from the latex gloves worn by the carer. If a rubber allergy is suspected, the carer should wear vinyl gloves to treat the patient. A further source of rubber may come from compression hosiery and it is essential that the hosiery manufacturers are contacted to identify whether there is rubber in the hosiery before it is prescribed for a sensitized patient (Cameron 1990, Gupta & Powell 1999, Wilson et al 1991).

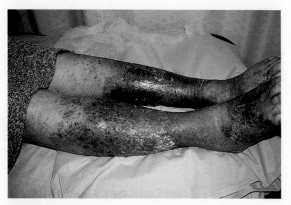

Figure 10.3
Allergic contact dermatitis to rubber

Topical antibiotics

The most commonly reported sensitizers in leg ulcer patients are neomycin and framycetin (Rudzki et al 1988). Sensitivity to neomycin may be masked in products where the antibiotic is combined with a topical corticosteroid, the latter suppressing the sensitivity reaction. In addition, a high incidence of sensitivity to bacitracin has been reported by Zaki et al (1994).

Emulsifiers – cetylstearyl alcohols

These are used in creams and some ointments as a stiffening agent and emulsion stabilizer. Consequently, these allergens are particularly difficult to avoid (Cameron & Powell 1992).

Lanolin (wool alcohols)

Wool alcohols are emulsifying agents and emulsion stabilizers used in the preparation of creams and ointments. Although not a potent sensitizer on normal skin, lanolin has been found to be a sensitizer in patients with venous stasis eczema and leg ulcers (Wilson et al 1991, Zaki et al 1994). Although there is good evidence that some of the newer lanolins are less likely to sensitize, it is difficult to distinguish the different lanolins from the ingredient labelling. It is therefore recommended that products containing lanolin should be avoided in this group of patients.

continued

**Box 10.2
continued**

Preservatives – parabens (hydroxybenzoates)
The parabens group possesses antibacterial and antifungal properties and is widely used as a preservative in topical medicaments, moisturizers and some paste bandages (Cameron 1990, Wilson et al 1991).

Adhesives – colophony/ester of rosin
Colophony and its derivatives can be found in some adhesive tapes and dressings.

Perfume–fragrance mix
Found in many over-the-counter preparations such as moisturizers, bath additives and baby products.

OEDEMA

It is essential that the cause of the oedema is understood so that the appropriate interventions can be implemented. Oedema may be associated with inflammation, limb dependency, venous insufficiency, malnutrition, cardiac disease and hypoalbuminaemia. Stasis eczema may be present in chronic oedematous legs. Treatment of this condition consists mainly of emollients to the skin and compression bandaging. However, care must be taken when treating oedematous tissue because it tends to be fragile and therefore vulnerable to shearing forces and pressure.

Table 10.1
Potential sources of leg ulcer allergens

Allergens	Potential sources
Rubber accelerators/anti-oxidants	
Thiuram/mercapto/carba mix	Elastic bandages, stockings and supports, latex gloves worn by carer
Vehicles/emulsifiers	
Wool alcohols	Creams and emollients, bath additives, skin barriers, baby preparations
Cetyl alcohol, stearyl alcohol, cetylstearyl alcohol	Most creams, including corticosteroid creams and aqueous cream, emulsifying ointment, some paste bandages and medicaments
Preservatives/antimicrobials	
Parabens	Some medicaments and creams, and some paste bandages
Adhesives	
Colophony, ester gum resin	Some adhesive-backed bandages and dressings
Antibiotics	
Neomycin, framycetin, tetracycline, gentamycin, chlortetracycline	Medicaments, creams, tulles, powders
Perfumes	
Fragrance mix, balsam of Peru	Bath oils, over-the-counter moisturizers and some baby products

MALIGNANCY

Fungating wounds are caused by the infiltration of the skin and its supporting blood and lymph vessels by a local tumour or as a result of metastatic spread from a primary tumour (Grocott 1999). As the tumour extends, capillaries rupture and adjacent tissue is destroyed. Anaerobic and aerobic bacteria proliferate causing the characteristic malodour, and profuse amounts of exudate are produced. Fungating wounds also produce pain, have an increased risk of bleeding and infection and can be particularly distressing for the patient (Twycross 1995). Management is essentially palliative and with a multidisciplinary approach focuses on symptom control (Grocott 1999). Appropriate dressings, which do not adhere to the tumour, maintain humidity at the wound interface, absorb exudate, and control bleeding and odour need to be considered for the different stages of tumour progression.

Occasionally, healthcare professionals are presented with wounds that fail to heal, despite appropriate treatment regimes being employed, or with wounds that present with an unknown aetiology. In such cases it is important to exclude the presence of malignant changes. Basal cell carcinomas affect the basal layer of the epidermis and are common in people with a high exposure to ultraviolet radiation. They present as an open, ulcerated lesion or as a reddened patch, which then forms a crust and fails to heal. Surgical intervention is usually the treatment of choice although photodynamic therapy has been shown to produce maximum tumour destruction with minimal cosmetic disfigurement (Morton et al 1996).

Squamous cell carcinomas arise from the keratinocytes of the epidermis and, if left untreated, can metastasize to the lymph nodes. They present as red, scaly indurated areas that have a potential to bleed easily, ulcerate and fail to heal (Newton & Jefferson 2001). Surgical excision is the recommended treatment.

Malignancy is often missed as a cause of non-healing leg ulcers and should be considered in patients who are not responding to conventional therapy after 3 months (Cameron et al 2001).

OVERGRANULATION

Overgranulation is the term given to an overabundance of granulation tissue progressing beyond the level of the wound bed (Dunford 1999). It has also been described as hypergranulation, proud tissue or hypertrophic granulation and can occasionally be mistaken for tumour formation. Although the cause is unknown it would appear that it is closely linked with a prolonged inflammatory response (Dealey 1999). Overgranulation will slow the healing process by inhibiting the migration of epithelial cells across the wound surface. In time, overgranulation often resolves itself, although some clinicians still feel the need to remove it.

The use of silver nitrate sticks is a traditional practice, which directly reduces fibroblast proliferation. It is known to be caustic and is not recommended for prolonged or excessive use (Dealey 1999, Morison 1992). Topical application of corticosteroids reduces the inflammatory response, although they might retard wound closure and alter wound quality (Kloth 1990). A popular treatment option is the use of a polyurethane foam applied directly over the overgranulation tissue with light pressure. This provides a non-traumatic treatment option in the absence of clear evidence to support the alternative methods.

PYODERMA GANGRENOSUM

Pyoderma gangrenosum is often described as an inflammatory ulcer. Its patho-genesis, although unknown, is thought to be immunological rather than bac-terial (Samuel & William 1996). The disease is characterized by the develop-ment of skin lesions, which start as deep-seated painful nodules, haemorrhagic plaques or pustules, which then ulcerate (Young 1997). They are commonly found on the lower limbs, although they can occur on any part of the body. Once ulcerated, the wound bed becomes necrotic and sloughy. The wound margins become raised and irregular with a purple, discoloured edge surround-ed by a halo of erythema. Most cases of pyoderma gangrenosum are associated with other underlying medical conditions such as ulcerative colitis, Crohn's disease or diverticulitis, although they can arise following trauma or surgery (Young 1997).

Pyoderma gangrenosum does not respond to antibiotic therapy, therefore once diagnosed the treatment of choice is the use of systemic steroids. Topical wound treatments need to reflect the characteristics of the wound and are secondary to the systemic treatment. Early referral to a dermatologist is advis-able to ensure accurate, timely diagnosis and an appropriate treatment plan.

PRESSURE DAMAGE

Any area of the body exposed to constant high pressure is at risk of tissue damage. One group of particularly vulnerable patients is those undergoing treatment for venous disease using compression bandaging. To reverse venous hypertension, the degree of pressure required at the ankle is 40 mmHg (Stemmer 1969). However, for some patients with small ankle circumferences and vulner-able bony prominences these high pressures can cause both superficial and deep tissue damage, depending on the duration and intensity of the pressure. The skin can develop blue/purple discoloration, particularly along the tibial crest, around the malleoli and at the join between the patient's ankle and lower leg. Accurate assessment of the patient and the vascular supply of the lower limb can identify potential risks. The use of orthopaedic wool padding assists in the protection of vulnerable areas and can be used to reshape the leg to allow the bandages to be applied effectively.

Pressure damage can also arise from ill-fitting compression hosiery or antiembolism stockings (Fig. 10.4). It is important that patients are measured

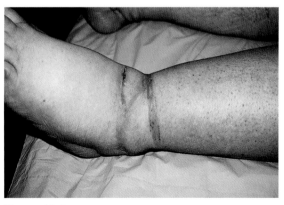

Figure 10.4
Skin damage from a poorly fitting compression stocking

accurately to avoid potential areas of high pressure. Tissues can become oedematous following lower limb surgery and patients may need to have their legs remeasured and the stocking size altered accordingly to reduce this risk of pressure damage. Patients who have plaster of Paris applied are also at risk of tissue damage, particularly if the limb is at risk of swelling. The application of adequate padding to protect these vulnerable areas is strongly recommended and patients should be advised to seek assistance if the plaster becomes uncomfortable.

EPIDERMAL STRIPPING

Epidermal stripping is the inadvertent removal of the epidermis by mechanical means, usually as a result of using tape or adhesive wound dressings (Bryant 1992). The resulting skin damage can present as tension blisters, epidermal stripping or chemical injury. Tension blisters can occur at either end of a taped surface, particularly if the tape is applied too tightly or if the tissues become oedematous following injury or surgery (Fig. 10.5).

Removal of some adhesive dressings and tapes causes minor skin damage to the superficial stratum corneum (Dykes et al 2001). Epidermal stripping can occur particularly where the skin is vulnerable. Elderly patients and neonates are particularly at risk due to the thinning of the dermis and a weakening/immaturity of the projections linking the epidermis with the dermis. Patients on long-term steroid therapy are also at risk, as are those patients whose skin integrity has already been damaged by pressure, maceration or excoriation.

Chemical injury results from irritating chemicals being trapped between the skin and the adhesive layer of dressing products (Blaylock et al 1995). This can be caused by skin preparations used during surgery or during clinical procedures.

In all cases, a comprehensive assessment of the patient's skin integrity together with the identification of potential risks can greatly influence the incidence of this type of skin damage.

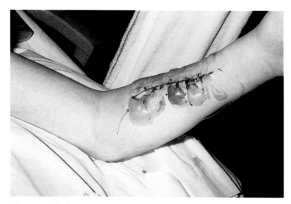

Figure 10.5
Skin damage from postoperative swelling of the limb

LYMPHOEDEMA

Chronic venous hypertension and damage to the lymphatic vessels can result in gross thickening of the dermis with increased skin scale (Ryan 1987). Treatment of this dry skin condition is by liberal application of emollients and massage. Acute inflammatory episodes are treated with topical corticosteroids as described above in the management of acute eczema.

FUNGAL INFECTIONS

Superficial mycoses affect the keratinous tissues of the skin and are sometimes seen on the skin around a leg ulcer. Correct diagnosis is required because clinical signs associated with a fungal infection in the skin around a leg ulcer are similar to eczema with red, scaly, macerated, irritated skin. Pustules and skin erosions might also be present. Fungal infections can be tested for by mycological examination of skin scrapings for hyphae and their culture (Fry & Cornell 1985). Following identification, treatment is by appropriate antifungal preparations.

CELLULITIS

Cellulitis is an acute rapidly swelling inflammation of the skin and soft tissues (Grey 1998) and often occurs following a break in the skin barrier. It is characterized by local erythema, heat, swelling and pain, and the patient may feel systemically unwell and develop a fever, or occasionally septicaemia. *Staphylococcus aureus* and *Streptococcus pyogenes* are the two main causative microorganisms and treatment is generally based on the type of presenting organism.

Cellulitis can sometimes be confused with an acute varicose eczema due to the resulting erythematous inflammation (Quartey-Papafio 1999). Fever, pain and tenderness are signs of cellulitis, whereas itching and crusting are signs of eczema.

Cellulitis is treated with broad-spectrum antibiotics, usually penicillin, with the route depending on the severity of the infection. Patients with cellulitis of the lower limb should be encouraged to elevate the leg as much as possible to reduce oedema and promote venous return. The application of an emollient encourages rehydration of the damaged tissues and any wound area should be dressed with an appropriate dressing.

EVALUATION OF TREATMENT

Ongoing evaluation should be undertaken to measure the effectiveness of the treatment plan and determine the modifications that may need to be made if any conditions change. However, if there has been little or no response to treatment, it is important to check that all appropriate interventions have been implemented. If, despite appropriate treatment, there is still failure to respond, consider referral to a dermatology department for further investigations.

CONCLUSIONS

Care of the skin and maintenance of skin integrity is an important part of wound management and failure in this area can result in extension of the wound, discomfort for the patient and increased costs from healthcare resources, particularly nursing and pharmacy costs. A thorough skin assessment will identify any existing problems and potential risk factors and enable a plan of care to be implemented with confidence. Ongoing evaluation will ensure that appropriate changes are made in the light of changing conditions and should be based on the best available evidence.

REFERENCES

Baer R L 1986 The mechanism of allergic contact hypersensitivity. In: Fisher A A (ed) Contact dermatitis, 3rd edn. Lea and Febiger, Philadelphia

Blaylock B, Murray M, O'Connell K, Rex J 1995 Tape injury in the patient with total hip replacement. Orthopaedic Nursing 14(3):25–28

Bryant R 1992 Skin. In: Bryant R (ed) Acute and chronic wounds: nursing management. Mosby Year Book, St Louis, MO

Cameron J 1990 Patch testing for leg ulcer patients. Nursing Times 86(25):63–64

Cameron J 1995 The importance of contact dermatitis in the management of leg ulcers. Journal of Tissue Viability 5(2):52–55

Cameron J 1997 Dermatological aspects of wound healing. In: Morison M, Moffat C, Bridel-Nixon J, Bale S (eds) Nursing management of chronic wounds, 2nd edn. Mosby, London

Cameron J 1998 Skin care for patients with chronic leg ulcers. Journal of Wound Care 7(9):459–462

Cameron J, Powell S M 1992 Contact dermatitis: its importance in leg ulcer management. Wound Management 2(3):12–13

Cameron J, Hofman D, Cherry G 2001 Malignancy and pre-malignancy in leg ulceration. EWMA Journal 1(1):18–19

Davies I 1992 The mechanisms of ageing. In: Graham-Brown R A C, Monk B E (eds) Skin disorders in the elderly. Blackwell Scientific Publications, Oxford

Dealey C 1999 The care of wounds, 2nd edn. Blackwell Science, Oxford

Dunford C 1999 Hypergranulation tissue. Journal of Wound Care 8(10):506–507

Dykes P J, Heggle R, Hill S A 2001 Effects of adhesive dressings on the stratum corneum. Journal of Wound Care 10(2):7–10

Ebbling F J B 1992 Functions of the skin. In: Rook A, Wilkinson D S, Ebbling F J (eds). Textbook of dermatology, 5th edn. Blackwell Scientific Publications, Oxford

Ebbling F J B, Eady R A J, Leigh I M 1992 Anatomy and organisation of human skin. In: Rook A, Wilkinson D S, Ebbling F J (eds). Textbook of dermatology, 5th edn. Blackwell Scientific Publications, Oxford

Fisher A A, Pascher F, Kanof N B 1971 Allergic contact dermatitis due to ingredients of vehicles. Archives of Dermatology 104:286–290

Flannagan M 2001 Should burn blisters be left intact or debrided? Journal of Wound Care 10(1):41–44

Frosch P J 1992 Cutaneous irritation. In: Rycroft R J G, Menne T, Frosch P J, Benezra C (eds) Textbook of contact dermatitis. Springer-Verlag, Berlin

Fry L, Cornell M 1985 Bacterial infections. In: Fry J, Lancaster–Smith M J (eds). Dermatology. Management of common skin diseases in family practice. MTP Press, Lancaster, UK

Grey J E 1998 Cellulitis associated with wounds. Journal of Wound Care 7(7):338–339

Grocott P 1999 The management of fungating wounds. Journal of Wound Care 8(5):232–234

Gupta C, Powell S M 1999 The problems of rubber hypersensitivity (types I and IV) in chronic leg ulcer and stasis eczema patients. Contact Dermatitis 41:89–93

Hunter J A A, Savin J A 1983 Common diseases of the skin. Blackwell Scientific Publications, Oxford

Hunter J A A, Savin J A, Dahl M V 1989 Clinical dermatology. Blackwell Scientific Publications, Oxford

Kloth L E 1990 Wound healing: alternatives in management. F.A. Davis, Philadelphia

Lahti A 1992 Immediate contact reactions. In: Rycroft R J G, Menne T, Frosch P J, Benezra C (eds) Textbook of contact dermatitis. Springer-Verlag, Berlin

McOsker D E, Beck L W 1967 Characteristics of accommodated (hardened) skin. Journal of Investigative Dermatology 48:372–383

Morison M 1992 A colour guide to the nursing management of wounds. Wolke, London

Morton C A, Whitehurst C, Mosely H et al 1996 Comparison of photodynamic therapy with cryotherapy in the treatment of Bowen's disease. British Journal of Dermatology 135:766–771

Newton H, Jefferson H 2001 What a difference the sun makes. Exposing the risks. Nurse 2 Nurse 1(12):46–47

Pasche-Koo F, Piletta P A, Hunziker N, Hauser C 1994 High sensitisation rate to emulsifiers in patients with chronic leg ulcers. Contact Dermatitis 31:226–228

Patti J, Cazzaniga A, Marshall D A et al 1990 An analysis of dermal irritation of several OTC first aid treatments. Wounds 2:35–42

Quartey-Papafio C M 1999 Importance of distinguishing between cellulitis and varicose eczema of the leg. British Medical Journal 318:1672–1673

Rudzki E, Zakrzewski Z, Rebadel P et al 1988 Cross reactions between aminoglycoside antibiotics. Contact Dermatitis 18:314–316

Ryan T J 1987 Management of leg ulcers, 2nd edn. Oxford University Press, Oxford

Samuel J, Williams C 1996 Pyoderma gangrenosum: an inflammatory ulcer. Journal of Wound Care 5(7):314–318

Scheper R J, von Blomberg M 1992 Cellular mechanisms in allergic contact dermatitis. In: Rycroft R G J, Menne T, Frosch P J, Benezra C (eds) Textbook of contact dermatitis. Springer-Verlag, Berlin

Stemmer R 1969 Ambulatory elasto-compressive treatment of the lower extremities particularly with elastic stockings. Der Kassenatzt 9:1–8

Stolze R 1966 Dermatitis medicamentosa in eczema of the leg. Acta Dermato-venereologica 46:54–61

Thomas S 1997 Assessment and management of wound exudate in the healing process. Journal of Wound Care 6(7):327–330

Twycross R 1995 Symptom management in advanced cancer. Radcliffe Medical Press, Oxford

Wilson C L, Cameron J, Powell S M et al 1991 High incidence of contact dermatitis in leg ulcer patients – implications for management. Clinical and Experimental Dermatology 16:250–253

Young T 1997 Identity crisis. Nursing Times 93(46):70–73

Zaki I, Shall L, Dalziel K L 1994 Bacitracin: a significant sensitiser in leg ulcer patients? Contact Dermatitis 31:92–94

CHAPTER 11

Nutritional screening, assessment and support

Susan McLaren

INTRODUCTION

In recent years, mounting evidence has suggested that malnutrition is relatively common, affecting up to 40% of patients at the point of admission to hospital, around 10% of those discharged home or consulting their general practitioner and between 10 and 85% of nursing home residents (Edington et al 1996, 1997, McWhirter & Pennington 1994). In these settings, and in diverse medical conditions, malnutrition has been associated with an increased morbidity and mortality. A rationale for the negative impact of malnutrition on recovery has been provided by the evidence for adverse effects on mood, organ function, functional capacity, work capacity, wound healing, immunity and resistance to infection (Green 1999). Potential relationships between malnutrition, organ function and wound healing are summarized in Fig. 11.1. Although it is acknowledged that many non-nutritional variables can affect outcomes, prospective clinical studies have linked inadequate dietary intakes and poor nutritional status with the development of pressure sores (Breslow & Bergstrom 1994, Gilmore et al 1995). In surgical populations, malnutrition has also been associated with impaired wound healing and inadequate preoperative dietary intakes (Haydock & Hill 1986, Windsor et al 1988).

Extensive reviews of the research literature evaluating the impact of nutritional support, either oral, enteral or parenteral, on functional capacity and clinical outcomes have shown that appropriately timed and targeted interventions can exert beneficial effects in diverse diagnostic groups, although not all findings are in agreement (Green 1999, Klein et al 1997, Lobo & Allison 2000, Stratton & Elia 1999). In surgical populations, an analysis of prospective

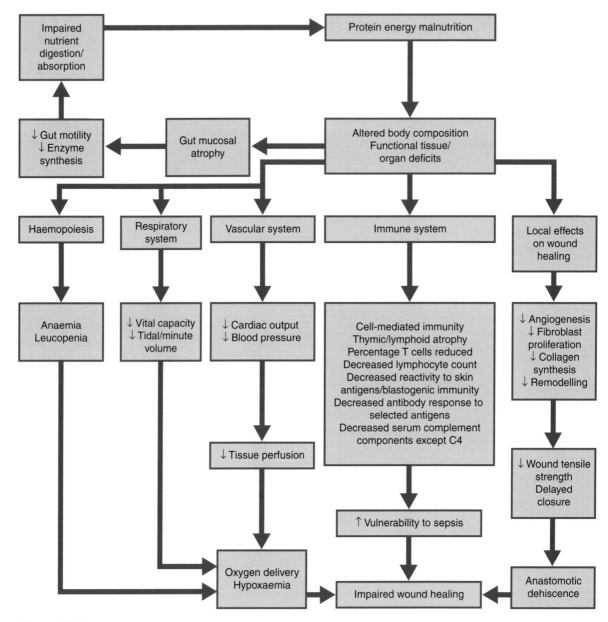

Figure 11.1
Effects of malnutrition on wound healing (reproduced from 'Nutrition and Wound Healing'. Proceedings of the 1st European Conference on Advances in Wound Management, by kind permission of MacMillan Magazines)

randomized controlled clinical trials suggests that nutritional support given for 7 days can reduce complications, including wound sepsis and anastomotic leakage, and that severely malnourished patients may derive greater clinical benefits (Satyanarayana & Klein 1998). The crucial questions are how to identify those at risk from malnutrition so that they can be referred for nutritional support in the hope of reaping benefits on both functional and clinical outcomes, and what specific types of interventions are of benefit in different situations?

Herein lies the challenge, to develop effective methods of nutritional screening, assessment and support and to implement these as part of a quality nutrition service in acute and community settings.

GENERAL PRINCIPLES AND THE BENEFITS OF NUTRITIONAL SUPPORT TEAMS

Five key stages can be distinguished in the management of nutritional support (Fig. 11.2). All five involve effective communication and decision making by different groups of health professionals. Ideally, these should be organized to form a 'nutritional support team' (NST) that, in conjunction with other clinical staff, has the principal responsibility for implementing nutrition support in accordance with evidence-based standards and guidelines for screening assessment, delivery and evaluation. A recent survey by the British Artificial Nutrition Survey (BANS 1999) found that NSTs had been established in 163 (41%) of UK centres (teaching and non-teaching hospitals); membership of teams included predominantly pharmacists, dietitians, medical consultants and specialist nurses, with other professional groups less commonly represented. Leadership was largely devolved upon medical consultants, a crucial role in encouraging work across professional boundaries and in ensuring clarity in accountability during operation.

How effective are nutrition support teams? Early evaluation suggests benefits encompass safer nutrition support, which when effectively targeted can reduce costs. A study by Maurer et al (1996) conducted on medical and surgical units found that consultation with a multidisciplinary team reduced the inappropriate

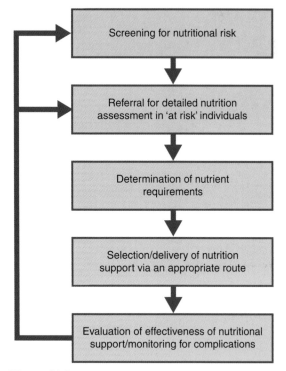

Figure 11.2
Management of nutritional support; key stages

use of total parenteral nutrition, evident in a decline in usage from > 500 to < 100 patient days monthly. Later investigations by Pattison & Young (1997) confirmed other benefits of teamwork in the development and implementation of guidelines for the management of gastrostomy feeding in acute care settings. Audit of practice prior to and following the implementation of standards found that the total number of patients with complications significantly decreased, evident in a decline in site sepsis and failure. Further studies are needed to establish whether patients managed at home on artificial nutrition have fewer complications and better clinical outcomes when managed by an NST (BANS 1999).

The focus of screening and assessment is to identify individuals who have malnutrition or are at high risk of becoming undernourished. On the basis of medical diagnosis alone, vulnerable groups for malnutrition are summarized in Table 11.1. Older adults are particularly vulnerable because of the changes in body composition, appetite and sensory impairment that can accompany ageing (McLaren 1999, Morley 1995). Social, psychological, pharmacological and financial problems can exacerbate these, hence their inclusion in the content of many screening and assessment instruments and in dietary histories.

Green (1999) has identified a number of iatrogenic factors that may contribute to the problem of disease-related malnutrition in hospitalized patients. These include lack of resources for nutrition support, inadequate education of nursing and medical staff and the absence of strategic policies and guidelines, which could improve the quality of service delivery.

Table 11.1 Diseases that may result in protein-energy malnutrition (reproduced from 'Eating Matters' by kind permission of the Centre for Health Services Research, University of Newcastle-upon-Tyne)	**Reduced nutrient intake** Reduced mobility and/or cognition, sensation, perception impairing food purchase and/or preparation (e.g. stroke, Parkinson's disease, dementia, cardiac failure, pulmonary disease, musculoskeletal trauma, osteo/rheumatoid arthritis) Loss of functional independence in eating, motor skills (e.g. stroke, Parkinson's disease, osteo/rheumatoid arthritis, dementia, musculoskeletal trauma) Loss of appetitie (e.g. depression, anxiety, cancer, infection (any cause), pain (any cause), renal and liver diseases) Nausea and vomiting (e.g. some types of cancer, renal, liver disease) Impaired oral food retention/ingestion, chewing, swallowing (e.g. dementia, stroke, cancer of the oesophagus, pharynx, oral cavity) **Decreased nutrient digestion/absorption** Chronic gut inflammation (e.g. ulcerative colitis, Crohn's disease, enteropathies, malabsorption syndromes, gastrointestinal infection, cancer) Liver disease Pernicious anaemia (reduced vitamin B_{12} absorption) **Increased metabolic utilization of nutrients/disposal** Metabolic responses to injury (e.g. burns, sepsis, orthopaedic trauma, grade IV pressure ulcers complicated by sepsis) Cancer cachexia syndrome Hyperthyroidism Chronic obstructive pulmonary disease (COPD) associated with hyperventilation

AIMS OF SCREENING AND ASSESSMENT

Nutritional screening is a vital, preliminary process that aims to identify individuals who are already malnourished or at high risk of becoming so (McLaren & Green 1999). Effective screening should result in the clear delineation of at risk groups who can be referred for further detailed assessment, which has the following aims (Taylor & McLaren 1992):

- to define nutritional status and evaluate the adequacy of recent nutritional intakes
- to identify individuals who require nutritional support
- to evaluate the efficacy of nutritional support by comparing serial measurements made over time.

Both screening and assessment can be based on protocols containing guidelines and standards developed by professional bodies and expert groups, for example The Kings Fund (1992), The Royal College of Nursing (1993) and the British Association for Parenteral and Enteral Nutrition (1996). As shown in Table 11.2, these focus on procedures (e.g. when used and by whom), utilizing predictors of malnutrition and emphasizing the need for systematic care planning and maintenance of accurate records.

Distinct from protocols are instruments or tools that attempt to quantify risk in the process of screening and/or assessment. Although several have been published, relatively few have completed the necessary stages of validity and reliability testing that are the essential prerequisites for their implementation in practice. In marked contrast to the relative paucity of risk assessment instruments available to the health professional are the many anthropometric, biochemical, functional, morphological and immunological techniques that are available for nutritional assessment. With the exception of certain research techniques that are not widely available, many are affected by non-nutritional variables and none constitutes a 'gold standard' for assessment. To overcome

Table 11.2
Key points: protocols containing guidelines and standards for screening and assessment

Kings Fund Report (1992)	RCN (1993)	BAPEN (1996)
• Initial assessment should question recent patterns in food intake, food avoidance; normal weight/recent losses; diarrhoea; vomiting; gut or weakness	• Initial assessment made of food/ fluid intake; eating/drinking patterns	• Primary assessment of nutritional status/risk includes height/weight; weight loss; reduced appetite; eating/digestion difficulties; weakness; infection; recent surgery
• Adult weight recorded once in general practice/hospital. Patients weighed regularly to evaluate changes	• Ward staff responsible to/meet individual requirements for eating/ drinking	• Nursing medical staff conduct assessments; patients referred to nutrition team on specific criteria
• Nutritional status should be recorded in medical and nursing records	• A plan of care is devised based on assessment that enables the patient/client to eat/drink	• Nutritional requirements of patients assessed/reviewed; protocol recommended for ongoing nutritional assessment
• Where malnutrition is detected, cause should be established, a plan of care devised and monitored	• Nutritional goals are continually evaluated and revised	• Records maintained of changes in nutritional status

deficiencies in any single measurement, it is usual to select three based on different techniques and to compare serial results made over time in any individual patient.

Screening instruments

Screening instruments are typically based on known predictors of malnutrition in a given population. Their content can encompass questions on dietary history, anthropometric measurements and details of medical conditions with associated symptoms. Exemplars of screening instruments summarized in Table 11.3 generate ordinal scores that are summed to give a total score indicative of low, medium or high risk and, in some cases, necessary actions for each level of risk are identified.

Which criteria should inform selection of a screening instrument? The following questions should be answerable based on the information provided in scientific reports or journal publications:

- Is the instrument user friendly? With appropriate training, would staff find it simple to use, easy to interpret? How long does it take to complete?
- Is the instrument costly? Could it be easily assimilated into medical/nursing recording systems?
- Would patients/clients find it non-intrusive and acceptable?
- Have different aspects of validity testing been addressed. Does the content adequately represent predictors of malnutrition? To what extent do screening scores correlate with external criteria (e.g. dietary intakes)? Do the scores show acceptable convergence with another method of assessing risk?
- Has reliability (i.e. consistency) in use been tested? Are levels of agreement acceptable between independent raters who screen the same patients at the same time?
- What is the sensitivity of the instrument? (i.e. to what extent does it detect true cases of malnutrition?)
- What is the specificity of the instrument? (i.e. to what extent does it detect true negative cases without malnutrition?)

To what extent can the adoption of screening impact on patient outcomes? A recent study that evaluated the implementation of dysphagia screening found that the time dysphagia patients spent nil orally prior to receiving nutritional support was significantly reduced, as was the incidence of chest infection and sepsis of unknown origin (Perry & McLaren 2000). To date, data on the impact of using other types of screening are sparse.

Dietary assessment

Assessment of dietary intakes can provide important information on the quality and quantity of food consumed. Key stages in this form of assessment identified by Gibson (1993) includes the following:

- Recording and measurement of food consumption; analysis of nutrient content and estimation of 24-h intakes of energy, macro- and micronutrients using computer software.
- Evaluation of the adequacy of daily nutrient intakes by comparison with the recommendations of expert groups (e.g. Department of Health 1991, 1992).

Table 11.3
Screening instruments: exemplars

Author/related publications	Name of instrument/target population	Content	Comments
Guigoz et al (1997)	Mini-nutritional Assessment Older adults (69–90 years)	• Screening component of instrument includes six categories focused on food intake, weight loss, mobility, stress, body mass index and neuropsychological problems • Assessment component contains 12 categories covering dietary intakes, anthropometry, drug prescriptions, presence of pressure ulcers and independence in living • Responses linked to weighted ordinal scores. Totals for low, moderate, high risk	• Content, criterion-related/convergent validity established • Instrument translated into other languages, used in different cultures and care settings
Wolinsky et al (1986, 1990)	Nutritional Risk Index Older adults (> 55 years)	• A 16-item questionnaire covers altered dietary intakes/habits; factors affecting food ingestion and other variables • Responses linked to weighted ordinal scores summed for low, moderate, high risk	• Early validity testing on males only • Content criterion related validity tested • Inter-rater reliability established
Nutrition Screening Initiative USA (1991) Barrocas et al (1995) Grindel & Costello (1996)	Determine (checklist/ awareness instrument) Older adults	• Utilizes three levels of risk screening/assessment in a 10-item checklist, 3-item questionnaire and interview encompassing physical, biochemical, functional capacity and other data	• Content validity addressed • Very detailed approach to screening/assessment
Reilly et al (1995)	Nutrition Risk Score Adults, children	• A 5-item questionnaire encompassing body mass index, history of weight loss, factors affecting food intake and recent stress • Responses generate low-, medium-, high- risk groups	• Content and convergent validity tested • Reliability evaluated between nurses versus dietitians and dietitians versus dietitians
Malnutrition Advisory Group (MAG; 2000) Standing Committee of British Association of Parenteral and Enteral Nutrition	Screening Tool for Adults at Risk of Malnutrition	• Step 1: measurement of body mass index, weight loss, clinical factors • Step 2: categorization of risk of malnutrition by summation across categories gives high, medium, low overall risk of malnutrition • Step 3: care plan determined; action plan noted	• Content validity • Inter-rater reliability • Ease in use established • Instrument is in process of development; further validity/reliability testing in progress

Both quantitative and qualitative approaches can be used; exemplars of the former include 24-h recall and 3-day food records. In contrast, food frequency questionnaires and dietary histories provide more qualitative or semiquantitative information. Use of rigorous recording protocols and dietetic weighing scales accurate to 0.5 g is essential in the approaches described below. A very detailed consideration of the validity and reliability of different dietary assessment methods is provided in Wolper et al (1997).

3-day food records

Normally conducted over two weekdays and one weekend day to account for different patterns of consumption, this method can include assessment of portion sizes using household measures, food models or weighing scales (Bingham et al 1994, Ministry of Agriculture, Fisheries and Food 1997). Procedures require all food and beverages consumed during the 3-day period to be recorded, including any snacks, condiments, sauces and supplements used. In addition, the method of preparation, brand names and label information on packaging should be described. Where composite products are used, access to original recipes can be necessary. Weighing food using dietary scales offers greater accuracy but it takes time, necessitating weighing of a serving dish, recording sequential weights as food items are added, weighing leftovers and deducting from the original weights. Care must be taken to ensure food does not cool to the extent that palatability is affected. When patients/clients are involved in recording, the possibility of bias can arise. Training in the techniques is also necessary to minimize error.

24-hour recall method

In fact, recall methods can encompass periods ranging from 1 day to 1 month. Reliant on memory, patients/clients are interviewed and asked to recall information on food/drink consumption over the desired time interval. It is important that the professional conducting the interview selects a calm, quiet setting to aid concentration, provides an explanation about the information needed and stresses its confidential nature. It is vital that a non-judgemental approach is adopted in which verbal or non-verbal behaviour by the interviewer, which could lead to bias, is avoided. The importance of interviewer training cannot be underestimated (Wolper et al 1997).

The information required includes descriptions of all food/drinks consumed, method of cooking, portion sizes, brand names and waste. At the conclusion of the interview, information is checked with the patient/client. Advantages of the method are the low cost, rapid completion (about 20 min), simplicity and limited burden placed on those interviewed. Set against these are disadvantages that arise from erroneous memory and the non-inclusion of infrequently consumed foods. The interviewer should check with the patient/client at the outset whether the period recalled was typical for dietary consumption. The method is unsuitable for use in individuals suffering from cognitive deficits.

Food frequency questionnaires

Using precoded forms, these can provide retrospective information on patterns of food intake covering periods of weeks/months. Frequency of consumption of a wide range of food items is recorded, for example in categories stating never eaten, once per month or less, once per fortnight or less and number of days per week. It is important to ensure that the content of the questionnaires considers vegetarians and other ethnic groups in design. The amount eaten, described in amounts using either household measures or photographs, is also recorded (Ministry of Agriculture, Fisheries and Food 1997). This method has the advantage that it assesses usual patterns of food intake and is neither costly nor excessively burdensome, but bias and memory deficits can still cause error.

Dietary history

A dietary history is also reliant on skilled interview techniques using a recording proforma containing a mix of closed and open questions. Content focuses on daily eating patterns and any factors that have caused a divergence from this, such as changes in health status. Frequency, types of foods consumed and portion sizes are recorded, in conjunction with methods of preparation. Socioeconomic background in relation to diet is addressed in questions about independence in shopping for food, kinship networks, financial resources for food purchase, storage and preparation. Any use of support services in the community, such as 'meals-on-wheels' should be noted, or where care assistants help with shopping and preparation. The impact of medical conditions and their treatments in causing distressing symptoms that impair food intake should be recorded, for example anorexia, dyspnoea, diarrhoea, pain, dysgeusia, dysphagia, impaired mobility and posture (McLaren et al 1997). Other vital information encompasses a history of weight loss, use of special diets in chronic conditions (renal, vascular, liver disease) and prescribed drugs, which can exert adverse effect on dietary intakes by causing nausea, vomiting, mucosal ulceration and pain.

Anthropometric assessment

According to the *Oxford English Dictionary* anthropometry is 'the measurement of the human body with a view to determine its average dimensions at different ages and in different classes or races'. A wealth of historical and contemporary survey data are available illustrating the diversity of anthropometric measurements – body weight, height, skinfold thickness, limb muscle circumference – in different populations, for example the National Diet and Nutrition Survey in the UK, conducted by Finch et al (1998) in older adults aged 65 and over. Fundamentally, serial anthropometry provides information on changes in body composition, extrapolated from weight (fat + fat-free mass) that approximates to total body energy stores, subcutaneous fat (skinfolds) and skeletal muscle (limb muscle circumference). In a healthy adult, fat provides the major energy store; total body fat weighing 5–15 kg can yield 50 000–140 000 kcal of energy that can be utilized in periods of negative energy balance. In contrast, the fat-free mass that comprises protein, water, bone mineral and glycogen weighs approximately 40–60 kg and can provide only 40 000–60 000 kcal of usable energy as a reserve, of which 15 000–20 000 kcal are contained within skeletal muscle (Wright & Heymsfield 1984).

Body weight provides one of the simplest anthropometric measures required in a nutritional assessment. It should be recorded using equipment that has been calibrated against standard weights, accurate to within ± 0.1 kg. A recent survey by Chu et al (1999) found that information on calibration and servicing weighing equipment available in 79 clinical sites within 22 NHS Trusts was not available in 45% of sites. Although all had access to at least one set of scales, only 17% possessed a stadiometer for measuring height. It is vital that equipment maintenance and provision for nutritional assessment should be regularly audited against standards and guidelines for service provision. Calibration of skinfold calipers should be included in such audits.

Table 11.4 summarizes key anthropometric measurements that can be used within an assessment, together with their advantages and limitations. Attention is drawn to the many non-nutritional variables that can influence measurements, including that of body weight, which is affected by oedema, ascites, tumour growth and fluid gains or losses.

Caution should also be exercised in comparing measurements with tables of reference standards that have been obtained from surveys of healthy populations within defined parameters of age, gender and ethnicity. These may not be applicable to individual patients in whom serial measurements made over time can offer useful information on changes in body composition. Readers will find more detailed information on the applications of anthropometry in Gibson (1993) and Downs & Hafferjee (1998).

Subjective global assessment

Subjective global assessment (SGA) combines six features of an individual's history to provide a composite evaluation of nutritional status (Detsky et al 1987). These encompass weight change, dietary intake, gastrointestinal symptoms, functional capacity, disease and a physical examination. Overall, the SGA classifies patients as either well-nourished, suffering from moderate or suspected malnutrition, or severely malnourished. Downs & Hafferjee (1998) have suggested that, although relatively reliable, this instrument may not be sufficiently sensitive to detect early responses to nutritional support.

A number of modifications to the original SGA have been published that are specific to diagnostic groups, for example Persson et al (1999) in oncology patients. This found that the SGA categories correlated well with biochemical predictors of nutritional status and patient reports of eating problems. In this study, patients completed part of the assessment themselves; the remainder was completed by a dietitian or a doctor.

Physical examination

Traditionally, physical examination is one of the most frequently used methods of nutritional assessment. This relies on diverse physical manifestations of malnutrition identified by a trained observer. Apart from a wasted, malnourished appearance, an array of features can indicate vitamin deficiencies. The problem of interpreting these features is that they can be caused by other non-nutritional manifestations of disease or, indeed, are side-effects of drugs. The possibility of drug–nutrient interaction also should be borne in mind (Downs & Hafferjee (1998).

Biochemical assessment

Biochemical tests can reflect either the total body content of a nutrient or the size of the tissue store most sensitive to depletion. An array of methods is available to measure either the levels of nutrients in biological fluids or tissues (e.g. blood, serum, urine, hair, saliva) or the urinary excretion rates of nutrients or

Table 11.4
Anthropometric indices

Parameter	Uses	Advantages	Limitations	Comments
Body mass index (BMI)				
$\dfrac{\text{Weight (kg)}}{\text{Height (m)}^2}$	• Index of weight in proportion to height – lean body mass to skeletal size BMI: < 19 underweight 20–25 normal 26–30 overweight > 30 obese	• Indicates changes in body fat stores • Easy to perform • Sensitive indicator of malnutrition	• High BMI does not preclude malnutrition in existing obesity where lean tissue may have been lost • In older people lean body mass declines due to ageing – reduces validity • Standing upright may be difficult for some older people	• BMI and health risks may differ in young versus older age groups[a] • Low BMI (< 19) associated with increased mortality in older and young age groups • Interpretation of high BMI values > 30 in relation to morbidity unclear in older populations[b]
Demispan				
Distance from web between middle and ring fingers along out-stretched arm to sternal notch (cm)	• Alternative to height measurement • Range in men aged 65–74; 81.6 ± 4.05; 75–91; 80.4 ± 4.1. In women aged 65–74; 73.8 ± 3.6 cm; 75–91; 72.7 ± 3.5 cm[c]	• Can be measured in seated elderly individuals • Total arm length and span change less with age than height • Easy to perform; use non-stretchable tape measure	• Unsuitable for use in older people who cannot raise arms due to chronic inflammatory or neurological diseases	• Further large-scale population studies necessary to clarify norms • Knee height an alternative where demispan cannot be measured • Useful assessment of skeletal size
Demiquet				
$\dfrac{\text{Weight (kg)}}{\text{Demispan m}^2}$	• Index of body mass in relation to skeletal size	• Useful index of body mass where height cannot be used • Easy to perform	• See above	• Range of norms for elderly populations not available
Percentage ideal body weight (IBW)				
$\dfrac{\text{Current weight}}{\text{ideal body weight (kg)}} \times 100/$	• Compares weight with ideal values obtained from surveys • < 60% IBW equated with severe malnutrition 61–80% IBW equated with moderate malnutrition	• Easy to perform • Reference tables available	• Actuarial data applicable to populations of specific age range, gender, frame size, ethnic group • May be inaccurate in ectomorphs and obese individuals	• Some actuarial data out of date • Not applicable to some elderly groups; > 74 years: caution needed in checking survey data age ranges • Limited discrimination between good and poor levels of nutritional status with this measure

Percentage usual body weight (UBW)

Current weight (kg) × 100/ usual body weight (kg)	• Provides information on recent weight loss • < 75% usual body weight may indicate severe malnutrition; 76–84% usual weight may indicate moderate malnutrition	• Weight change considered on an individual basis • Relates weight loss with organ dysfunction	• Poor memory of usual weight may introduce error • Presence of oedema, organomegaly, tumour growth may result in error	• Crude discrimination between levels of malnutrition • Weight losses of 1–2% UBW/1 week; 5% in 1 month; 10% in 6 months significant in terms of recovery

Triceps skin-fold thickness (TSF)

Thickness of fat fold at midpoint of non-dominant upper arm (mm)	• Index of changes in body fat stores • Use high-resolution callipers with scale reading accurate to ± 0.1 mm and standard pressure of 10 g/mm² • Average of three measurements	• TSF in upper arm easily accessible • Useful in long-term monitoring • Non-invasive; inexpensive	• Subcutaneous fat in upper arm is not absolutely proportional to total body fat[d] • Not useful in detecting short-term changes (< 4 weeks) • Training required	• Variations in subcutaneous fat produced by non-nutritional variables such as hydration status, age, sex, ethnic group

Mid-arm muscle circumference (MAMC)

MAMC (cm) = Mid-arm circumference (cm) − 0.3142 × TSF (mm)	• Index of changes in skeletal muscle protein reserve (indirect) • Based on TSF and mid-arm circumference measured using non-stretchable tape measure • Average of three measurements taken	• Accessible measure, non-invasive, inexpensive content	• Assumes muscle mass proportional to protein content • Protein may decrease and fat and water increase in muscle • Assumes circular limb, constant areas of bone, continuous layers of muscle and fat	• Mass and composition of muscle can be affected by disease • Assumptions are all sources of error; care needed in interpretation

[a]Kushner R F 1993 Body weight and mortality. Nutrition Reviews 51(5):127–136

[b]Lehman A B, Bassey E J, Morgan K, Dalluso H M 1991 Normal values for weight, skeletal size and body mass indices in 890 men and women aged >65 years. Clinical Nutrition 10:18–22

[c]Tayback M, Kumanyika S, Chee E 1990 Body weight as a risk factor in the elderly. Archives of Internal Medicine 150(5):1065–1072

[d]Heymsfield S, McManus C B, Seitz S B et al 1984 Anthropometric assessment of adult protein energy malnutrition. In: Wright R A, Heymsfield S (eds) Nutritional assessment. Blackwell Scientific, Oxford, p 27–82

Reproduced by kind permission of 'Professional Nurse', EMAP Healthcare.

their metabolites (Gibson 1993). In considering the selection, use and interpretation of biochemical tests, the following points that should be borne in mind are summarized in Box 11.1.

Box 11.1 ***Factors influencing the selection, use and interpretation of biochemical tests***	• Sampling and collection procedures should minimize the risk of injury, contamination or haemolysis. • Expert advice on accuracy, precision, sensitivity and specificity of analytical methods, together with availability and cost should be sought from a consultant biochemist. • Circadian rhythms, age and gender can affect measurements; use of appropriate reference ranges is therefore necessary. • Certain drugs, diseases, injury and stress can affect the concentrations of some biochemical indicators of nutritional status in body fluids. • Rates of biosynthesis, body pool size and half-life can affect the concentrations of serum proteins and their sensitivity to malnutrition. The ideal protein marker has a rapid rate of biosynthesis, small body pool and short half-life. • Serum protein concentrations can be reduced by shifts from the intravascular to extravascular compartment when vascular permeability is increased. • Diluting or concentrating effects caused by expansion or contraction of the extracellular fluid volume can reduce or elevate concentrations of several serum components including proteins.

The most common biochemical methods used in nutritional assessment are serum proteins and urinary nitrogen balance studies. For detailed information on the assessment of vitamins, mineral and trace element status, see the publications by Shenkin (1997, 1999).

Serum proteins

Characteristics of serum proteins are summarized in Table 11.5. Serum protein concentrations are dependent on the balance between hepatic synthesis, biological half-life and rate of catabolism. In malnutrition concentrations decline due to lack of substrate for hepatic synthesis. However, a number of non-nutritional variables can influence serum concentrations (Box 11.2).

The long half-life of albumin precludes its use as a reliable indicator of nutritional status in the short term, where prealbumin and retinol-binding protein are more useful.

Nitrogen balance studies

Estimates of nitrogen balance can provide useful information on the adequacy of dietary protein intakes, based on the precept that 6.25 kg of protein contains 1.0 g of nitrogen:

$$\text{Nitrogen balance (g/24 h)} > \text{protein intake (g)}/6.25 - \text{urinary nitrogen (g)} + \text{extrarenal losses (4 g)}$$

Table 11.5
Serum proteins: characteristics (reproduced by kind permission of Wolfe Publishing)

Serum protein	Body pool size (mg per kg body weight)	Half-life	Normal ranges in serum (g/L)	Protein-energy malnutrition (g/L)	
				Moderate	Severe
Albumin	5000	19 days	35–45	21–27	< 21
Transferrin	100	9 days	2.5–3.0	1.0–1.5	< 1.0
Thyroxine-binding prealbumin	10	2 days	0.16–0.30	0.05–0.1	< 0.05
Retinol-binding protein	2	12 h	0.026–0.1	< 0.02	

Box 11.2
The influence of non-nutritional variables on serum proteins

- **Albumin:** hepatic disease, metabolic injury responses and excessive losses in wound exudate can lower serum concentrations.
- **Transferrin:** serum concentrations rise in pregnancy, hypoxaemic iron-deficiency anaemia and chronic blood loss. A decrease occurs in hepatic disease and in protein-losing nephropathies.
- **Prealbumin:** metabolic injury responses, hepatic disease and hyperthyroidism result in a decrease in serum concentrations. A rise occurs in chronic renal failure or haemodialysis.
- **Retinol-binding protein:** vitamin A and zinc deficiency and hyperthyroidism lead to a decrease, and vice versa, in chronic renal failure and the use of oral contraception.

Extrarenal losses (hair, sweat, skin, faeces) can be markedly increased by leaking gut fistulae, wound exudate and diarrhoea. In these conditions, collection of fluids is essential for accurate measurement of nitrogen balance. Normally, nitrogen balance studies are concentrated over three consecutive days and results averaged to provide 24-h estimates; this requires serial 24-h urine collections. In non-catabolic individuals nitrogen balance may be achieved by increasing dietary nitrogen intakes to exceed losses by 3–5 g. In catabolic individuals there are limits regarding the extent to which nitrogen input can balance output. Beyond 20–22 g/24 h, excessive nitrogen intakes can lead to uraemia and other problems. Thus, in very severe catabolism it might not be possible to balance intake and output.

ASSESSMENT OF NUTRIENT REQUIREMENTS

If the results of screening and assessment confirm that an individual is already malnourished, or at high risk of becoming so, the third stage of management requires referral to a dietitian for assessment of both macro- and micronutrient requirements:

- Energy requirements can be determined with the greatest degree of accuracy using predictive equations, nomograms and reference tables. Upwards adjustments are necessary based on metabolic responses to trauma, injury and sepsis, needs for repletion of malnourished states, wound healing and level of physical activity. These are intrinsically weighted in calculations arising from calorimetry, predictive equations and nomograms (Reid & Carlson 1998, Rombeau & Rolandelli 1997, Silbermann 1989).
- Nitrogen requirements can be established, as previously described, using nitrogen balance studies or reference tables that provide ranges of nitrogen intakes in g/24-h based on metabolic status.
- Micronutrient requirements can be estimated using reference tables (Shenkin 1997, 1999).

Patients with acute and chronic wounds can represent a range of medical conditions and metabolic states. Care should be taken in the assessment of nutrient requirements to establish metabolic status, because the potential impact of an extensive pressure ulcer can be easily overlooked. Some reference tables, for example Department of Health (1991), do not consider the nutrient requirements of metabolically unstable individuals and should be applied only to the healthy.

NUTRITIONAL SUPPORT

Considered against the background of diverse medical conditions and their treatment, nutritional support has three principal aims (Klein et al 1997):

1. Maintenance of lean body mass, organ function and immunocompetence.
2. Repletion of body composition in malnourished states.
3. Prevention of malnutrition-associated morbidity and mortality (including wound-related complications).

From the outset, decision making encompasses available routes of administration, timing regarding initiation and expected duration of support, patient/client preferences, ethical aspects of delivery and formulation of dietary regimens based on assessed requirements for nutrients. It is beyond the scope of this text to give a detailed account of these aspects of delivery. For this, readers are referred to the comprehensive texts of Rombeau & Rolandelli (1997) and the British Association of Parenteral and Enteral Nutrition series of publications.

In general, the maxim that 'if the gut functions, use it' guides the initial stage of decision making, as both oral and enteral tube feeding are associated with fewer complications than parenteral feeding. Another important consideration is that using the functioning gut prevents disuse atrophy, marked by loss of villous architecture in the mucosa, loss of enzyme secretion and biliary sludging. It is vital that decision making on nutritional support is not delayed unless there are good reasons to do so, because a deterioration in nutritional status could bring about adverse consequences. Prior to commencing nutritional support – enteral or parenteral – haemodynamic stability should be secured and major fluid and electrolyte imbalances corrected. Refeeding syndrome, marked by hypophosphataemia, electrolyte imbalances and an array of potentially dangerous respiratory and vascular complications, is a risk in treating chronically malnourished, wasted individuals. Preliminary correction of fluid and electrolyte balances, particularly with regard to phosphate replacement, aligned with slow initial rates of nutrient delivery is advised (Pennington et al 1996).

Oral nutrient supplements

A variety of commercial supplements is available, designed to complement dietary intakes, although they can occasionally be used to replace the normal diet (McLaren et al 1997). Normally, supplements are prescribed by a dietitian in conjunction with an assessment of nutrient needs and palatability. Although supplements vary in content, they usually take the form of milk-based, fruit-flavoured, nutrient-dense beverages. Accurate timing and recording of supplement ingestion is vital, as is attention to storage instructions and expiry dates.

A recent systematic review of the literature on supplement use in the community by Stratton & Elia (1999) concluded that weight gain depended on duration and amount of supplementation used and disease status. Individuals who benefited most in terms of weight gain were those with a body mass index (BMI) $< 20 \, \text{kg/m}^2$. Improved functional benefits were noted in some categories of chronic illness. Problems associated with supplement use included poor palatability and gastrointestinal side-effects. A study by Breslow et al (1993) involving 8 weeks' supplementation found a decline in truncal pressure ulcer surface area, specifically in stage IV ulcers; other investigations evaluating the impact of supplement use in healing are urgently needed.

Enteral nutrition

This form of artificial feeding is advocated for patients who have a functioning gut but are unable to meet their nutritional requirements via normal food ingestion (McAteer et al 1999). Fundamentally, the route for enteral nutrition (EN) is dependent on the level of alimentary tract function, accessibility, ease in use and the preference of patients (Taylor & McLaren 1992). Administration is via a catheter that delivers nutrients distal to any gastrointestinal tract abnormally and proximal enough to enable complete absorption to occur. Essentially, patients can be divided into two categories; those with an acute illness, requiring enteral feeding for < 4 weeks and those with chronic illnesses who require feeding for longer periods of time, occasionally permanently. Nasogastric, nasoduodenal or nasojejunal fine-bore tubes can be used in the short term, while percutaneous catheters sited through pharyngostomy, oesophagostomy, gastrostomy or jejunostomy can be used for longer-term feeding. Indications for using EN include pharyngeal or oesophageal obstruction due to cancer; dysphagia due to neurological diseases; hypercatabolic states associated with injury, trauma and sepsis; mild inflammatory bowel disease and following radiotherapy or chemotherapy. Although generally regarded as safer in terms of complications than total parenteral nutrition (TPN), mechanical, infective, vascular, metabolic and other problems can occur with EN (Table 11.6).

EN: impact on outcomes

Meta-analyses and reviews by Klein et al (1997), Satyanarayana & Klein (1998) have evaluated the use of EN in prospective, randomized controlled trials (PRCTs). Findings were that:

- Two PRCTs evaluating EN administered for 10 days preoperatively via nasogastric tube in comparison with an oral diet. Both found a reduction in major complications, one of which reached statistical significance.

Table 11.6
Artificial nutrition; potential problems associated with EN and TPN

Type of problem	Enteral nutrition	Total parenteral nutrition
Psychological	• Depression, anxiety, disturbed body image in long-term use	• See EN
Mechanical, physical	• Gastro-oesophageal reflux, aspiration pneumonia (nasoenteral catheters) • Stoma site leakage, pneumoperitoneum • Tube obstruction, soft tissue damage • Pressure necrosis at enterostomy site (fixation device related)	• Pneumothorax, air embolism • Catheter breakage, embolism, extravasation • Neural damage arising from catheter misplacement • Catheter obstruction, origin thrombotic, crystalline drug debris, lipid • Biliary sludging, atrophy of gut mucosa
Infective, inflammatory	• Enteral feed contamination • Stoma site sepsis • Intra-abdominal abcess, peritonitis • Necrotizing fascitis	• Sepsis at exit site/tunnel, catheter-related sepsis (CRS) • Endocarditis, osteomyelitis following CRS • Hypersensitivity reactions
Vasular	• Bleeding following insertion, accidental perforation	• Central vein thrombosis, thrombophlebitis • Haemorrhage following insertion
Metabolic	• Disequilibrium of electrolytes in extracellular fluid, osmotic disturbances • Refeeding syndrome • Metabolic acidosis, alkalosis	• Substrate overload, hepatic steatosis • Hyperglycaemia, hypoglycaemia • Zinc, copper, magnesium, chromium, selenium deficiencies (long-term use) • See also EN

The above table lists exemplars; it is not a comprehensive list.

- Postoperative EN administered for 5–10 days via nasojejeunal tube or needle-catheter jejeunostomy. In comparison with an oral diet there was a reduction in major complications in three of four PRCTs.
- Considerable interest has focused on the potential benefits of feeding regimens containing novel nutrients, e.g. arginine, glutamine, n3-fatty acids and micronutrients. Wound healing benefits could arise from the following (McLaren & Green 2001):
  - arginine: enhanced protein synthesis mediated via increased growth hormone, insulin and glucagon secretion
  - glutamine: fuels fibroblast, macrophage and lymphocyte metabolism; reduces free-radical tissue damage via enhanced glutathione synthesis; precursor of proline and, thereby, collagen in fibroblasts
  - n3-fatty acids: precursors of prostaglandin E3 and leukotrienes that exert anti-inflammatory and vasodilatory effects.

Meta-analyses by Heys et al (1999) and Beale et al (1999) of PRCTs comparing standard enteral feeds with those enhanced with novel nutrients found that, while mortality was not significantly affected, reductions in sepsis occurred in the EN intervention groups. Exemplar PRCTs conducted by Kudsk et al (1996) and Senkal et al (1997) compared outcomes in surgical patients receiving isocaloric, isonitrogenous commercially prepared standard feeds with those enhanced with arginine, nucleotides and n3-fatty acids. Lower rates of postoperative infections and wound complications were found in the intervention groups.

Parenteral nutrition

Intravenous feeding via a peripheral or central catheter can be a life-saving intervention in conditions where the gut is non-functional or when enteral feeding alone is insufficient to meet nutritional needs. In the short term, parenteral nutrition (PN) can be used in severe pancreatitis, mucositis following chemotherapy, multi-organ failure and following major surgery (Pennington et al 1996). Longer-term PN is indicated in severe inflammatory bowel disease, radiation enteritis, short bowel syndrome and gut motility disorders.

Use of TPN involves the creation of a portal through which a biocompatible catheter is inserted attached to a sterile infusate via an administration set; a potential for ineffective, mechanical and other problems is therefore apparent (see Table 11.6). Rigorous daily monitoring and use of preventive strategies are necessary to ensure risks are minimized. In the short term, TPN can be administered through a central or peripheral vein and via a number of access devices (e.g. a subcutaneously implanted reservoir). Tunnelling of long-term catheters has been undertaken to reduce sepsis and provide a secure fixation.

TPN: impact on outcomes

Selected findings arising from the analyses of Klein et al (1997) and Satyanarayana & Klein (1998) were as follows:

- In 13 PRCTs evaluating preoperative TPN conducted predominately in malnourished patients, pooled data analyses found a 10% reduction in overall complications in comparison with controls that reached significance in five studies; two PRCTs identified benefits relating to reduced anastomotic leakage and healing timescale.
- In contrast, 9 PRCTs evaluating postoperative TPN alone, predominately in malnourished patients, found a 10% increase in postoperative complications, from 30% to 40%, on analysis of pooled data.

CONCLUSIONS

Because malnutrition can exert negative effects on wound healing and other clinical outcomes, screening for nutritional risk and assessment of nutritional status are both vital steps in the identification of individuals who require nutritional support. A range of techniques accessible with training is available; these can be effective when linked to clear referral systems for specialist review. Nutritional interventions, both oral and artificial, can be used to support patients following identification of their needs. Rigorous monitoring is then necessary to ensure needs continue to be met and to identify any complications at an early stage. Although few would dispute that artificial nutrition has proved to be a valuable and in some cases life-saving intervention, it is not risk free and should not be used indiscriminately. Appropriate quality mechanisms can ensure, for example through evidence-based standards linked to audit and feedback, that the nutritional support provided achieves its aims and improves outcomes for patients, who are at the heart of service delivery.

REFERENCES

Barrocas A, Belcher D, Champagne C, Jastram C 1995 Nutrition assessment: practical approaches. Clinics in Geriatric Medicine 11(4):675–712

Beale R, Bryg D J, Bihari D J 1999 Immuno-nutrition in the critically ill: a systematic review of clinical outcome. Critical Medical Care 27:2799–2805

Bingham S A, Gill C, Welch A et al 1994 Comparison of dietary assessment methods in nutritional epidemiology; weighed food records versus 24 hour recalls, food frequency questionnaires and estimated dietary records. British Journal of Nutrition 72(4):619–643

Breslow R A, Bergstrom N 1994 Nutritional prediction of pressure sores. Journal of the Dietetic Association 94(11):1301–1304

Breslow R A, Hallfrisch J, Guy D G 1993 The importance of dietary protein in healing pressure ulcers. Journal of the American Geriatric Society 41:357–362

British Artificial Nutrition Survey 1999 Trends in home artificial nutrition support in the UK during 1996–1999. British Association for the Parenteral and Enteral Nutrition, Maidenhead, UK

British Association for Parenteral and Enteral Nutrition 1996 Standards and guidelines for nutrition supports of patients in hospitals. BAPEN, Maidenhead, UK

Chu L, Eberhardie C, Forte D et al 1999 An audit of measuring equipment in elderly care. Professional Nurse 14(7):463–466

Department of Health 1991 Dietary reference values for food energy and nutrients for the United Kingdom. Report on Health and Social Subjects No. 41. HMSO, London

Department of Health 1992 The nutrition of elderly people. Report on Health and Social Subjects No. 43. HMSO, London

Detsky A S, McLaughlin J R, Baker J P 1987 What is subjective global assessment of nutritional status? Journal of Parenteral and Enteral Nutrition 11(1):8–13

Downs J H, Hafferjee A 1998 Nutritional assessment in the critically ill. Current Opinion in Clinical Nutrition and Metabolic Care 1(3):275–279

Edington J, Kon P, Martyn C N 1996 Prevalence of malnutrition in patients in general practice. Clinical Nutrition 15:60–63

Edington J, Kon P, Martyn C N 1997 Prevalence of malnutrition after major surgery. Journal of Human Nutrition and Dietetics 10:111–116

Finch S, Doyle W, Lowe C et al 1998 National diet and nutrition survey in people aged > 65 years. HMSO, London

Gibson R S 1993 Principles of nutritional assessment. Oxford University Press, Oxford

Gilmore S A, Robinson G, Posthauer M E, Raymond J 1995 Clinical healthcare associated with unintentional weight loss and pressure ulcers in elderly residents of nursing home facilities. Journal of the American Dietetic Association 95:984–992

Green C J 1999 Existence, causes and consequences of disease-related malnutrition in the hospital and the community and clinical and financial benefits of nutritional intervention. Clinical Nutrition 18(2):3–28

Grindel C G, Costello M C 1996 Nutrition screening: an essential assessment parameter. Medical-Surgical Nursing 5(3):145–156

Guigoz Y, Velles B, Garry P J 1997 Mini-nutritional assessment: a practical assessment tool for grading the nutritional state of elderly patients. Facts, research and intervention in geriatrics. Serdi, Paris, p 15–59

Haydock D A, Hill G L 1986 Impaired wound healing in surgical patients with varying degrees of malnutrition. Journal of Parenteral and Enteral Nutrition 10:550–554

Heys S D, Walker L G, Smith I, Eremin O 1999 Enteral nutritional supplementation with key nutrients in patients with critical illness and cancer: a meta-analysis of randomised controlled clinical trials. Annals of Surgery 229:467–477

Klein S, Kinney J, Jeejeebhoy K et al 1997 Nutritional support in clinical practice: review of published data and recommendations for future research directions. Journal of Parenteral and Enteral Nutrition 21(3):133–156

Kudsk K A, Minard G, Croce M A et al 1996 A randomised trial of isonitrogenous enteral diets after severe trauma: an immune-enhancing diet reduces septic complications. Annals of Surgery 224:531–540

Lobo D N, Allison S P 2000 Nutritional support and functional recovery. Clinical Nutrition 3:129–134

Malnutrition Advisory Group 2000 A screening tool for adults at risk of malnutrition. British Association for Parenteral and Enteral Nutrition, Maidenhead, UK

Maurer J, Weibaum F, Turner J 1996 Reducing the inappropriate use of parenteral nutrition in an acute care teaching hospital. Journal of Parenteral and Enteral Nutrition 20(4):272–274

McAteer C A, Arrowsmith H, McWhirter J et al 1999 Current perspectives on enteral nutrition in adults. BAPEN Publications, Maidenhead, UK

McLaren S 1999 Eating and drinking. In: Ross F, Redfern S (eds) Nursing and older people. Churchill Livingstone, Edinburgh, p 363–394

McLaren S, Green S 1999 Nutritional assessment and screening: instrument selection. British Journal of Community Nursing 3(5):233–242

McLaren S, Green S 2001 Nutritional factors in the aetiology, development and healing of pressure ulcers. In: Morison M (ed) The prevention and treatment of pressure ulcers. Mosby, London

McLaren S, Holmes S, Green S, Bond S 1997 An overview of nutritional issues relating to the care of older people in hospital. In: Bond S (ed) Eating matters. The Centre for Health Services Research, University of Newcastle upon Tyne Publications, UK

McWhirter J P, Pennington C R 1994 Evidence and recognition of malnutrition in hospital. British Medical Journal 308:945–948

Ministry of Agriculture, Fisheries and Food 1997 A photographic atlas of food portion sizes. HMSO, London

Morison M (ed) 2001 The prevention and treatment of pressure ulcers. Mosby, London

Morley J E 1995 Anorexia of ageing and protein-energy malnutrition. In: Morley J E, Glick Z, Rubinstein L Z (eds) Geriatric nutrition: a comprehensive review. Raven Press, New York, p 75–78

Nutrition Screening Initiative (NSI) 1991 Nutritional screening manual for professionals caring for older Americans. NSI, Washington DC

Pattison D, Young A 1997 Effects of a multidisciplinary care team on the management of gastrostomy feeding. Journal of Human Nutrition and Dietetics 10:103–109

Pennington C, Fawcett H, Macfie J et al 1996 Current perspectives on parenteral nutrition in adults. British Association For Parenteral and Enteral Nutrition. BAPEN Publications, Maidenhead, UK

Perry L, McLaren S 2000 An evaluation of implementation of evidence-based guidelines for dysphagia screening and assessment following acute stroke: phase 2 of an evidence-based practice project. Journal of Clinical Excellence 2:147–156

Persson C, Sjoden P O, Glimelius B 1999 The Swedish version of the patient generated subjective global assessment of nutritional status: gastrological versus urological cancers. Clinical Nutrition 18(2):71–77

Reid C L, Carlson G 1998 Indirect calorimetry; a review of recent clinical applications. Current Opinion in Clinical Nutrition and Metabolic Care 1(3):281–286

Reilly H, Martineau J K, Moran A, Kennedy H 1995 Nutritional screening: evaluation and implementation of a simple risk score. Clinical Nutrition 14:269–273

Rombeau J L, Rolandelli R H 1997 Clinical nutrition; enteral and tube feeding, 3rd edn. W B Saunders, London

Satyanarayana R, Klein S 1998 Clinical efficacy of perioperative nutritional support. Current Opinion in Clinical Nutrition and Metabolic Care 1:51–58

Senkal M, Mumme A, Eickoff U et al 1997 Early post-operative enteral immunonutrition: clinical outcome and cost-comparison analysis in surgical patients. Critical Care Medicine 25:1489–1496

Shenkin A 1997 Micronutrients. In: Rombeau J L, Rolandelli R H (eds) Clinical nutrition: enteral and tube feeding, 3rd edn. W B Saunders, London, p 96–111

Shenkin A 1999 Why are vitamins and trace elements needed? Proceedings of the 21st ESPEN Congress. Stockholm, Sweden, p 75–79

Silbermann J 1989 Parenteral and enteral nutrition. Appleton & Lange, New York

Stratton R J, Elia M 1999 A critical systematic analysis of the use of oral nutritional supplements in the community. Clinical Nutrition 18:29–84

Taylor S, McLaren S 1992 Nutritional support: a team approach. Wolfe Publishing, London

The Kings Fund Centre 1992 A positive approach to nutrition as treatment. Report of a Working Party Chaired by Professor J Lennard Jones. Multiplex Ltd, Medway, UK

The Royal College of Nursing (RCN) 1993 Dynamic quality improvement programme: nutrition standards and the older adult. RCN, London

Windsor J A, Knight G S, Hill G L 1988 Wound healing response in surgical patients: recent food intake is more important than nutritional states. British Journal of Surgery 75:133–137

Wolinsky F D, Coe R M, Chavez M N et al 1986 Further assessment of the reliability and validity of a nutritional risk index: analysis of a 3-wave panel study of elderly adults. Health Services Research 20(6):977–998

Wolinsky F D, Coe R M, Chavez M N et al 1990 Progress of the development of a nutritional risk index. Journal of Nutrition 120(11):1549–1553

Wolper C, Heshka S, Heymsfield S B 1997 Measuring food intake: an overview. In: Allison D B (ed) Handbook of assessment methods for eating behaviours and weight related problems. Sage, London, p 215–240

Wright R A, Heymsfield S 1984 Nutritional assessment. Blackwell Scientific Publications, Oxford

FURTHER READING

Allison S 1999 Hospital food as treatment. BAPEN Publications, Maidenhead, UK. *Essential practical guide geared to quality service delivery in nutritional support.*

Bond S 1997 Eating matters. Centre for Health Services Research, University of Newcastle upon Tyne, Newcastle upon Tyne. *Provides a review of practical issues that can be considered in all the stages of nutritional support management.*

Gibson R 1993 Nutritional assessment: a laboratory manual. Oxford University Press, Oxford. *One of the classic texts, which despite the publication date is still relevant and eminently practical.*

Lennard Jones J E 1998 Ethical and legal aspects of clinical hydration and nutritional support. BAPEN Publications, Maidenhead, UK. *Essential reading on the moral aspects of intervention and non-intervention.*

Rombeau J L, Rolandelli R H 1997 Clinical nutrition: enteral and tube feeding, 3rd edn. W B Saunders, London. *The authoritative text on artificial, enteral nutrition.*

CHAPTER

12

Pain assessment and management

David M McNaughton and Sheila M Nimmo

INTRODUCTION

As some degree of pain accompanies most wound healing, achieving the most effective pain control becomes an essential component of holistic care. There is good evidence that poor pain management in a patient with a leg ulcer can adversely affect many aspects of quality of life. In any context, prolonged, unrelieved pain can lead to stress, anger, tiredness and the inability to sleep and rest, and can result in lack of compliance with treatment. This chapter reviews the physiology and assessment of pain and various pharmacological and non-pharmacological treatment options.

THE PHYSIOLOGY OF PAIN

Injury to the body, whether through trauma, underlying disease, or planned surgery, generally results in pain. The body has complex and multisynaptic pathways carrying the pain sensation from the wound site to the brain. These pathways are mediated by neurotransmitters, with suppression and augmentation taking place before the experience of pain is processed by the cerebral cortex and is experienced and can be described.

Nociceptive versus neuropathic pain

There are two distinct types of pain: nociceptive and neuropathic pain. Nociceptive pain is defined as pain generated as a result of injury to body tissues. Neuropathic pain is caused by actual damage to the nerve fibres carrying the pain impulse, the rogue signals generated passing by the same pathways as nociceptive pain to be processed by the brain, before pain is experienced. The use of valid assessment tools can enable clinicians to differentiate the type of pain being experienced and this influences the treatment options.

Algesic substances

Injury to the body causes the manufacture and release of a number of chemicals at the site of injury. The chemicals are called algesic, algogenic or pain-producing substances, and are released into the extracellular fluid that surrounds the nociceptors. These substances include potassium, serotonin, histamine, prostaglandins, bradykinin and substance P. They either stimulate nerve endings at the site of injury or render these nerve endings more sensitive to stimulation. The net result is the generation of a pain impulse, which travels to the dorsal horn of the spinal column and from there via a number of relays to the cerebral cortex where the pain is experienced. This type of pain is termed nociceptive pain.

The different algesics have markedly different ways of generating pain (Table 12.1). They are associated with inflammation, trauma, bone tumours, ischaemia, and a variety of other conditions. In addition to direct excitatory action on the membrane of nociceptors, these agents may have an indirect action by altering the local microcirculation. Some of the analgesics used in everyday practice have an effect on these chemicals and reduce the painful experience by interfering with their release and/or synthesis, as is described later in this chapter.

Pain of mixed aetiology

With some wounds there may be both nociceptive and neuropathic pain. In the case study given in Box 12.1, a diabetic patient reports a stabbing pain with delayed onset. In diabetic patients, the nerves transmitting the painful stimulus can be damaged and this gives rise to neuropathic pain, with the local damage causing the release of a 'soup' of chemicals and stimulating the nociceptors – resulting in nociceptive pain. This is an example of pain of mixed aetiology.

Table 12.1
The effects of algesics on pain receptors

Algesic	Source	Effect on nociceptors
Potassium	Damaged cells	Activates
Serotonin	Platelets	Activates
Bradykinin	Plasma	Activates
Histamine	Mast cells	Activates
Prostaglandins	Arachidonic acid	Sensitizes damaged cells
Leukotrienes	Arachidonic acid	Sensitizes damaged cells
Substance P	C fibre terminals	Sensitizes

Box 12.1
Case study of a diabetic patient with a leg ulcer

Mrs Smith is 88 years old and has a past medical history of diabetes, hypertension and stroke. She is currently taking the following medication: glipizide, atenolol 100 mg, aspirin 150 mg, and nitrazepam 5 mg. She presents at her GP's surgery with a leg ulcer 5 cm in diameter and reports that the pain has been getting worse for a month and is becoming unbearable. She cannot bear cloth touching the wound and any slight pressure gives a shooting pain up her leg after a short delay.

The second case study (Box 12.2) involves a young woman who is suffering from neuropathic pain following amputation, as a result of nerve endings being trapped in the scar tissue.

Box 12.2
Case study of a young adult with a below-knee amputation, following a traumatic road traffic accident

Ms Logan is a 28-year-old student with a past medical history of asthma precipitated by aspirin. 18 months ago she fell badly while walking home from a night-club and landed on the roadway. When trying to crawl back onto the pavement the lower part of her left leg was run over by a car. This caused a crush injury of such severity that the only recourse was a below-knee amputation. She reports pain that she says 'feels like it is coming from my foot – but it can't be – my foot is not there.'

She is currently taking the following medication: salbutamol, beclometasone, and co-proxamol.

The third case study (Box 12.3) illustrates how pain can result from adhesions.

Box 12.3
Case study of an elderly man with pain resulting from adhesions

Mr West is 72 years old and has a past medical history of acute and frequent chest pain and repeated surgery for coronary artery bypass grafting with a total of four operations in the chest cavity. He is currently taking the following medication: digoxin 0.125 mg, isosorbide mononitrate 40 mg b.d., nicorandil 30 mg b.d., co-proxamol 2 q.d.s., furosemide (frusemide) 80 mg. He presents at his GP's surgery for a routine visit reporting pain of angina but also pain on movement, which has been getting worse. The pain is localized to an area under the scar tissue and on questioning is described as shooting on occasion with a burning pain underlying at all times.

THE PAIN PATHWAY

The pain pathways should be understood in the context of the complex of peripheral nerve fibres. The peripheral sensory system is classified into three groups of neurons: A, B and C. This classification is based on their cross-sectional area. Table 12.2 illustrates the functions and characteristics of the nerve fibres.

Table 12.2
The functions and characteristics of nerve fibres

Type of fibre	Where they work	Mean diameter (μm)	Mean conductivity velocity (m/s)
A-alpha (efferent)	Activate skeletal muscle	12–20	70–120
A-beta (afferent)	Touch and pressure on the skin	5–15	30–70
A-gamma (efferent)	Activate muscle	6–8	15–30
A-delta (afferent)	The feeling of cold/ heat and pain	1–4	12–30
B	Sympathetic nervous system	1–3	3–15
C (afferent)	The feeling of heat/ cold and pain (but these are slow fibres)	0.5–1.5	0.5–2

The activation of nociceptors results in electrical activity in both the A-delta and C fibres. These fibres connect to the dorsal horn of the spinal cord and then to the medulla. The neurotransmitters for these primary nociceptive afferents are peptides such as substance P and calcitonin-gene-related peptide (CGRP).

Two sets of nerve fibre are involved in passing the painful impulse to the dorsal horn of the spinal column, which explains why two types of pain are experienced when injury occurs. The first pain occurs immediately after injury and is transmitted by the A-delta fibres. This pain is often described as being sharp and localized, and lasts for 3 to 5 min. This is generally followed by a pain-free interval of 5 to 10 min. At about 10 min the second pain begins and is often described as dull, aching and burning. The C fibres transmit this pain.

Nociceptive afferents described in Table 12.2 terminate on second-order neurons in the dorsal horn of the spinal cord or medulla. The second-order neurons ascend the spinal cord to synapse on third-order neurons in the brain. The second-order neurons in the spinal cord are grouped into layers called rexed laminae. There are ten rexed laminae; six in the dorsal horn, three in the ventral horn, and one in the central canal of the spinal cord. The A-delta fibres terminate primarily in laminae I and V, the C fibres primarily in lamina II and the A-beta fibres primarily in laminae III and IV.

Inhibitory interneurons and a rich diversity of neurotransmitters are present in the dorsal horn. The dorsal horn thus serves as a modulated gate through which all pain impulses must travel. It plays a prominent role in pain processing. Thus there is a balance of painful impulses passing up through the dorsal horn to the medulla and an inhibitory process taking place, which suppresses these impulses from progressing upwards.

The 'gate theory' of pain

The most influential theory to explain the balance of painful excitation and inhibition was propounded by Melzack & Wall (1965). Their 'gate theory' is a useful way of explaining the cognitive and multidimensional aspects of the pain experience and also goes a long way to explain the successes of some of the complementary therapies.

Figure 12.1 shows a simplistic view of the gate theory. When a painful area is massaged or a TENs machine is used the A-beta fibres are stimulated. There are cells in the dorsal horn that inhibit and facilitate pain transmission.

Referring back to the three case studies in Boxes 12.1–12.3, it is now possible to explain how the pain impulse is transmitted from receptors to the brain and how it can be modified. The A-delta and the C fibres carry pain information. Stimulation of the A-beta fibres has an excitatory effect on the substantia gelatinosa (SG) cells and this in turn inhibits the T cells located in lamina V that transmit impulses to the contralateral thalamus. This effect is called 'closing the gate' to pain.

GENERAL PRINCIPLES OF PAIN ASSESSMENT

In any painful condition, and particularly in wound pain, it is important to help patients to describe their pain. This provides a baseline for gauging the effects of any analgesia offered, and is also valuable in allowing some measure of control to be retained by the patient.

The main objectives of a good assessment are to:

- identify the cause of the pain, as a precursor to deciding on appropriate treatment

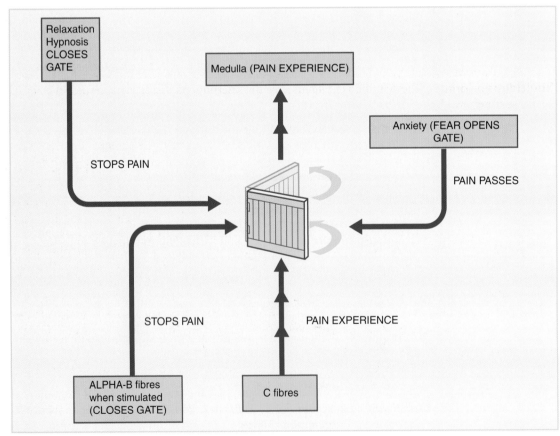

Figure 12.1
A simplistic view of the gate theory of pain

- gain objective understanding of a subjective experience
- encourage communication, trust and patient participation
- promote a systematic approach, to assist in the identification of a possible pattern of pain experience.

Lack of appropriate assessment tools and skills can lead to the following problems:

- collection of inaccurate data, which then leads to the possible omission of critical information
- making assumptions and stereotyping – pain is an individual experience
- making decisions too quickly, resulting in inappropriate treatment options.

Atkinsanya (1985) argues that, as pain is a totally subjective experience, it is questionable whether it is sensible to attempt a verbal definition that will be universally acceptable. However, there are a variety of ways in which the health-care professional can attempt to gain an accurate picture of the patient's pain experience, including:

- direct observation of the patient
- using pain assessment tools
- interviewing the patient and discussing the patient's interpretation of the causes of pain, exacerbating factors and their coping strategies.

These approaches should not be used in isolation but should be holistic, a 'combination of coordination, communication and liaison' (Munafo & Trim 2000).

Pain as a 'multidimensional experience'

Any approach to pain assessment and management should take into account the definition of pain used by the International Association for the Study of Pain (1979, 1982), which is:

> An unpleasant sensory and emotional experience associated with actual or potential tissue damage, or described in terms of such damage.

Far from being a simple physiological process, pain is a complex 'multidimensional' experience. It is important to take account of a number of factors in pain management, and the patient's emotional state is as important as the extent and type of wound giving rise to the pain. Consideration should also be given in the assessment process to the inclusion of factors, such as social and psychological issues, for example the activities that have been given up because of pain and the presence of other stressful life events, as these factors may exacerbate pain.

Pain varies according to the site and extent of the wound. For example, surgical wounds to the joints, abdomen and chest are usually quite painful in the early postoperative period. However, patients with a similar cause for their pain may actually report pain of widely differing intensities. Pain is therefore what patients say they feel:

> pain is whatever the experiencing person says it is, existing whenever he says it does. (McCaffery & Beebe 1994)

The assessment of pain involves recording patient perceptions of pain, which can be modulated by many factors.

The significance of the wound can affect the emotional and psychological response to the pain experience. For example, a mastectomy wound can induce physical and psychological problems for the patient, which can in turn influence the pain experience. A surgical scar can be a constant reminder of an underlying life-threatening disease, such as cancer. Scars from burns or accidents can be a reminder of a traumatic event or perhaps the loss of a loved one. Awareness of these problems enables the practitioner to develop sympathetic and supportive counselling skills that will assist in the achievement of effective pain control.

Essentials of the pain assessment process

In the assessment process, consideration of the following factors should enable the collection of relevant data by the healthcare professional in order to gain an accurate assessment of the patient's individual pain experience:

- Patient empowerment can have a positive effect on pain relief, therefore include and work with the patient to plan realistic goals that will improve quality of life.
- When appropriate, and specifically in the arena of chronic pain, try to involve the family in the assessment process. Relatives and carers can often report a more realistic picture of the patient's daily pain experience.
- Always take into account pre-existing medical problems and medication regimes, which may influence the pain experience and possible treatment regimes.
- Consider a multidisciplinary approach to pain relief, the participation of staff from other disciplines can contribute to a more successful outcome.
- Avoid the 'pain/fear of pain' cycle. If a procedure such as a dressing change is likely to be painful, analgesia should be offered before the procedure is carried out. This will also help to reduce any pain in the wound after the dressing has been changed.

Effective communication in the assessment process

Effective communication between professionals is important to facilitate the 'smooth' running of a multidisciplinary approach to pain control. It is also important to reflect on factors that might interfere with patient/practitioner communication.

Hawthorn & Redmond (1998) consider that the following factors can contribute to poor communication:

- ward duty rotas, which can compromise continuity of the staff/patient relationship
- using medical jargon inappropriately with patients, which can lead to misunderstandings and lack of comprehension
- language problems, which mean that not all patients find it easy to express themselves, and English may not be their first language
- general physical discomfort accompanied by stress and anxiety, which can have a detrimental effect on the patient's level of concentration during assessment
- impaired cognitive ability, which can adversely affect the patient's ability to express and describe their pain.

It is also important to remember to use open questions when asking about a patient's pain: 'Can you rate your pain today from 0 to 10 – with 10 the most severe?' gives a much more useful and real measure of the patient's experience of pain than 'How is the pain today?'. The healthcare professional should also ask specific questions to address the following dimensions of the pain:

- location
- intensity
- pattern
- onset
- is the pain intermittent or continuous?
- what makes the pain better or worse?
- the effects of the pain on the patient's ability to fulfil activities of living.

The healthcare professional should also be aware of non-verbal behaviour, which may indicate pain. Acute pain can often be manifested by restlessness, sweating, pallor and raised pulse.

The use of validated pain assessment tools

A number of assessment tools can be used to measure pain and some are suitable for use in assessing pain related to a wound. Some of these tools are described below. They can enable patients to express their individual pain experience more easily and in a manner that is understood by both the practitioner and client.

The McGill Pain Questionnaire

The McGill Pain Questionnaire (MPQ) was developed at the McGill University, Canada, by Melzack and Torgerson (1971); a short form of the questionnaire was developed some 16 years later for more general use (Melzack 1987) (Figure 12.2). The MPQ is a multidimensional pain scale that offers a validated tool for evaluating mainly chronic pain. It is the gold standard against which other pain-scoring models are compared and can be administered to patients whose wound pain has moved from acute to chronic (duration more than 6 months).

The MPQ is based on 78 adjectives from which patients can chose combinations that describe their pain experience. These adjectives are assigned numerical values and patients receive pain scores according to the number of adjectives chosen and the strength of pain they have described. The short form of the MPQ contains the following 15 adjectives:

- throbbing
- shooting
- stabbing
- sharp
- cramping
- gnawing
- hot – burning
- aching
- heavy
- tender
- splitting
- tiring – exhausting
- sickening
- fearful
- punishing – cruel.

McGill - Melzack Pain Questionnaire

Patient's name: _____ Date _____ Time: _____ AM/PM

Analgesic(s): _____ Dosage _____ Time given: _____ AM/PM

Dosage: _____ Time given: _____ AM/PM

Analgesic Time Difference (Hours): +4   +1   +2   +3

PRI: S _____   A _____   E _____   M(S) _____   M(AE) _____   M(T) _____   PR(T) _____
       (1-10)   (11-15)   (16)   (17-19)   (20)   (17-20)   (1-20)

1 FLICKERING	11 TIRING
QUIVERING	EXHAUSTING
PULSING	12 SICKENING
THROBBING	SUFFOCATING
BEATING	13 FEARFUL
POUNDING	FRIGHTFUL
2 JUMPING	TERRIFYING
FLASHING	14 PUNISHING
SHOOTING	GRUELLING
3 PRICKING	CRUEL
BORING	VISCIOUS
DRILLING	KILLING
STABBING	15 WRETCHED
LANCINATING	BLINDING
4 SHARP	16 ANNOYING
CUTTING	TROUBLESOME
LACERATING	MISERABLE
5 PINCHING	INTENSE
PRESSING	UNBEARABLE
GNAWING	17 SPREADING
CRAMPING	RADIATING
CRUSHING	PENETRATING
6 TUGGING	PIERCING
PULLING	18 TIGHT
WRENCHING	NUMB
7 HOT	DRAWING
BURNING	SQUEEZING
SCALDING	TEARING
SEARING	19 COOL
8 TINGLING	COLD
ITCHY	FREEZING
SMARTING	20 NAGGING
STINGING	NAUSEATING
9 DULL	AGONISING
SORE	DREADFUL
HURTING	TORTURING
ACHING	
HEAVY	PPI
10 TENDER	0 NO PAIN
TAUT	1 MILD
RASPING	2 DISCOMFORTING
SPLITTING	3 DISTRESSING
	4 HORRIBLE
	5 EXCRUCIATING

PPI: _____   COMMENTS:

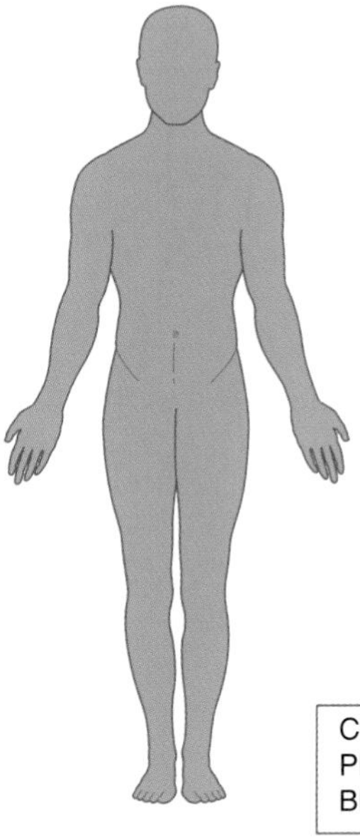

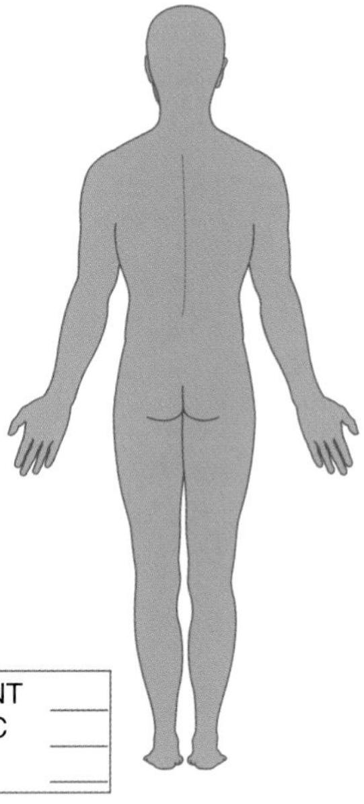

CONSTANT _____
PERIODIC _____
BRIEF _____

ACCOMPANYING
SYMPTOMS:
NAUSEA _____
HEADACHE _____
DIZZINESS _____
DROWSINESS _____
CONSTIPATION _____
DIARRHOEA _____
COMMENTS:

SLEEP:
GOOD _____
FITFUL _____
CAN'T SLEEP _____
COMMENTS:

ACTIVITY:
GOOD _____
SOME _____
LITTLE _____
NONE _____

FOOD INTAKE:
GOOD _____
SOME _____
LITTLE _____
NONE _____
COMMENTS:

Figure 12.2
The McGill–Melzack pain questionnaire

These in turn are rated on a scale of intensity: 0 = no pain, 1 = mild pain, 2 = moderate pain and 3 = severe pain. The severity of pain can be calculated by weighting the adjectives and, in turn, by the weighting applied to each term.

Although the MPQ can take about half an hour to complete, the short-form MPQ can be completed in a couple of minutes and has been shown to be comparable to the MPQ in its results (Melzack 1987). It is important to stress that the values achieved for the Pain Rating Index (the total of the scores) is not important as such but is relevant on repeat assessments to monitor change in pain experienced. Both the MPQ and the short form, however, do require a developed vocabulary and for many patients the use of a much simpler tool is required.

Visual analogue scales

This is one of the simplest pain assessment methods and allows a patient to score by marking a point on a continuous line from no pain to worst pain imaginable. This has been modified by using faces from sad to happy as the end points and by using colours to describe pain, for example white to red.

Professor Swanston and colleagues at the University of Abertay, Dundee, (Swanston et al 1993), have developed a graphic tool (WindowPain) that uses computer technology to present moveable graphics to represent different types of pain. There are graphics to represent pressure, burning, throbbing and piercing pain, and the graphics automatically record a value between (0 and 100) for each type of pain (Fig. 12.3). There is also a computer-generated visual analogue scale incorporated in the package. This program is being used extensively in the pain clinics supported by the Abertay Pain Management Research Centre and is particularly useful for patients whose first language is not English. The WindowPain program has been successfully validated using the MPQ as a comparator.

Pain diaries

Pain diaries represent another useful tool in the armoury of pain management. These diaries can help patients best understand their own progress through healing and, when medication is recorded alongside the pain, provide valuable clues to the medical and nursing staff as to the success of the treatment prescribed.

Differential diagnosis using pain-assessment tools

The use of descriptors in both the MPQ and in the WindowPain assessment tools allows some degree of differential diagnosis to be carried out. It is possible to differentiate neuropathic pain from nociceptive pain and to adjust the treatment options accordingly. When terms like 'burning pain' and 'shooting pain' are rated with large numeric values there is the probability of pain being neurogenic in origin. If it is suspected that a pain is predominantly neuropathic it has a marked effect on the choice of medication used. The treatment options are discussed later in the chapter.

Assessment tools as a means of treatment evaluation

Although it is important that the practitioner is aware of the strengths and limitations of different assessment tools, the utilization of such tools in the assessment process should be considered as an effective way of monitoring the results of interventions and can be used to titrate analgesic doses.

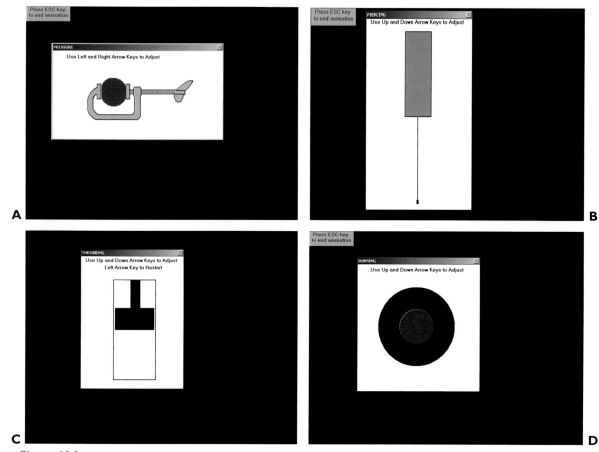

Figure 12.3
(A) WindowPain: pressure; (B) WindowPain: piercing; (C) WindowPain: throbbing; (D) WindowPain: burning.
(From Swanston et al 1993)

TREATMENT OPTIONS IN PAIN MANAGEMENT

A number of pharmacological and non-pharmacological treatment options are described below. It should be borne in mind that pain is a very personal experience, which is influenced by emotional, cognitive and environmental factors, the degree of stress and anxiety the patient is experiencing and previous experience of pain. This is why pharmacological treatments are just one aspect of pain management. A reduction in anxiety and in stress can help patients cope with a painful episode. Research has shown that pain can be reduced by information-giving and patient empowerment. This is why a holistic approach to treatment, based on a sound assessment of the patient, is so important.

Pharmacological treatment options

Medications used in pain management can be broadly divided into two major groups: narcotic medications and non-steroidal anti-inflammatory drugs (NSAIDs).

Narcotic analgesics

Narcotic analgesics may be classified as follows:

- Opiate analgesics: often used in acute pain management following injury. They fall into two broad categories:
  (i) those derived from opium alkaloids, e.g. morphine and codeine
  (ii) semisynthetic congeners of morphine, e.g. diamorphine, dihydrocodeine and pholcodine.
- Non-opiate, morphine-like analgesics: e.g. pethidine, methadone, dipipanone, dextromoramide, dextropropoxyphene, pentazocine, diphenoxylate, tramadol.

Mechanism of action. In the central nervous system (CNS), opiate analgesics bind to specific opioid receptors and act as partial and complete agonists, mimicking the effects of the endogenous encephalins that normally bind to those receptors. This results in a variety of different effects, each of which depends on the area of brain affected and the physiological function of that area. For example, the analgesic effects are thought to be mediated by the binding of opiate analgesics to those areas involved in the perception of pain in the spinal cord, spinal trigeminal nucleus, periaqueductal and periventricular grey matter. A multiplicity of CNS effects results from the actions of opiates on various areas of the brain and spinal cord, including:

- analgesia
- drowsiness
- mood change – usually euphoria
- respiratory depression
- nausea and vomiting
- lowering of temperature
- decreased sympathetic outflow
- pupillary constriction.

Codeine, dihydrocodeine and dextropropoxyphene are weak opioid analgesics and are commonly administered in fixed-dose combinations with paracetamol. They can form a convenient step-up from simple analgesics such as paracetamol alone. While usually safe, problems can occur when patients take additional paracetamol. Dextropropoxyphene-induced respiratory depression is only poorly reversed by the opioid antagonist naloxone.

The opioid drugs offer a good choice in pain relief by suppressing the pain pathway. It is possible to give large doses of opioids and these medications are a mainstay in the treatment of pain of all types.

The non-steroidal anti-inflammatory drugs (NSAIDs)

The NSAIDs comprise a group of medications used for mild to moderate pain. NSAIDs are most effective in providing analgesia in pain syndromes that are associated with inflammatory conditions. It is important to note that NSAIDs do not give rise to tolerance or physical dependence. This offers an important advantage over the narcotic analgesics. Although the NSAIDs are often used alone in treating pain they can be used in combination with the opioid analgesics and indeed with tricyclic antidepressants (which are used in the treatment of neuropathic pain; see the following section).

Mechanism of action. The NSAIDs produce analgesia by decreasing the production of prostaglandin, particularly PGE_2, through inhibition of the enzyme called cyclo-oxygenase. With inflammatory conditions (such as rheumatoid arthritis), prostaglandins are among the cellular products that are produced and released. The prostaglandins that are released subsequently sensitize the peripheral nociceptors and thereby elicit the pain response. By inhibiting prostaglandin synthesis, the NSAIDs inhibit peripheral nociceptor sensitization and this results in decrease pain perception.

The inhibition of cyclo-oxygenase has a mixed bag of effects, including pain reduction. However, a raft of adverse effects is also attributable to the traditional NSAIDs. Side-effects of NSAIDs include:

- gastric irritation
- prolongation of bleeding time
- CNS stimulation – with salicylate overdose, e.g. tinnitus
- renal dysfunction
- allergic hypersensitivity reactions, e.g. urticaria
- hepatic dysfunction usually reversible
- fluid retention and oedema.

The main classes of NSAIDs are summarized in Table 12.3. The most dangerous side-effect of the traditional NSAIDs is the propensity to cause gastric erosion and bleeding. In recent years, much work has focused on this adverse effect and the mode of action of the NSAIDs in both pain reduction and gastric erosion. It has been found that there are at least two distinct types of prostaglandin involved when cyclo-oxygenase is inhibited by an NSAID (Needleman & Isakson 1998). The cyclo-oxygenase found in the gastric tract (COX_1) is involved in the synthesis of prostaglandin PGE_1, which is a constituent prostaglandin involved in the maintenance of the gastric mucosa. Thus it is intrinsically involved in protecting the stomach wall from acid attack. When traditional NSAIDs are used, this COX_1 is also inhibited and the production of PGE_1 reduced. This renders the gastric wall more susceptible to acid attack and can result in a serious gastric bleed. The cyclo-oxygenase identified as associated with the inflammatory process is synthesized only when injury occurs and has been identified as cyclo-oxygenase 2 (COX_2). It has been possible for COX_2-specific NSAIDs to be developed and these new drugs seem likely to provide a big step towards the goal of an effective anti-inflammatory analgesic with no gastric effects.

Pharmacokinetics of NSAIDs. The different NSAIDs possess similar absorption characteristics. They are absorbed rapidly after both oral and rectal administration, are highly protein bound and are metabolized primarily in the liver. There are marked differences in duration of action, however. Drugs such as ibuprofen require a dose every 4–6 h to retain a therapeutic level, whereas piroxicam is administered once a day.

The NSAIDs are particularly valuable in treating wounds with an inflammatory aspect. They can be used in combination with the opioids and with other therapies.

Paracetamol is a centrally acting cyclo-oxygenase inhibitor that is an effective and widely used analgesic in mild and moderate pain, but the peripheral anti-inflammatory properties of the drug are minimal. Paracetamol is generally safe, with an absence of gastric and haematological effects, and it is suitable for all age groups ≥ 3 months. Major problems arise with overdosage: metabolic pathways are easily saturated, resulting in the formation of hepatotoxic metabolites. The early administration of acetylcysteine can substantially reduce the incidence of fatal hepatic necrosis in paracetamol overdose.

Table 12.3
Classes of NSAIDs

Aspirin	
Acetic acid derivatives	Diclofenac, indometacin, sulindac
Propionic acid derivatives	Ibuprofen, fenoprofen, ketoprofen, flurbiprofen, naproxen
Oxicam derivatives	Piroxicam
Pyrazolone derivatives	Phenylbutazone
Anthranilic acid derivatives	Mefenamic acid
Naphthyl-alkanones	Nabumetone
Coxibs	Celecoxib, rofecoxib

Patient-controlled analgesia

The use of patient-controlled analgesia (PCA) gives control of postoperative and other pain to the patient (Ballantyne et al 1993). Because the patient is in control, any anxiety about availability of analgesia can be banished. PCA usually utilizes a syringe driver filled with medication, which is connected to a subcutaneous or intravenous catheter. The syringe is programmed to deliver a small bolus dose of medication on the patient's command (by pressing a button). To prevent overdosage a 'lock-out' period is set before the button press will deliver medication again. Provided patients are well informed about how to use such analgesia, this type of opiate administration can give effective and reliable pain relief, especially in the arena of postoperative wound care, when patients may be on nil orally. It is important, however, that patients receiving such pain relief are monitored regularly for the effects of sedation, respiratory depression, nausea and vomiting. As successful pain relief with PCA is dependent on effective patient education, it is of benefit only after elective surgery. The use of PCA allows a cocktail of medications to be used in the syringe driver. Medications can be added to act as antinauseants to counteract the nausea associated with the use of opioids. Adjunctive therapies can be added in the form of anaesthetic agents to assist in pain control and opioid antagonists can be used in low doses to counteract the adverse effects of the opioids.

Inhaled analgesia

An inhaled analgesic, such as Entonox, may be administered for burns patients, during dressing changes or if the patient requires to be moved. The constituents in Entonox are nitrous oxide 50% and oxygen 50%. Nitrous oxide is a weak anaesthetic with strong analgesic properties. It is absorbed rapidly on inhalation and, because the blood/gas coefficient is low, most of the inhaled nitrous oxide is rapidly eliminated through the lungs. It thus has a very short half-life so is only suitable for short-term use. It is the medication of choice for use at the scenes of accidents, where paramedical staff can administer it to the injured to give immediate pain relief.

General principles to consider in the selection of appropriate analgesia

The choice of analgesic will depend on a number of factors, which include:

- type and source of pain (neuropathic versus nociceptive)
- degree of pain reported
- degree of inflammation
- medical history and condition of the patient
- pain history
- cognitive control.

Neuropathic pain

For the treatment of neuropathic pain, a mainstay has been the use of tricyclic antidepressant (TCA) medications, with other treatments such as antiepileptic drugs also being used. The rationale for the use of TCAs and antiepileptics is to suppress the inappropriate nerve transmission of painful stimuli that is the hallmark of damaged nerves. The most common example of pain of neuropathic origin is post-herpetic neuralgia. This is a pain associated with shingles that does not disappear after the shingles attack is over. The cause is damage to the nerves that is still present even after the causative agent (the herpes virus) has been eradicated. Another example is the pain associated with diabetic ulcers, where tissue and nerve damage overlays the nociceptive pain experienced by the local inflammatory process. These types of pain can respond very well to TCAs and antiepileptic medications. Often, diabetic ulcers need to be treated as pain of mixed aetiology with a regimen of opioid medication and TCAs used.

Nocioceptive pain

Most wound pain will be nociceptive in origin and the World Health Organization (1996) has published an analgesic ladder that forms the backbone of any treatment protocol. Starting with simple analgesia on the first step (paracetamol), and with the addition of an NSAID, the next step is a mild opioid (codeine, dihydrocodeine), often in combination with paracetamol, and the third step is a strong opioid (morphine, diamorphine, etc.).

Healthcare professionals working in specialist areas, using a flow chart and continuous assessment guidelines, may develop similar analgesic ladders appropriate to their specialism. The implementation of analgesic ladders and stepwise management guidelines can facilitate the planning and implementation of more appropriate individualized pain control. It should be stressed, however, that the developments of specific pain management algorithms for specialist areas should be evidence-based and refer to relevant existing guidelines and protocols.

OTHER METHODS OF PAIN RELIEF

It is important that healthcare professionals remember simple measures, which may well assist in the alleviation of pain. Such measures include repositioning, warm or cold packs, relaxation techniques, massage or diversion techniques. As indicated earlier, information-giving can also reduce patient anxiety and can lessen the pain experience. Pressure-relieving aids are also effective in lessening physical discomfort when patients have considerable exudate from wounds, such as those with extensive burns.

Complementary therapies can also have a part to play. Further sources of information on these therapies are given in Box 12.4.

Box 12.4
Some useful sources of information about complementary and other therapies

British Acupuncture Council
63 Jeddo Road, London W12 9HQ
   e-mail: info@acupuncture.org.uk
   website: www.acupuncture.org.uk

British Homeopathic Association
27 Devonshire Street, London W1N 1RJ
   website: www.nhsconfed.net/bha/

continued

Box 12.4
continued

General Chiropractic Council
334–354 Grays Inn Road, London WCIX 8BP
website:www.gcc-uk.org

General Osteopathic Council
176 Tower Bridge Road, London SE1 3LU
website: www.osteopathy.org.uk

The following are specialist web-based sources
www.iasp-pain.org
The International Association for the Study of Pain is an international, multidisciplinary, non-profit professional association dedicated to furthering research on pain and improving the care of patients with pain. Membership of IASP is open to scientists, physicians, dentists, psychologists, healthcare professionals, physical therapists and other health professionals actively engaged in pain research, and to those who have special interest in the diagnosis and treatment of pain.

www.pain.com
An American pain site with excellent references.

The following gateways are a useful approach to searching the internet for healthcare-related matters:
CliniWeb: www.ohsu.edu/cliniweb/
Healthgate: www3.healthgate.com
Medical Matrix: www.medmatrix.org/index.asp

CONCLUSIONS

This chapter has provided an overview of the many issues that should be addressed in the achievement of effective pain control. The following key points should assist the reader to reflect on the general principles of good pain control, which are applicable in any context:

- comprehensive assessment is imperative to enable effective interventions to be selected
- pain is a multidimensional experience
- the patient's own interpretation of pain is important
- measurement tools provide useful objective data
- patients should be encouraged to take part in their own care, this may improve their general well-being
- if possible, an inclusive approach should be adopted towards relatives and carers
- pain control should be monitored regularly
- management of pain in children and elderly requires special consideration.

As healthcare professionals, it is our responsibility to plan and implement the most effective pain control possible for patients and to employ a multidisciplinary approach to care, whenever possible.

A glossary of terms used in pain management is given in Box 12.5, for reference.

Box 12.5 *A glossary of terms used in pain management*

Acute pain, pain of recent and limited duration

Afferent pathways, carry information to the brain

Agonist, a substance that acts at a cell receptor

Algesic substances, substances produced in the body as a result of injury, they either stimulate or potentiate the nociceptors

Analgesia, pain relief

Antagonist, a substance that blocks a cell receptor

Autonomic nervous system, the nervous system that is *not* under cognitive control

Bradykinin, an algesic substance

Chronic pain, pain lasting for a long period of time – persisting beyond the time of normal healing

Dysphoria, reduced feeling of well-being

Efferent pathways, carry information to the periphery and organ groups

Euphoria, enhanced feeling of well-being

Fascia, connective tissue

Histamine, algesic and inflammatory substance

Mydriasis, dilated optic pupil

Neuropathic pain, pain caused by injury to the nerve pathways (peripheral or central)

Nociceptive pain, pain arising from stimulation of the peripheral nociceptors

NSAIDs, drugs that inhibit the enzyme cyclo-oxygenase and in turn reduce the production of protanoids (which sensitize nociceptors after injury)

Opioid, a term used for substances that act like morphine

Periosteum, tissue covering a bone

Prostaglandins, produced as a result of tissue damage – algesic substances

Topical rubefacients, act by counterirritation of the skin, often useful in muscular–skeletal pain

Serotonin, an algesic substance and neurotransmitter

SP, substance P, an algesic substance

REFERENCES

Ballantyne J C, Carr D B, Chalmers T C et al 1993 Postoperative patient controlled analgesia: meta analysis of initial randomised controlled trials. Journal of Clinical Anaesthesia 5:182–193

Hawthorn J, Redmond K 1998 Pain causes and management. Blackwell Science, Oxford

Hutchcroft B M 1999 The patient's perception of chronic pain. Professional Healthcare Professional 15(1):26

McCaffery M, Beebe A 1994 Pain: clinic manual for nursing practice. C V Mosby, London

Melzack R 1987 The short-form McGill Pain Questionnaire. Pain 30:191–197

Melzack R, Wall P 1965 Pain mechanisms: a new theory. Science 150:971–979

Melzack R, Torgerson W S 1971 On the language of pain. Anaesthesiology 34:40–49

Munafo M, Trim J 2000 Chronic pain, a handbook for healthcare professionals. Butterworth Heinmann, Oxford

Needleman P, Isakson P C 1998 Selective inhibition of cyclo-oxygenase 2. Science and Medicine Jan/Feb:26–35

Swanston M, Abraham C, Macrae W A et al 1993 Pain 53(3):347–351

World Health Organization 1996 Cancer pain relief, 2nd edn. World Health Organization, Geneva

CHAPTER

13

Health promotion and patient education

Nancy Tomaselli

INTRODUCTION

Despite the significant growth in health education driven by rising healthcare costs and managed care organizations, education in wound prevention and treatment is lacking. Part of the problem is that wound care is not considered a specialty, so patients often do not know where to turn to find information. Many healthcare providers are not taught specifics about prevention and treatment of wounds and, consequently, do not educate patients in this area. Physicians readily admit that wound care is not part of their residency education and often rely on nurses to educate them and their patients.

Patient education is essential for wound care. However, with limited time and resources, making sure patients get the appropriate information to ensure positive outcomes remains a challenge. It is critical that the information provided helps prevent complications, promotes self care and independence, empowers the caregiver and reduces readmissions. The time available for patient education will vary in different care settings from a few days in acute care, a few minutes in outpatient care to an hour in a home care setting.

For patient teaching to be effective, modalities must be used to ensure patients comprehend the material and apply it to their individual needs. The charge for healthcare professionals is to provide innovative teaching strategies that are easily understood, cost-effective and adaptable for all care settings. How quickly information can be delivered depends on the patient or caregiver's level of comprehension and ability to understand and demonstrate the tasks. Caregivers provide a large percentage of care for home care services. Many of these caregivers are elderly and have their own health problems or are reluctant to assist with care.

Patient education requires more than one teaching tool and can include written instructions along with diagrams and reinforcement with verbal instruction.

Other tools may include the internet, computer software programs, TV, newspaper, videos, tape players, written materials, community-based programmes or websites and local experts among others. The challenge is to find patient education materials that are credible.

Patient teaching is also driven by guidelines from payer, regulator and accreditor standards and policies. Therefore, documentation is essential and should include the content of the teaching sessions, description of education materials provided, and the learner's response to instruction (Twitchell 1999). Education is endorsed by managed care organizations and is considered critical to prevention of illness.

HEALTH PROMOTION

The main goal of health promotion is to encourage individuals to take responsibility for improving their own health. People of all ages, including those with chronic comorbidities and disabilities, can achieve a high level of wellness. The focus of health promotion is on optimal mental and physical health rather than specific disorders.

Health promotion is emphasized by the media and schools, and by community programmes, which empower individuals to take charge of their own health. However, healthcare professionals can be challenged by patients and/or caregivers, who question them regarding conflicting information in the media. In addition, individuals may be unmotivated to achieve mutually set goals.

Primary prevention is similar to heath promotion but focuses on specific disorders. Bietz (1998) proports the emphasis of primary prevention to be protection of the body from specific disease entities such as diabetes. This process requires active participation by the patient. To seek out this participation, healthcare providers must convince people that it is worth it to make the effort to stay healthy. Healthcare professionals must develop effective teaching strategies for specific specialty areas of practice. This requires specific skills on the part of the educator. These skills are enumerated later in this chapter. This is certainly an area where prevention modalities for wounds can be instituted in a teaching programme. For instance, a patient might prevent a diabetic ulcer if they participate actively in maintaining normal blood glucose levels.

PATIENT EDUCATION

The nursing process is an ideal format for patient education. This framework can be used to:

- assess the need for education
- assess readiness to learn
- plan and develop an individualized programme
- implement the programme
- document and evaluate patient education.

Assessment

Assessing the need for education depends upon the patient problems. Factors associated with these problems are discussed below.

The assessment of readiness to learn is the most difficult, as the programme will not be effective if the patient is not ready to learn. Factors to assess include:

- awareness of risk factors and diagnosis
- previous knowledge and experience

- intellectual level
- motivation level
- physical condition
- psychological state
- perceived need to learn.

Nurses must also understand how physiological changes in ageing affect learning. Older patients will fatigue more easily, and have decreased energy levels, strength and speed, which all affect endurance. They also have visual changes, such as loss of visual acuity and peripheral vision, and problems with glare. Make sure the lighting is good, reduce glare and use materials with large print. Hearing loss is also very common, and they may need more time to process the information. Speak slowly, distinctly and face the patient.

Some patients have problems with short-term memory, which creates anxiety and exacerbates the problem affecting their ability to learn. Written instructions and calendars can assist with memory loss. Patients will remember what they consider to be important or of interest to them.

Psychological aspects must also be considered. If patients experience stress or anxiety, they will often not be able to focus on teaching and will be unable to retain the information being presented.

Cultural aspects must also be addressed. Toward that end, healthcare professionals must be skilled in verbal and non-verbal commmunication, such as touch and listening, in addition to addressing personal cultural needs (Ojanlatva et al 1997). Work with patients to identify their cultural norms and practices, such as nutritional needs or other aspects of their lifestyle. They may have health beliefs, folk practices or communication styles that differ from the healthcare providers. Other considerations include dressing and habits of cleanliness, marriage and sexuality, and honour. An interpreter may be needed and instructional materials should be obtained in different languages. Contact local religious organizations, community centres, schools or minority health resource centres for more information.

Plan Before teaching can commence, strategies must be implemented to motivate the individual to learn. Redman (1997) describes several principles of motivation that affect how people learn:

- Internal motivation is longer lasting than external motivation reinforced by rewards.
- Well-organized education materials increase motivation and decrease learner frustration.
- The learning environment influences the focus of the learner.
- Achievable goals must be set.
- A mild level of anxiety is a motivator for learning.
- Affiliation and approval enhance motivation.
- Learning results from a combination of motives.

The focus for the learner must be based on individual goals. Patients will want to know why they need to learn something new, and many of them will enjoy learning. The nurse must be sensitive to characteristics such as the patient's life experiences, habits, tastes, pride, preoccupations, ability to change and the desire to learn what they can use now (Knowles 1990). Also, not all individuals can attain or desire to attain self care and some may require assistance from a caregiver.

Implementation

The plan should include the content, method of learning to be used and methods of evaluation. The objectives of the plan must be realistic and measurable with specific time lines.

Katz (1997) discusses techniques for healthcare providers to incorporate in their teaching styles:

- Maintain the patient's attention:
  1. make points clear – speak in layman's terms
  2. vary the tone of voice
  3. use several teaching methods (visual aids, lists, charts)
  4. use practical, everyday terms.
- Keep it basic:
  1. limit instruction to three or four points each session
  2. present key points of what the patient needs to know
  3. use simple, everyday language.
- Use time wisely:
  1. teach the patient when delivering patient care
  2. involve significant others in the patient's care
  3. provide the patient with written information.
- Reinforce the teaching:
  1. serve as a role model
  2. provide positive reinforcement
  3. teach small amounts of information over time.
- Evaluate the patient's understanding:
  1. have the patient perform a return demonstration
  2. ask the patient to keep a written log of activities performed
  3. review written materials with the patient.
- Address barriers to learning:
  1. physical barriers: pain, altered level of consciousness, hearing loss, poor vision
  2. emotional barriers: stress, anxiety
  3. language and cultural: does not speak English, different cultural norms or practices
  4. low reading level: low literacy or illiteracy; written materials should be at the level for 10-year-olds.

Evaluation and documentation

Basic principles of teaching and learning must be incorporated in the evaluation. These include:

- cognitive: body of knowledge that is grasped by the learner
- affective: emotional response to the learning situation
- psychomotor: skill or actions the person takes with the new knowledge.

Therefore, it is important for the nurse to evaluate if patients have grasped and accepted the information and have changed their behaviour. The above categories must be used to establish short- and long-term goals, which are used to evaluate the effectiveness of the plan.

The general information presented thus far provides the student with necessary background to begin the problem-based learning process for patient education.

EVIDENCE-BASED PRACTICE

With problem-based learning, the student will identify steps for problem-solving and research the issues to produce solutions. Research should be directed towards evidence-based practice for acquisition of scientific information. Learners can then apply what they have learned to understand and resolve the problem.

Many of the practice patterns for wound care are based upon expert opinion, consensus or habit rather than evidence-based practice. Hence, there is an ongoing need in the wound-care field to improve practice patterns based on implementation of the results of clinical and basic research. Evaluation of current research patterns will support actions that improve patient outcomes, and help to eliminate practice patterns that provide no benefit or harm to wound healing. Nursing research should generate well-controlled clinical trials that confirm, change or revolutionize our practice. For uncommon wounds, case studies and clinical series can provide information regarding our experiences with such wounds rather than just expert opinion. This information can provide suggestions for more definitive clinical research. Therefore, the nurse must review, evaluate and publish the best available evidence for wound care practice (Gray 1997).

The Agency for Health Care Policy and Research (AHCPR), now known as the Agency for Health Care Research and Quality (AHRQ), has developed guidelines for prevention and treatment of pressure ulcers for clinicians and consumers (Bergstrom et al 1994, Panel for Prediction and Prevention of Pressure Ulcers in Adults 1992). These guidelines emphasize the need and importance for continuous patient education and are based on what is available in the scientific literature. They were developed to reduce the morbidity, mortality and financial costs of pressure ulcers and to educate lay people as well as professionals in the treatment and prevention of pressure ulcers (Wilson 1995). Ayello (1995) critiqued the consumer guidelines and suggested revisions to improve them. She also discussed the criteria for selecting patient education materials:

- relates to a majority of people with the problem
- developed by credible sources
- written at the appropriate reading level
- appropriate breadth and scope of content
- organized, logical sequence
- content is accurate, clear, concise, up-to-date and contains essential material
- visuals are informative
- appropriate size of type
- no healthcare jargon or cliches
- provides an extra dimension to teaching
- promotes consumer interaction
- attractive to the reader
- provides purpose, objectives and summary
- cost-effective and easily accessible.

Several guidelines have been developed for the treatment of diabetic ulcers. Groups involved in this process are the American Diabetes Association (ADA) (1999), the American College of Foot and Ankle Surgeons (Frykberg et al 1999), the American Pharmaceutical Association (Albrant & AphA 2000), and the Wound Healing Society and the Wound, Ostomy and Continence Nurses Society (WOCN); their guidelines are posted on their websites (see Web-based resources at the end of this chapter). These groups identified the need for education for healthcare providers for the care of diabetic ulcers. They all agree that there is little scientific evidence to support appro-priate care of diabetic ulcers, however, they have identified enough similarities to hold them as a standard of care.

CASE STUDIES

The reader now has a basic understanding of patient education and the process needed to identify pertinent scientific literature. The case studies presented in Boxes 13.1 – 13.3 provide the student with the opportunity to solve patient education needs for specific wound types.

For the cases described below, a format described by Delise (1997) is a useful tool to assimilate data for problem-based learning in a class setting:

Possible solutions	Facts known about the issue	Gaps in student knowledge; questions that direct research	Places and people to contact for information

Once the information is complete, the findings are presented to the class. The class then evaluates the options in column 1 to determine which solution is most reasonable for the case presented.

The following learning objectives for all three cases are:

- Identify patient-related factors affecting wound healing.
- Discuss disease-related factors affecting wound healing.
- Describe wound-related factors affecting wound healing.
- List education strategies for wound healing.

For the above objectives, the student would enter facts that were obtained from the information presented in the case studies and which were relevant for each objective into the grid. Gaps and questions for each objective would then be entered. The student would then search for the information needed to answer the questions. Some examples of resources are provided with the case studies below. There is often more than one solution to solve each problem.

General information for case studies

For all cases presented, patients and caregivers must understand that healing the ulcers is a team effort, and they are the most important members of the team. The team will work with them to develop a plan of care. Team members may include doctors, nurses, wound-care specialists, dietitians, social workers, pharmacists, and occupational and physical therapists. The caregiver role includes learning how to perform care, knowing what to report to the doctor, knowing how to tell if the treatment works and helping to change the treatment plan as needed.

To ascertain information for the treatment plan, the patient will need to share information with the team, such as general health, illnesses that may slow healing, medications and the emotional and physical support provided by significant others. The treatment plan will then be developed from the health history, physical exam, individual circumstances and the wound assessment. The healthcare professional will then provide information to the patient and/or caregiver regarding the actual care of the wound and nutritional needs, such as calories, protein, vitamins and minerals. Other areas to consider for teaching include management of pain and infection.

Education for the care of healthy skin to prevent further breakdown should be provided for the patient and/or caregiver:

- bathe when needed for cleanliness
- use mild soap and warm water
- use moisturizers to prevent dry skin
- inspect skin daily for changes
- for incontinence, cleanse the skin immediately after soiling occurs, use protective barrier cream or ointment for protection, use incontinence pads or briefs to absorb excrement if incontinence cannot be treated.

The patient and/or caregiver should be instructed in signs to report to the physician including:

- increase in size or depth of the wound
- increased drainage from the wound
- absence of healing in 2 to 4 weeks
- signs of infection (yellow or green drainage, foul odour, redness and/or warmth around the wound, tenderness around the wound, swelling, fever)
- inability to eat a well-balanced diet
- difficulty following the treatment plan
- change in general health.

Box 13.1
Case study of a patient with a pressure ulcer in an acute care setting

A 36-year-old female, paraplegic from a motor vehicle accident 2 years ago, is admitted from home to an acute care facility with bilateral stage IV ischial pressure ulcers and incontinence of bowel and bladder. Both of the ulcers have necrotic tissue and are draining copious amounts of foul-smelling, purulent drainage. Her family is extremely supportive and she has a specialty bed and cushion to reduce pressure to the ulcers. She is depressed about being on bedrest to prevent the ulcers from worsening.

Comment

- Patient-related factors:
  1. inability to perform self- care, necessitating need for assistance from caregiver
  2. isolation and depression due to bedrest to heal pressure ulcers.
- Disease-related factors:
  1. paraplegia increases the risk for pressure ulcers due to immobility, friction, shear, decreased sensation, incontinence.
- Wound-related factors:
  1. bilateral stage IV ulcers of the ischium
  2. possible wound infection
  3. inadequate pressure-reducing devices.

Resources. The AHCPR guidelines for prevention and treatment of pressure ulcers are an excellent resource to guide healthcare professionals in the care of patients with pressure ulcers. They also have guidelines for patients and caregivers (Bergstrom et al 1994, Panel for Prediction and Prevention of Pressure Ulcers in Adults 1992). Patients with pressure ulcers are often incontinent. The AHCPR also has guidelines for incontinence. All of the guidelines can be accessed on the AHCPR website (see Web-based resources at the end of this chapter).

WOCN also has guidelines for pressure ulcers (WOCN 1992), which can be obtained from their website.

Educational needs. In this case, the caregivers are responsible for the prevention and treatment of the pressure ulcers. They will need to be educated in the care of the patient while encouraging the patient to participate as much as possible. The key areas for education would relate to the patient-related factors, disease-related factors and wound-related factors.

Patient-related factors. In this case, the caregivers were feeling guilty about the occurrence of the ischial ulcers. They had initial instruction in the care and prevention of pressure ulcers in the hospital but did not have significant follow-up instruction. However, the fact that the patient has now developed ulcers illustrates the need for more in-depth teaching regarding prevention and treatment modalities. Additional resources will need to be mobilized to reinforce this teaching, such as visiting nurse services.

The patient can be encouraged to take an active role in the plan. The quicker the ulcers begin to heal, the sooner she will be able to get back in the wheelchair and socialize, thus reducing her depression. Her participation will also give her a sense of control over her situation.

Disease-related factors. Risk factors of immobility, friction, shear, decreased sensation and incontinence must be addressed. Immobility is heightened by the fact that she cannot sit on the ulcers. The family will need education in the reduction of friction and shear when moving the patient in bed and transferring her to the wheelchair, such as a transfer board or lift.

The patient cannot feel from the waist down and therefore does not change position when she feels pressure. Education for pressure relief is paramount to prevention and treatment of pressure ulcers and includes:

- Understanding of pressure points when lying on back or side and when sitting.
- Reducing pressure with support surfaces such as specialty beds, mattresses or overlay mattresses and seat cushions.
- Proper positioning in bed:
  1. do not lie on ulcer
  2. turn every 2 hours
  3. do not lie directly on a hip bone (use 30° side-lying position)
  4. keep heels off the bed with a pillow or foam
  5. do not use doughnut-shaped rings
  6. keep knees and ankles from touching with pillows
  7. keep the head of the bed no higher than 30° if the patient can tolerate it.
- Proper positioning in chair or wheelchair:
  1. use good posture to prevent friction and shear
  2. do not sit on ulcer
  3. change position at least every hour
  4. do not use doughnut-shaped rings.

Incontinence must also be addressed. At this point, the patient is using a moisture barrier ointment to protect her skin and diapers to contain the excrement, which is also absorbed by the dressings on her ulcers. This patient is a candidate for a bowel and bladder programme. Caregivers can be taught how to perform intermittent self-catheterization and use suppositories for bowel control.

Wound-related factors.   The patient has bilateral stage IV ischial pressure ulcers with necrotic tissue and copious amounts of foul-smelling, purulent drainage. During her hospital stay, both the ulcers are surgically debrided and she is treated with an antibiotic for her wound infection. The caregivers will need education regarding appropriate wound-care dressings and signs of infection. In addition, signs to report to the physician (listed earlier) should be included in the teaching plan.

An assessment of her wheelchair cushion by the physical therapy department reveals inadequate pressure reduction. She is fitted with a new cushion. The family needs instruction in hand checks to be sure the cushion is providing adequate pressure reduction. They also need to contact the specialty bed company that provides the bed at home for periodic inspections.

Box 13.2 **Case study of a patient with a venous ulcer in an outpatient wound care centre**	An 82-year-old Hispanic male with a 6-month history of a venous ulcer on his right lower extremity visits the wound-care centre weekly for treatment. He does not speak English. The ulcer is partial thickness with granulation tissue but has not decreased in size since his initial visit 3 weeks ago. The ulcer produces a large amount of serous drainage. He changes the dressing when he gets around to it, which is about twice a week. The skin surrounding the ulcer is dry and scaly with brown discoloration and 2+ pitting oedema. He says he is unable to tolerate compression therapy, which is the cornerstone of treatment for venous disease.

Comment
- Patient-related factors:
  1. age
  2. language barrier.
- Disease-related factors:
  1. venous disease
  2. previous history of venous ulcers.
- Wound-related factors:
  1. non-healing ulcer
  2. intolerance of compression therapy.

Resources. WOCN has guidelines and fact sheets for the care of venous ulcers (WOCN 1993, 1996a).

Many education companies print booklets for prevention and treatment of venous ulcers. Companies who make compression devices provide written information and also have videos. Healthcare providers can also provide information.

Educational needs. In this case, prevention measures are key to healing the present ulcer and preventing future ulcers. Education for prevention includes:

- no smoking
- adequate nutrition
- keep skin clean and well lubricated
- elevate the legs above the heart
- avoid sitting with the legs crossed
- avoid standing for prolonged periods
- ambulate as tolerated several times a day
- take medications as prescribed
- use compression therapy
- follow-up with healthcare provider.

Patient-related factors. The patient is at risk for ulcers because of his advanced age. Therefore, teaching prevention strategies is even more important for him. Before teaching can commence, an interpreter will be needed to translate the information into Spanish. There are also many written materials that can be obtained in Spanish.

Disease-related factors. The patient has a previous history of venous ulcers, which eventually healed. With the progression of his venous disease, he has developed oedema, and dry, scaly skin with brown discoloration, which has resulted in another ulcer. Instruction is needed for emollients to prevent dry skin. Education to reduce oedema would include:

- strategies listed for prevention
- raise the foot of the bed while sleeping
- exercise feet and ankles while elevating legs
- avoid constrictive clothing.

Wound-related factors. The non-healing ulcer is associated with lack of appropriate dressing changes and inability to tolerate compression. The dressing should be one that absorbs the drainage to keep the wound from being too moist and to prevent maceration of the surrounding skin (see Chapter 8). Different types of compression therapy should be discussed with the patient to determine if he could tolerate another system (see Chapter 15). He would then need to be educated in the proper wound-care dressing and compression therapy.

Box 13.3 *Case study of a patient with a diabetic ulcer in home care*	A 78-year-old obese male with a 10-year history of insulin-dependent type II diabetes with neuropathy and retinopathy is being treated at home for a diabetic ulcer on the plantar surface of his left foot. The wound bed is full thickness with pale pink, dry tissue. A callous surrounds the ulcer. Pedal pulses are palpable but weak. He does not follow his diabetic diet and his blood sugar levels are consistently elevated. Due to the above comorbidities, he cannot reach, see or feel his feet. He lives alone but has a supportive girlfriend who has agreed to act as his caregiver.

Comment

- Patient-related factors:
  1. age
  2. non-compliance with glucose control.
- Disease-related factors:
  1. uncontrolled diabetes
  2. diabetic retinopathy and neuropathy
  3. obesity.
- Wound-related factors:
  1. decreased blood supply
  2. dry tissue
  3. callous surrounds ulcer.

Resources.   WOCN has guidelines and fact sheets for the care of diabetic ulcers (WOCN 1993, 1996b) and other guidelines are available from the websites of the American Diabetes Association (ADA), the American College of Foot and Ankle Surgeons, the American Pharmaceutical Association, and the Wound Healing Society (see Web-based resources).

Educational needs.   In this case, the patient cannot perform self care because of his poor eyesight and obesity. His neuropathy impairs his ability to identify any type of skin breakdown.

Patients with diabetes need the following education to help them prevent diabetic ulcers:

- no smoking
- control the diabetes
- avoid exposure to cold, friction, moisture between toes, bare feet
- daily foot care (inspection, wash and dry well between toes, wear clean socks)

- keeping the feet dry by applying a thin coat of lubricating oil (baby oil) after drying feet; do not apply between toes
- avoid soaking the feet
- avoid garters; wear properly fitted stockings, avoid mended stockings or stockings with seams; change stockings daily
- avoid wearing shoes without stockings or socks
- avoid sandals with thongs between toes
- cut the toenails straight across
- seek professional foot care for toenails, corns and callouses
- avoid over-the-counter medications for corns and callouses, antiseptic solutions, adhesive tape
- well fitting footwear (made of leather)
- inspect inside of shoe for foreign objects, nail points, torn linings, rough areas
- orthotic footwear for altered gait or orthopaedic deformities
- avoid crossing the legs
- pressure reduction for bony prominences
- avoid temperature extremes
- avoid external heat (heating pad, hot water bottle, hydrotherapy, hot surfaces)
- follow-up with healthcare provider regularly
- notify physician immediately if sore, blister, cut or scratch develops.

Patient-related factors.   The patient's advanced age is a risk factor for diabetic ulcers. This is compounded by the fact that he does not follow his diabetic diet. Diet teaching could be provided by a dietitian or visiting nurse to help control his blood sugar levels. Modifications would be needed to help satisfy his 'sweet tooth'. His girlfriend will need to be taught how to prepare meals that meet the requirements of the diet but also satisfy the needs of the patient.

Disease-related factors.   Because the patient's eyesight is poor and he has difficulty reading the numbers on the syringe, the girlfriend has agreed to learn how to give the insulin injections. She will need written instructions and return demonstrations because she has short-term memory loss. She will also need instruction in foot care, as outlined in prevention. Due to his neuropathy and retinopathy, the patient has not been able to perform this assessment properly.

Once the diabetes is under control, the patient might begin to lose weight. He presently has difficulty lifting his foot for wound care because of his obesity.

Wound-related factors.   Three factors are currently delaying wound healing: decreased blood supply, the dry wound and the callous surrounding the wound. The patient is not a candidate for bypass surgery to increase circulation to the area.

His caregiver can be instructed in the appropriate wound care using a dressing to hydrate the wound to promote moist wound healing. Written instructions for wound care would be needed, with return demonstrations with the visiting nurse or wound-care nurse.

The callous surrounding the ulcer needs to be surgically removed. The patient would then need to be fitted for a special orthotic shoe to off-load the pressure from the ulcer. The girlfriend would then have to inspect for further callous formation and inform the doctor if it reoccurs.

CONCLUSIONS

Understanding patient education needs for wound care is multifactorial, requiring a strong patient focus. The professional must search for scientific evidence and develop problem-solving and clinical reasoning skills. A diversity of resources is required to solve complex teaching needs encountered in the real world.

REFERENCES

Albrant D H, AphA Diabetic Foot Ulcer Protocol Panel 2000 AphA drug treatment protocols: management of foot ulcers in patients with diabetes. Journal of the American Pharmaceutical Association 40(4):467–474

American Diabetes Association 1999 Consensus development conference on diabetic foot wound care. Diabetes Care 22(8):1354–1360

Ayello E A 1995 Critique of AHCPR's consumer guide: "Treating Pressure Ulcers". Advances in Wound Care 8(5):18–32

Beitz J M 1998 Education for health promotion and disease prevention: convince them, don't confuse them. Ostomy/Wound Management 44(3A):71S–77S

Bergstrom N, Bennett M A, Carlson C E et al 1994 Treating pressure sores. Consumer version clinical practice guideline, number 15. AHCPR publication no. 95-0654. Rockville, MD

Delise R 1997 How to use problem-based learning in the classroom. Association for Supervision and Curriculum Development, Alexandria, VA

Frykberg R G, Armstrong D G, Giurini J et al 1999 Diabetic foot disorders: a clinical practice guideline. The Journal of Foot and Ankle Surgery 39(5): S1–S60

Gray M 1997 The demand for evidence-based practice. Journal of Wound, Ostomy and Continence Nursing 24:291–292

Katz J R 1997 Back to basics: providing effective patient teaching. American Journal of Nursing 97(5):33–36

Knowles M 1990 The adult learner: a neglected species. Gulf, Houston

Ojanlatva A, Vandenbussche C, Heldt H 1997 The use of problem-based learning in dealing with cultural minority groups. Patient Education and Counseling 31:171–176

Panel for Prediction and Prevention of Pressure Ulcers in Adults 1992 Preventing pressure ulcers: a patient guide. Consumer version clinical practice guideline, Number 3. AHCPR publication no. 92-0048. Rockville, MD

Redman B K 1997 The practice of patient education, 8th edn. CV Mosby, St Louis

Twitchell E 1999 Patient education: use it to save visits and dollars. Success in Home Care III(1): 12–16

Wilson R 1995 Commentary: using AHCPR's consumer guide on treating pressure ulcers. Ostomy/Wound Management 41(5):54–55

Wound Ostomy and Continence Nurses Society (WOCN) 1992 Standards of care: patients with dermal wounds: pressure ulcers. WOCN, Laguna Beach, CA

Wound Ostomy and Continence Nurses Society (WOCN) 1993 Standards of care: patients with dermal wounds: lower extremity ulcers. WOCN, Laguna Beach, CA

Wound Ostomy and Continence Nurses Society (WOCN) 1996a Clinical fact sheets: venous insufficiency (stasis). WOCN, Laguna Beach, CA

Wound Ostomy and Continence Nurses Society (WOCN) 1996b Clinical fact sheets: peripheral neuropathy. WOCN, Laguna Beach, CA

FURTHER READING

Bryant R A 2000 Acute and chronic wounds: nursing management, 2nd edn. Mosby, St Louis

Cuddigan J, Ayello E A, Sussman C and the National Pressure Ulcer Advisory Panel 2001 Pressure ulcers in America: prevention, incidence, and implications for the future. NPUAP, Reston, VA

Foltz A 1998 Get real: clinical testing of patients' reading abilities. Cancer Nursing 21(3):162–166

Hess C T 1999 Nurse's clinical guide. Wound care, 3rd edn. Springhouse Corporation, Springhouse, PA

Krasner D, Kane D 2001 Chronic wound care: a clinical source book for healthcare professionals 3rd edn. Health Management Publications, Wayne, PA

Motta G 2001 Kestrel Wound Product Sourcebook, 4(1). Kestrel Health Information, Williston, VT

Sussman C, Bates-Jensen B M 1998 Wound care: a collaborative practice manual for physical therapists and nurses. Aspen Publishers, Gaithersburg, MD

Wound Ostomy and Continence Nurses Society (WOCN) 1996 Clinical fact sheets: Arterial insufficiency. WOCN, Laguna Beach, CA

**WEB-BASED
RESOURCES**

http://campus.fortunecity.com/medicine/975/pbl/pbleindex.html

Wound, Ostomy and Continence Nurses Society (WOCN): www.wocn.org

Agency for Healthcare Research and Quality (AHRQ): www.ahrq.gov

National Pressure Ulcer Advisory Panel (NPUAP): www.npuap.org

Wound Healing Society (WHS): www.woundheal.org

Association for Advancement of Wound Care (AAWC): www.aawc1.com

Wound management principles and resources

Wound types

CHAPTER 14

Pressure Ulcers

Jane Nixon

INTRODUCTION

The European Pressure Ulcer Advisory Panel (EPUAP 1999) has described pressure ulcers as 'an area of localized damage to the skin and underlying tissue caused by pressure, shear, friction and or a combination of these'. They are complex lesions of the skin and underlying structures and vary in size and severity of tissue layer affected, ranging from skin erythema to damage to muscle and underlying bone (Witkowski & Parish 1982).

The majority of pressure ulcers occur below the waist, with particularly vulnerable areas being the sacrum, buttocks and heels. They are associated with increased mortality rates and are a marker for underlying disease severity and other comorbidities (Thomas et al 1996). Pressure ulcers have both cost and quality implications for health services and they are increasingly seen as preventable rather than a tolerable complication of illness.

The emphasis is on identifying patients at risk and implementing appropriate interventions to prevent pressure ulcer occurrence. However, many practice recommendations are not based on good research evidence. In particular, the evidence base associated with assessment of risk is limited and the effectiveness of preventative interventions has not been demonstrated using robust research methodologies (Cullum et al 1995).

This chapter provides a brief summary of key areas of the literature including the definition and classification of pressure ulcers, prevalence, pathophysiology, aetiology, principles of prevention and treatment.

DEFINITION AND CLASSIFICATION

Various terms have been used to describe pressure ulcers, including 'pressure sores', 'bed sores' and 'decubitus ulcers'. However, following publication of international guidelines (AHCPR 1992, EPUAP 1998), there is consensus amongst researchers and clinical experts in the field to refer to such lesions as 'pressure ulcers'.

The severity of pressure ulcers varies from erythema of intact skin to tissue destruction involving skin, subcutaneous fat, muscle and bone, and a number of classification systems have been developed. At an international level, attempts to standardize classification have resulted in good consensus – the American (AHCPR 1992) and European (EPUAP 1999) classifications are detailed in Table 14.1.

However, there remain practical difficulties regarding the use of classification scales. From a professional accountability perspective it is as important that a record is made that no skin damage has been observed as it is to record the grade of ulcer where one is present. It is also recognized that when eschar is present, accurate staging is not possible until the eschar is desloughed or the wound debrided (AHCPR 1992). To address the problems associated with record keeping, researchers and clinicians complement the basic classification systems

Table 14.1
AHCPR (1992) and EPUAP (1999) skin classification

AHCPR classification	EPUAP classification
Stage I Non-blanchable erythema of intact skin; the heralding lesion of skin ulceration	**Grade 1** Non-blanchable erythema of intact skin. Discoloration of the skin, warmth, oedema, induration or hardness may also be used as indicators, particularly on individuals with darker skin
Stage II Partial thickness skin loss involving epidermis and/or dermis. The ulcer is superficial and presents clinically as an abrasion, blister, or shallow crater	**Grade 2** Partial thickness skin loss involving epidermis, dermis, or both. The ulcer is superficial and presents clinically as an abrasion or blister
Stage III Full thickness skin loss involving damage or necrosis of subcutaneous tissue that may extend down to, but not through, underlying fascia. The ulcer presents clinically as a deep crater with or without undermining of adjacent tissue	**Grade 3** Full thickness skin loss involving damage to or necrosis of subcutaneous tissue that may extend down to, but not through, underlying fascia
Stage IV Full thickness skin loss with extensive destruction, tissue necrosis or damage to muscle, bone or supporting structures (for example, tendon or joint capsule). *Note:* undermining and sinus tracts may also be associated with stage IV pressure ulcers	**Grade 4** Extensive destruction, tissue necrosis, or damage to muscle, bone, or supporting structures with or without full thickness skin loss

with additional grades/stages, such as grade 0 to indicate 'normal skin' and grade 5 to document the presence of eschar (Nixon et al 1999).

Furthermore, there are difficulties associated with both the description, inclusion and clinical assessment of grade/stage 1 pressure ulcers. Erythema is difficult to assess clinically, particularly in patients with darkly pigmented skin and the American classification of stage 1 was revised in 1998 (NPUAP 1998) to address limitations of the original guideline document (Box 14.1).

Box 14.1
NPUAP (1998)
stage 1 pressure
ulcer

A stage 1 pressure ulcer is an observable pressure-related alteration of intact skin whose indicators as compared to the adjacent or opposite area on the body may include changes in one or more of the following:

skin temperature (warmth or coolness), tissue consistency (firm or boggy feel) and/or sensation (pain, itching).

The ulcer appears as a defined area of persistent redness in lightly pigmented skin, whereas in darker skin tones, the ulcer may appear with persistent red, blue or purple hues.

There also remains some debate in relation to the documentation of blanching erythema for both practice and research perspectives. Whilst on one level it is argued that it is not a pressure ulcer, on the other there is evidence that it is pathologically different from normal skin (Nixon 2001a, Witkowski & Parish 1982).

Despite the increasing consensus for the classification of pressure ulcers, there remain differences in the operational definitions used. For example, whilst recording and classifying alterations of intact skin (such as non-blanching erythema) as grade 1, for the purposes of audit and research the operational definition of the term 'pressure ulcer' may be specified as a grade/stage 2 ulcer or above, that is a superficial skin break or above (Nixon et al 1999). Historically there has been great variation in the definition of the term (including blanching erythema) and it is important when appraising any source of data to be mindful of the baseline definition used.

PREVALENCE

Pressure ulcers are common in hospital and nursing home facilities and are seen in homecare patients across Western Europe and North America. Multi-centre prevalence studies undertaken in America (Barczak et al 1997) and Western European countries, including the UK (O'Dea 1995), Netherlands (Bours et al 1999), Italy (O'Dea 1995), Germany (O'Dea 1995) and France (Barrois et al 1995) report prevalence rates ranging from 83.6% to 5.2%. Rates excluding grade 1 ulcers range from 22.9 to 4%.

Variation in methodology used and the populations studied account for some of the variation in rates and make comparisons difficult to appraise. However, results suggest that somewhere in the region of 1 in 10 hospital patients have a pressure ulcer at any given point in time.

PATHOPHYSIOLOGY

The three different types of pressure ulcer described by researchers are:

- necrosis of the epidermis or dermis, which may or may not progress to a deep sore
- deep or 'malignant' pressure ulcer where necrosis is first observed in the subcutaneous tissue (muscle or fat) and tracks outwards
- full-thickness wounds of dry black eschar.

The mechanisms leading to tissue breakdown are not entirely clear from the limited research undertaken to date but at least three pathophysiological processes are evident, including:

- occlusion of skin blood flow and subsequent injury due to abrupt reperfusion of the ischaemic vascular bed
- endothelial damage of arterioles and the microcirculation due to the application of disruptive and shearing forces
- direct occlusion of blood vessels by external pressure for a prolonged period resulting in cell death (Nixon 2001b).

It is not possible to determine a dominant pathological mechanism and all three may play a role in the development of pressure-induced skin lesions. The feature common to the three mechanisms is occlusion or disruption of the blood supply to the skin or underlying structures, resulting in ischaemia and tissue loss (Nixon 2001b).

Blood flow to the skin varies from individual to individual, is site dependent and is affected by a combination of systemic, local and disease-related factors. In addition, various autoregulatory mechanisms affect blood flow to protect or enable recovery both during and following pressure assault, including: raising of capillary pressure to maintain flow; intermittent flow at subcritical pressures; response to repetitive loading; and the reactive hyperaemic response following full or partial occlusion. The large number of baseline and autoregulatory factors that affect the localized tissue response explain the individualized nature of patients' response to external load (Nixon 2001b).

AETIOLOGY

A conceptual schema for the study of the aetiology of pressure ulcers was developed by Braden and Bergstrom (1987) and provides a useful framework. They identified the critical determinants of pressure-ulcer development as the intensity and duration of pressure and the tolerance of the skin and its supporting structure to pressure. At an individual level, pressure ulcers develop as a result of the interaction between these two elements.

A summary of key findings from two comprehensive reviews exploring the aetiology of pressure ulcers are provided (Bridel 1993, Nixon 2001b). The overview of mechanisms that protect the skin microvasculature from ischaemic assault and restore local tissue perfusion following occlusion illustrate clearly that there is an interaction between the pressure assault and the capacity of the skin to maintain and effectively restore skin blood flow. A number of autoregulatory mechanisms exist to protect the skin from pressure assault and these processes break down at pressure values that are highly variable. Pressure ulcer development is multidimensional and complex (Nixon 2001b).

Intensity and duration of pressure

The primary cause of pressure ulcers is the application of pressure in areas of skin and tissue not adapted to external pressure assault. Although no critical threshold values can be determined in relation to intensity and duration of pressure, previous review has established important principles.

Local versus uniform pressure

The nature of the pressure assault is important in the development of pressure ulcers. It is the effect of the application of a local or point pressure upon the skin that is of interest in pressure ulcer aetiology. Such localized pressure is complicated by shear forces, contact area, underlying bone, bone depth, pressure distribution, contact surface conditions and associated tissue distortion (Nixon 2001b).

Critical pressure thresholds

It appears that the autoregulation processes that maintain skin blood flow during pressure assault break down at pressure values that are highly variable and there is no universal capillary occlusion threshold level. The 'critical closing pressure' is the pressure within a vessel at which it collapses completely and blood flow ceases. It is determined by an interplay of forces, including intravascular pressure, muscle contraction and elastic forces of the blood vessel wall and externally applied pressure (Guyton 1992). That at least four variables are involved explains why no individual response is the same, although trends are apparent (Nixon 2001b).

Parabolic intensity–duration curve

Studies that examine the relationship between pressure and time report an inverse relationship between the amount and duration of pressure, that is, low pressure for long periods and high pressure for short periods both cause ulceration (Nixon 2001b).

Critical time threshold

Reappraisal of early studies suggests that once a critical pressure threshold and critical time value is exceeded then tissue damage will proceed at a similar rate regardless of the magnitude of the pressure applied (Bridel 1993).

Tolerance of the skin to pressure

Braden and Bergstrom (1987) use the term 'tissue tolerance' to 'denote the ability of both the skin and its supporting structures to endure the effects of pressure without adverse sequela'. They distinguish between extrinsic and intrinsic factors affecting tissue tolerance and describe intrinsic factors as 'those that influence the architecture and integrity of the skin's supporting structures and/or the vascular and lymphatic system that serves the skin and underlying structures'.

Extrinsic factors

The main extrinsic factor affecting skin tolerance to pressure is the application of frictional forces, which exacerbates the pressure assault by causing mechanical disruption of the epidermis. Other extrinsic factors commonly cited in the literature include moisture and skin irritants. It is noteworthy that urinary incontinence is not identified as a primary risk factor and skin irritants have been the subject of little research and their contribution is unknown.

Architecture of the skin

Many intrinsic variables associated with pressure ulcer development directly affect collagen, an important element within the structure of the skin and underlying tissues. Attention to this important structure has developed following observations, which revealed that the collagen content of the dermis is reduced following spinal cord injury. It appears that collagen prevents disruption to the microcirculation by buffering the interstitial fluid from external load, thereby maintaining the balance of hydrostatic and osmotic pressures (Krouskop 1983). The collagen theory interrelates with other predisposing factors such as age, nutrition, steroid administration and spinal cord injury, which affect the synthesis, maturation and degradation of the connective tissue (Bridel 1993).

Perfusion

A large number of intrinsic perfusion-related factors are associated with pressure ulcer development, including systemic blood pressure, extracorporeal circulation, serum protein, smoking, serum haemoglobin, diseases of the vascular system, vasoactive drug administration and increased body temperature (Bridel 1993). The literature suggests an overall trend. That is, the tolerance of the skin is affected by perfusion-related variables but there is no single cause–effect factor. This can be linked to the physiology of blood flow and the interplay of factors that determine capillary blood pressure, exchange mechanisms between capillaries and interstitial fluid (Guyton 1992) and factors affecting the availability of essential nutrients (particularly oxygen) to the local tissue.

The development of pressure ulcers is determined by various aetiological factors particular to individual patients that determine the ability of the skin to respond to external pressure and maintain skin integrity.

RISK FACTORS

Although there is a considerable pressure ulcer literature, only a small number of cohort studies have assessed the relationship of potential risk factors to pressure ulcer development (Table 14.2). An important feature of these studies is their use of multifactor statistical analyses to identify, rank and weight the risk factors that best predict or account for pressure ulcer development (Cullum et al 1995).

The studies cited have used a variety of possible risk factors, measured similar variables in different ways, included various population groups and do not utilize a common pressure ulcer definition. Despite these differences, five key themes emerge:

- mobility
- nutrition
- perfusion
- skin condition
- age.

These can be directly related to the aetiology of pressure-ulcer development where the interaction between the intensity and duration of pressure (mobility) and the tolerance of the skin (nutrition, perfusion and age) determines the skin response (skin condition).

Table 14.2

Risk factor cohort studies utilizing multifactorial statistical analyses

Study	Sample	Incidence	Risk factors	Statistical method
Clarke and Kadhom 1988	88 hospitalized (orthopaedic, elderly + ICU) bedfast/chairfast	29.5%	1. Change in condition of skin 2. Time on pressure area care 3. Appetite 4. Norton score 5. Diagnosis 6. Method of manual pressure relief 7. Observed skin condition 8. Age	Discriminant analysis
	30 community bedfast/chairfast	20%	1. Appetite 2. Condition of skin 3. Frequency of care 4. Norton score 5. Age 6. Diagnosis	
Guralnik et al 1988	5193 US nationwide cohort 55–75 years 10-year follow-up	2.2%	1. Heart disease (negative association) 2. Activity level 3. Self-assessed health 4. Smoking 5. Neurological abnormality 6. Dry or scaling skin 7. Anaemia (Hb < 12)	Multiple logistic regression
Berlowitz and Wilking 1989 (Record review)	185 chronic medical	10.8%	1. Cerebrovascular accident 2. Bed or chair bound 3. Impaired nutritional intake	Multiple logistic regression
Kemp et al 1990	125 surgical > 20 years stratified by operating time	12%	1. Age 2. Time on operating table 3. Extracorporeal circulation	Discriminant analysis
Ek et al 1991	495 long-term medical LOS > 3 weeks	10.1%	1. Albumin 2. Mobility 3. Activity 4. Food intake	Multiple regression
Marchette et al 1991	161 postoperative ICU > 59 years	39.1%	1. Skin redness 2. Days static air mattress for prevention 3. Faecal incontinence 4. Diarrhoea 5. Preoperative albumin	Discriminant analysis
Bergstrom and Braden 1992	200 nursing home > 65 years LOS > 10 days Braden < 18	73.5%	1. Braden scale 2. Diastolic blood pressure 3. Temperature 4. Dietary protein intake 5. Age	Logistic regression

continued

Table 14.2—cont'd
Risk factor cohort studies utilizing multifactorial statistical analyses

Study	Sample	Incidence	Risk factors	Statistical method
Hoshowsky and Schramm 1994	505 surgical	16.8%	1. Time on operating table 2. Vascular disease 3. Age over 40 years 4. Preoperative Hemphill scale	Logistic regression
Brandeis et al 1994	1322 nursing home	12.9%	1. Ambulation difficulty 2. Faecal incontinence 3. Diabetes mellitus 4. Difficulty feeding oneself	Logistic regression
Allman et al 1995	286 hospitalized > 55 years bed/chair > 5 days hip fracture length of stay > 5 days	12.9%	1. Non-blanchable erythema of intact sacral skin 2. Lymphopenia 3. Immobility 4. Dry sacral skin 5. Decreased body weight	Multivariate Cox regression
Bergstrom et al 1996	843 nursing home and acute	12.8%	Model 1: 1. Braden scale 2. Age 3. Race Model 2: 1. Mobility 2. Activity 3. Cardiovascular disease	Logistic regression
Schnelle et al 1997	100 nursing home incontinent	21%	1. Blanchable erythema severity	Stepwise multiple regression
Schue and Langemo 1998	170 male elderly rehabilitation	27.1%	1. Moisture 2. Nutrition 3. Friction and shear	Multiple logistic regression
Nixon et al 2000	416 surgical patients	15.6%	1. Hypotensive episodes 2. Mobility 3. Core temperature	Logistic regression
Halfens et al 2000	320 surgical, neurological, orthopaedic and medical hospitalized	14.7%	1. Sensory perception 2. Age 3. Friction and shear 4. Moisture	Stepwise logistic regression
Nixon 2001a	97 general, vascular and orthopaedic surgical	15.5%	1. Non-blanching erythema 2. Preoperative albumin 3. Weight loss 4. Diastolic blood pressure	

Mobility

The important relationship between reduced mobility and pressure-ulcer occurrence suggested by early prevalence surveys is confirmed by cohort studies, which identify mobility-related factors to be significant and independent predictors of pressure-ulcer development (see Table 14.2). Of the 16 studies detailed, 13 identify mobility-related factors as important determinants of pressure-ulcer development.

Factors affecting skin tolerance

Studies utilizing univariate analyses have identified a large number of factors affecting skin tolerance that are significantly associated with pressure ulcer development (Bridel 1993). However, the three themes emerging from multifactorial analyses both challenge and support some common assumptions made with regard to the relative importance of pressure ulcer risk factors.

Nutrition-related factors are identified by 10 of the 16 studies, although the exact relationship remains unclear. It is likely that reduced dietary intake is a general indicator of morbidity, as well as directly affecting tissue perfusion and skin structures, which reduce tolerance to pressure (Bridel 1993). The wide range of factors identified within such a small number of research studies reflects the absence of recognized indicators of nutritional status.

Factors affecting tissue perfusion are identified by nine studies. This is the most diverse area of the literature, reflecting the large number of variables that affect tissue perfusion. The existing research base cannot identify key factors more specific than 'perfusion related' and there is a clear need for further exploration of these variables in specialty-specific patient populations.

Five of the cohort studies determine age as associated with pressure-ulcer development. Other studies suggest that, in high-risk groups, age is less important than associated morbidity (Allman et al 1995, Berlowitz & Wilking 1989). The relationship is likely to be multifactorial and related to both increased morbidity and disease, which affect mobility- and age-related changes of the skin, and these in turn reduce tissue tolerance (Allman 1997).

It is noteworthy that only two studies identify moisture and two faecal incontinence as risk factors. This challenges the common assumption that incontinence is a central risk factor in pressure-ulcer development. It is likely that incontinence is strongly associated with both immobility and age, and these factors emerge as more important in the majority of multifactorial models.

Skin condition

Finally, skin condition is identified as a risk factor associated with subsequent skin loss by all six studies that included this variable as a potential risk factor. In particular, the observation of a non-blanching erythema indicates that the patient is at high risk of subsequent skin loss (Nixon 2001a).

PATIENT ASSESSMENT

Nursing assessment is a dynamic and continuous process involving synthesis of information from a variety of sources, including underpinning knowledge, previous experience, specialty-based knowledge, recognition of important indicators and knowledge of the patient. Nursing skill is required to select, weight and combine important factors so as to notice, understand and act (Nixon & McGough 2001).

It is essential from the outset to identify which patients require baseline skin assessment in order to determine the presence or absence of existing pressure ulcers. Subsequent assessment of individual patient risk is an ongoing and dynamic process (Nixon & McGough 2001).

Risk assessment step 1 – assessment of skin

Baseline nursing assessment is required to identify both actual and potential problems, which then inform individual planning and delivery of effective care. The main characteristic associated with the presence of pressure ulcers at baseline are reduced mobility and increased age (Barrois et al 1995, Berlowitz & Wilking 1989).

In addition, the literature identifies a number of high-risk patient groups, including elderly medical, nursing home, cardiovascular/vascular surgery, acute orthopaedic, intensive care, spinal cord injured, disabled and terminally ill patients (Nixon & McGough 2001).

It is suggested that baseline skin inspection to determine the presence or absence of a pressure ulcer, and to identify patients who require assessment of potential risk, is necessary if one or more of the following criteria apply:

- mobility/activity restrictions – confined to bed or chair
- aged over 75 years
- high-risk group (Nixon & McGough 2001).

Baseline skin assessment should establish one of three scenarios, specifically that the patient:

- has one or more existing pressure ulcer(s) of grade 2 or above
- has observable skin changes of intact skin
- the skin is observed as 'normal'.

When baseline skin assessment identifies that a patient has an existing pressure ulcer of grade 2 or above, the patient has an actual problem which requires treatment and that treatment will depend upon the severity of the ulcer and the individual patient circumstance. Patients with existing pressure ulcers are also at risk of further pressure ulcer development and require active prevention.

When baseline skin assessment identifies observable skin changes, best practice can be summarized as follows:

1. Observation of a non-blanching erythema indicates that the patient is at high risk of subsequent skin loss and requires active intervention to prevent skin loss.
2. Observation of blanching erythema or other skin changes indicates the need for informed judgement of its clinical relevance and further assessment of potential risk of pressure ulcer development.

When the skin is observed as 'normal' the purpose of further assessment is to identify any potential risk of pressure ulcer development so that preventative measures can be adopted.

Risk assessment step 2

Risk assessment scales have been developed in an attempt to provide a structure and consistency to patient assessment and provide a number of advantages.

They raise awareness of risk factors, prompt risk assessment and provide a minimum standard for assessment and documentation. However, they are limited in construction methods and validity and their use as a single instrument to assess risk in patients who are free from pressure ulcers is not supported on the basis of current evidence (Nixon & McGough 2001).

A major limitation of the majority of scales is that they fail to include the condition of the skin within the risk assessment framework, and yet this is a key risk factor. Further, risk assessment scales rarely take into consideration the local context, patient circumstance, patient prognosis, motivational factors and self-limiting factors (such as position favoured by patient).

Over 40 pressure ulcer risk assessment scales have been published and the majority were developed on the basis of expert opinion, literature review and/or adaptation of an existing scale with only seven original scales (McGough 1999). There is no statistical basis to the majority of risk assessment scales either in relation to the selection of risk factors or the scores allocated to elements within the scales. In most risk assessment scales using a simple ordinal scoring system, the weighting within the scale is equally allocated between risk factors. Thus any potential differences in the contribution or importance of one factor over another or the cumulative importance of two or more factors are not identified.

The absence of a statistical base is evident in the large number of variables found in risk assessment scales. McGough (1999) identified 23 different variables in 38 modified risk assessment scales, with most frequent inclusion of continence/moisture, nutrition/appetite and mobility. Given the large number of variables that are not key risk factors, but that *are* included within risk assessment scales, the validity of the scales in defining 'at risk' patients is immediately questionable.

Testing the validity of such scales poses difficult methodological problems because preventive interventions are frequently provided to the patients under study and the majority of studies undertake only a limited number of assessments and might not reflect the patient's condition at the time of pressure-ulcer development.

The most widely tested risk assessment scale across American and European communities and in a variety of clinical settings is the Braden scale (Fig. 14.1). This has shown good reliability when used by qualified nurses (Bergstrom et al 1987) and varying levels of sensitivity (64% to 100%) (Nixon & McGough 2001).

Despite the limitations of risk assessment scales (Cullum et al 1995, McGough 1999), their widespread utilization would suggest that clinical nurses value them and that their limitations are not necessarily important within the clinical environment. Evidence suggests that their introduction in conjunction with the establishment of skin-care teams, education programmes and care protocols may reduce the incidence of pressure ulcers (McGough 1999).

European guidelines reflect the emerging debate and evidence base associated with risk assessment scales (EPUAP 1998). The guidelines make the following recommendations:

> Risk assessment scales should be used as an adjunct to clinical judgment and not as a tool in isolation from other clinical features.

> Assessment of risk should be more than just the use of an appropriate risk assessment tool and should not lead to a prescriptive and inflexible approach to patient care.

SENSORY PERCEPTION Ability to respond meaningfully to pressure-related discomfort.	1. Completely limited: Unresponsive (does not moan, flinch or grasp) to painful stimuli, due to diminished level of consciousness or sedation OR limited ability to feel pain.	2. Very limited: Responds only to painful stimuli. Cannot communicate discomfort except by moaning or restlessness OR has a sensory impairment which limits the ability to feel pain or discomfort over 1/2 of body.	3. Slightly limited: Responds to verbal commands but cannot always communicate discomfort or need to be turned OR has some sensory impairment which limits ability to feel pain or discomfort in 1 or 2 extremities.	4. No impairment: Responds to verbal commands. Has no sensory deficit which would limit ability to feel or voice pain or discomfort.	
MOISTURE Degree to which skin is exposed to moisture.	1. Constantly moist: Skin is kept moist almost constantly by perspiration, urine, etc. Dampness is detected every time patient is moved or turned.	2. Very moist: Skin is often but not always moist. Linen must be changed at least once a shift.	3. Occasionally moist: Skin is occasionally moist, requiring an extra linen change approximately once a day.	4. Rarely moist: Skin is usually dry, linen only requires changing at routine intervals.	
ACTIVITY Degree of physical activity.	1. Bedfast: Confined to bed.	2. Chairfast: Ability to walk severely limited or non-existent. Cannot bear own weight and / or must be assisted into chair or wheelchair.	3. Walks occasionally: Walks occasionally during day but for very short distances, with or without assistance. Spends majority of each shift in bed or chair.	4. Walks frequently: Walks outside the room at least twice a day and inside room at least once every 2 hours during waking hours.	
MOBILITY Ability to change and control body position.	1. Completely immobile: Does not make even slight changes in body or extremity position without assistance.	2. Very limited: Makes occasional slight changes in body or extremity position but unable to make frequent or significant changes independently.	3. Slightly limited: Makes frequent though slight changes in body or extremity position independently.	4. No limitation: Makes major and frequent changes in position without assistance.	
NUTRITION Usual food intake pattern.	1. Very poor: Never eats a complete meal. Rarely eats more than 1/3 of any food offered. Eats 2 servings or less of protein (meat or dairy products) per day. Takes fluids poorly. Does not take a liquid dietary supplement OR is NPO and / or maintained on clear liquids or IVs for more than 5 days.	2. Probably inadequate: Rarely eats a complete meal and generally eats only about 1/2 of any food offered. Protein intake includes only 3 servings of meat or dairy products per day. Occasionally will take a dietary supplement OR receives less than optimum amount of liquid diet or tube feeding.	3. Adequate: Eats over half of most meals. Eats a total of 4 servings of protein (meat or dairy products) each day. Occasionally will refuse a meal but will usually take a supplement if offered OR is on a tube feeding or TPN regimen which probably meets most of nutritional needs.	4. Excellent: Eats most of every meal. Never refuses a meal. Usually eats a total of 4 or more servings of meat and dairy products. Occasionally eats between meals. Does not require supplementation.	
FRICTION AND SHEAR	1. Problem: Requires moderate to maximum assistance in moving. Complete lifting without sliding against sheets in impossible. Frequently slides down in bed or chair, requiring frequent repositioning with maximum assistance. Spasticity,contractures or agitation leads to almost constant friction.	2. Potential problems: Moves feebly or requires minimum assistance. During a move skin probably slides to some extent against sheets, chair, restraints or other devices. Maintains relatively good position in chair or bed most of the time but occasionally slides down.	3. No apparent problem: Moves in bed and in chair independently and has sufficient strength to lift up completely during move. Maintains good position in bed or chair at all times.		

Total Score

Figure 14.1
The Braden scale. (With permission of B Braden and N Bergstrom and Mosby Publishers.)

INTERVENTIONS TO PREVENT AND TREAT PRESSURE ULCERS

The conceptual schema for the study of the aetiology of pressure ulcers (Braden & Bergstrom 1987) provides a useful framework to establish principles for the prevention and treatment of pressure ulcers. That is, interventions need to address the intensity and duration of pressure and the tolerance of the skin, whether the patient has an existing pressure ulcer or may be at risk of pressure ulcer development.

Interventions should be evidence based and the components that inform evidence-based interventions combine best available research evidence, clinical experience, available resource and patient preference (Fleming & Kenton 2002). The best available research evidence encompasses basic principles established by aetiology, pathophysiology, epidemiology and risk factor research in addition to experimental intervention studies. Clinical experience may encompass specialty-based experience, training and local expertise in the use of specific treatments and equipment. Practitioners must also adapt best available evidence to the local environment and available resources (staff, carers, equipment and treatments) and take full account of patient preferences. Together, these factors – when consciously considered – enable informed and evidence-based practice interventions.

The following sections make specific reference to the best available evidence in relation to experimental intervention studies that have been summarized by systematic reviews, highlight the limitations of our knowledge base and emphasize the contribution that aetiology, pathophysiology, epidemiology and risk-factor research and clinical experience make to the evidence-based decision-making process.

There are various web-based sources of good-quality systematic reviews relating to the effectiveness of interventions for the treatment and prevention of pressure ulcers and various guidelines (AHCPR 1992, EPUAP 1998, NICE 2001), which recommend interventions based upon expert clinical opinion. These reviews and guidelines challenge myths, inform practice and re-emphasize the importance of clinical experience and expertise in the decision-making process.

Intensity and duration of pressure

The need for relief of pressure has long been established and various interventions are used in practice to reduce or relieve both the intensity and duration of pressure applied to skin areas at risk of tissue breakdown, including patient repositioning, equipment provision and patient education.

Positioning

Positioning is important in a number of ways. The position adopted can achieve complete pressure relief of an area, redistribute or reduce localized pressure, and minimize friction and shearing forces. Interventions include turning schedules at specified intervals such as 2–4 hourly, intermittent relief such as standing or elevation in chair fast patients and the use of positioning devices such as pillows and specific techniques such as the 30° tilt.

The relative effectiveness of the different strategies and optimum repositioning intervals have not been determined, reflecting the difficulties associated with research in this field including the operational problems of managing trials which require the cooperation of a large number of ward staff (Cullum et al 1995) and the ethical and professional accountability issues associated with withdrawing individualized patient care.

The absence of good evidence reflects a lack of evidence and conclusions can't be made regarding any lack of benefit (Cullum et al 2001). Indeed, experts across America and Europe continue to include repositioning as an intervention central to the prevention and treatment of pressure ulcers (AHCPR 1992, EPUAP 1998).

In terms of frequency, this should be determined on an individual patient basis and need will depend upon the support surface used, therapies and treatment for primary and secondary diagnoses, patient circumstance, prognosis and preference and ongoing evaluation of the patient's individual skin response.

Equipment

There is an increasingly diverse and expanding equipment market providing for pressure ulcer prevention needs. Support surfaces are generally categorized as:

- Constant low-pressure devices that aim to reduce the overall pressure applied by moulding to the patients, thereby increasing the contact surface area and providing a reduced and more evenly distributed pressure (Cullum et al 1995).
- Dynamic or alternating pressure devices that consist of inflatable cells that are programmed to inflate and deflate and provide intermittent relief of pressure.

Within these two categories, design and performance are greatly variable and comparing and contrasting equipment is difficult. For example, constant low-pressure supports include fibre-filled, foam, gel, and water as both overlay and mattress replacements, as well as complex low air-loss and air-fluidized systems. Similarly, a large number of dynamic overlay and mattress replacement systems are available, which vary in basic construction and design elements, including cell depth, cell cycle, fabric materials, automated pressure adjusters and whether they are pressure generated.

In assessing the clinical effectiveness of mattress and seating interventions, a systematic review of the literature illustrates the limitations of the research base in this area (Cullum et al 2000). However, this review establishes that, as a basic minimum, a high specification foam mattress should be provided for at-risk patients, and perhaps challenges arguments and myths about 'what's best'. The lack of evidence places individual patient need as the central focus to decision making. Key findings of the systematic review are summarized in Box 14.2.

Box 14.2 **Beds, mattresses and cushions for pressure ulcer prevention and treatment (Cullum et al 2000)**	**Prevention of pressure ulcers** High-specification foam alternatives are more effective than 'standard' hospital foam in moderate–high-risk patients Pressure-relieving mattresses in the operating theatre reduce pressure-ulcer incidence postoperatively The effectiveness of alternating pressure mattresses is unknown The effectiveness of constant low-pressure devices is unknown There is insufficient evidence on the effects of seat cushions There is insufficient evidence on the effects of low-tech, constant low-pressure supports such as fibre, gel and water **Treatment of pressure ulcers** Air-fluidized beds may improve healing rates

Patient education

The involvement of patients and carers in the prevention and treatment of pressure ulcers for both the inspection of skin and relief of pressure is advocated by American (AHCPR 1992) and European (EPUAP 1998) guidelines. Although the relative effectiveness of patient involvement has not been compared to other possible interventions, there is some evidence of its importance, particularly in home-care settings. In a small study of community patients, frequency of care (as delivered by carers) was found to be one of a number of factors that discriminated between the patients who did and did not develop pressure ulcers (Clarke & Kadhom 1988). In addition, the American guidelines (AHCPR 1992) cite three home-care programmes advocating patient and carer education and involvement on the basis of clinical experience.

Tolerance of skin Maintaining or improving the tolerance of the skin and its capacity to maintain integrity requires a holistic, comprehensive and multiprofessional team approach to patient care. In particular, intrinsic risk factors including nutrition and tissue perfusion require an approach that embraces the large number of potential factors associated with the development of pressure ulcers throughout episodes of care.

It is also a challenge for the multiprofessional team to ensure that treatment for a primary or secondary diagnosis does not exacerbate intrinsic or extrinsic risk factors associated with pressure-ulcer development. Examples are anecdotal but familiar and can include surgical techniques that generate friction, therapeutic hypotension, cooling and warming of patients, inadequate pain relief and treatment side-effects such as diarrhoea, incontinence, loss of appetite, dehydration, altered sensation, reduced dermal thickness and so on.

Interventions to promote tissue tolerance care largely established on the basis of clinical experience and expert opinion.

Skin care

Although the relationship between both urinary and faecal incontinence and pressure ulcer development remains unclear (as discussed above), all clinical guidelines advocate that skin cleansing and adequate skin hydration are important features in the prevention of pressure ulcers (AHCPR 1992, EPUAP 1998).

Skin cleansing and hydration has been the subject of little experimental research in relation to pressure ulcer development, and it is recommended that care should be individualized according to need and preference, taking into account the condition of the skin, patient age, dryness, ambient temperature and humidity (AHCPR 1992).

Friction and shear

A range of interventions minimize or reduce exposure to friction and shear, and include: effective positioning and equipment allocation that minimize forward slide; transferring and repositioning techniques that avoid drag; the use of protective dressings such as films; and the use of protective padding.

The evidence for such interventions is minimal and recommendations for practice are based upon clinical experience and expert opinion (AHCPR 1992, EPUAP 1998).

Nutritional care

Assessing the nutritional status of patients, both hospital and community, and addressing deficits is a key component of care in the prevention and treatment of pressure ulcers. A complex aspect of care, principles for practice are discussed in detail in Chapter 11.

Wound-care interventions

In practice, the majority of pressure ulcers remain superficial (grade 2) and heal with minimal or no dressing interventions. However, a range of therapeutic interventions can be used to promote the healing of pressure ulcers, although their effectiveness is largely unknown. A number of systematic reviews have been undertaken by The Cochrane Wounds Group and the NHS National Coordinating Centre for Health Technology Assessment, which summarize the evidence available in some areas of wound-care intervention in relation to the treatment of pressure ulcers. Key findings include:

- it is unclear whether wound debridement is a beneficial process that expedites healing (Bradley et al 1999a)
- there is insufficient evidence to promote the use of one debriding agent over another (Bradley et al 1999a)
- there is little evidence to indicate which dressings or topical agents are the most effective in the treatment of chronic wounds (Bradley et al 1999b)
- there is evidence that hydrocolloid dressings are better than wet-to-dry dressings for the treatment of pressure ulcers (Bradley et al 1999b)
- three randomized controlled trials comparing ultrasound versus non- or standard treatment found no difference (Flemming & Cullum 2001a)
- two studies comparing electromagnetic therapy versus control found no difference (Flemming & Cullum 2001b).

The limitations of the evidence base in relation to the clinical effectiveness of interventions reinforces the need to consider individual patient need and preference, accurate documentation of wound progression, regular evaluation of wound healing and local clinical expertise and experience.

EVALUATION AND REASSESSMENT

Evaluation of care interventions and ongoing reassessment of risk need to be focused upon patient comfort and the individual skin response to pressure. Where skin sites are free from pressure ulcers, observation of 'normal' skin at pressure sites should be recorded as a positive outcome of the interventions. Blanching erythema or other skin changes should prompt consideration as to whether the response observed is normal or abnormal and a judgement made regarding clinical importance. The observation of non-blanching erythema should prompt immediate review of the interventions provided and clinical judgement of their appropriateness.

In relation to healing of existing pressure ulcers, reverse staging has been widely criticized and various wound assessment tools developed, for example, Sessing scale, PSST (Pressure Sore Status Tool) and PUSH tool (Pressure Ulcer Scale for Healing) (Woodbury et al 1999). Issues such as validity, reliability and practicality of such tools are beyond the scope of this chapter but debate highlights the difficulties encountered in practice in evaluating wound progress, particularly for severe wounds.

CONCLUSIONS

Pressure-ulcer prevention and treatment requires a holistic and multidisciplinary approach. The evidence base provides a broad framework for baseline screening and individual assessment of patient risk and intervention needs. The framework combines consideration of the patient's exposure to pressure (intensity and duration), the tolerance of the skin and the skin's actual response and requires a dynamic, continuous process involving the synthesis of information from a variety of sources.

REFERENCES

AHCPR (Agency for Health Care Policy and Research) 1992 Pressure ulcers in adults: prediction and prevention: quick reference guide for clinicians. Department of Health and Human Services, Rockville, MD

Allman R M 1997 Pressure ulcer prevalence, incidence, risk factors and impact. Clinics in Geriatric Medicine 13:421–436

Allman R M, Goode P S, Patrick M M et al 1995 Pressure ulcer risk factors among hospitalized patients with activity limitation. Journal of the American Medical Association 273:865–870

Barczak C A, Barnett R I, Child E J, Bosley L M 1997 Fourth national pressure ulcer prevalence survey. Advances in Wound Care 10:18–26

Barrois B, Allaert F A, Colin D 1995 A survey of pressure sore prevalence in hospitals in the Greater Paris region. Journal of Wound Care 4:234–236

Bergstrom N, Braden B 1992 A prospective study of pressure sore risk among institutionalized elderly. Journal of the American Geriatrics Society 40:747–758

Bergstrom N, Braden B J, Laguzza A, Holman V 1987 The Braden scale for predicting pressure sore risk. Nursing Research 36:205–210

Bergstrom N, Braden B, Kemp M et al 1996 Multi-site study of incidence of pressure ulcers and the relationship between risk level, demographic characteristics, diagnosis and prescription of preventive interventions. Journal of the American Geriatrics Society 44:22–30

Berlowitz D R, Wilking S V B 1989 Risk factors for pressure sores: a comparison of cross-sectional and cohort-derived data. Journal of the American Geriatrics Society 37:1043–1050

Bours G J, Halfens R J, Lubbers M, Haalboom J R E 1999 The development of a national registration form to measure the prevalence of pressure ulcers in the Netherlands. Ostomy and Wound Management 45:28–40

Braden B, Bergstrom N 1987 A conceptual schema for the study of the etiology of pressure sores. Rehabilitation Nursing 12:8–16

Bradley M, Cullum N, Sheldon T 1999a The debridement of chronic wounds: a systematic review. 3(17) part 1. The National Coordinating Centre for Health Technology Assessment, Southampton

Bradley M, Cullum N, Nelson E A et al 1999b Systematic reviews of wound care management: (2) Dressings and topical agents used in the healing of chronic wounds. 3 (17) (part 2.) The National Coordinating Centre for Health Technology Assessment, Southampton

Brandeis G H, Ooi W L, Hossain M et al 1994 A longitudinal study of risk factors associated with the formation of pressure ulcers in nursing homes. Journal of the American Geriatrics Society 42:388–393

Bridel J 1993 The pathophysiology of pressure sores. Journal of Wound Care 2:230–238

Clarke M, Kadhom H M 1988 The nursing prevention of pressure sores in hospital and community patients. Journal of Advanced Nursing 13:365–373

Cullum N, Deeks J, Fletcher A et al 1995 The prevention and treatment of pressure sores: How effective are pressure-relieving interventions and risk assessment for the prevention and treatment of pressure sores? Effective Health Care Bulletin 2:1–16

Cullum N, Deeks J, Sheldon T A et al 2000 Beds, mattresses and cushions for pressure sore prevention and treatment. The Cochrane Library, issue 2. Update Software, Oxford

Cullum N, Nelson E A, Nixon J 2001 Pressure sores. In: Clinical evidence: a compendium of the best available evidence for effective healthcare. Issue 5 (June). BMJ Publishing Group, London, p 1357–1364

Ek A-C, Unosson M, Larsson J et al 1991 The development and healing of pressure sores related to the nutritional state. Clinical Nutrition 10:245–250

EPUAP (European Pressure Ulcer Advisory Panel) 1998 Pressure ulcer prevention guidelines. European Pressure Ulcer Advisory Panel, Oxford

EPUAP (European Pressure Ulcer Advisory Panel) 1999 Pressure ulcer treatment guidelines. European Pressure Ulcer Advisory Panel, Oxford

Flemming K, Cullum N 2001b Therapeutic ultrasound for pressure sores. The Cochrane Library, issue 4. Update Software, Oxford

Flemming K, Cullum N 2001a Electromagnetic therapy for treating pressure sores. The Cochrane Library, issue 4. Update Software, Oxford

Flemming K, Fenton M 2002 Making sense of research evidence to inform decision making. In: Thompson C, Dowding D (eds) Critical decision making and nursing judgement in nursing. Churchill Livingstone, Edinburgh

Guralnik J M, Harris T B, White L R, Cornoni-Huntley J C 1988 Occurrence and predictors of pressure sores in the National Health and nutrition examination survey follow-up. Journal of the American Geriatrics Society 36:807–812

Guyton A C 1992 Local control of blood flow by the tissues, and humoral regulation. In: Guyton A C (ed) Human physiology and mechanisms of disease. W B Saunders, Philadelphia, p 136–142

Halfens R J G, Van Achterberg T, Bal R M 2000 Validity and reliability of the Braden scale and the influence of other risk factors: a multi-centre prospective study. International Journal of Nursing Studies 37:313–319

Hoshowsky V M, Schramm C A 1994 Intraoperative pressure prevention: an analysis of bedding materials. Research in Nursing and Health 17:333–339

Kemp M G, Keithley J K, Smith D W, Morreale B 1990 Factors that contribute to pressure sores in surgical patients. Research in Nursing and Health 13:293–301

Krouskop T A 1983 A synthesis of the factors which contribute to pressure sore formation. Medical Hypotheses 11:255–267

Marchette L, Arnell I, Redick E 1991 Skin ulcers of elderly surgical patients in critical care units. Dimensions of Critical Care Nursing 10:321–329

McGough A J 1999 A systematic review of the effectiveness of risk assessment scales used in the prevention and management of pressure sores. University of York, MSc thesis

NICE (National Institute for Clinical Excellence) 2001 Pressure ulcer risk assessment and prevention. Online. Available: www.nice.org.uk

Nixon J E 2001a Predicting and preventing pressure sores in surgical patients. University of Newcastle-upon-Tyne, PhD thesis

Nixon J 2001b The pathophysiology and aetiology of pressure ulcers. In: Morison M (ed) The prevention and treatment of pressure ulcers. Mosby, Edinburgy, p 17–36

Nixon J, McGough A 2001 Principles of patient assessment: screening for pressure ulcers and potential risk. In: Morison M (ed) The prevention and treatment of pressure ulcers. Mosby, Edinburgh, p 55–74

Nixon J, Smye S, Scott J, Bond S 1999 The diagnosis of early pressure sores: report of the pilot study. Journal of Tissue Viability 9:62–66

Nixon J, Brown J, McElvenny D et al 2000 Prognostic factors associated with pressure sore development in the immediate post-operative period. International Journal of Nursing Studies 37:279–289

NPUAP 1998 Stage 1: assessment in darkly pigmented skin. Online. Available: www.npuap.org/positn4.htm

O'Dea K 1995 The prevalence of pressure sores in four European countries. Journal of Wound Care 4:192–195

Schnelle J F, Adamson G M, Cruise P A et al 1997 Skin disorders and moisture in incontinent nursing home residents: intervention implications. Journal of the American Geriatrics Society 45:1182–1188

Schue R M, Langemo D K 1998 Pressure ulcer prevalence and incidence and a modification of the Braden scale for a rehabilitation unit. Journal of Wound Ostomy and Continence Nurses 25:36–43

Thomas D R, Goode P S, Tarquine P H, Allman R M 1996 Hospital-acquired pressure ulcers and risk of death. Journal of the American Geriatrics Society 44:1435–1440

Witkowski J A, Parish L C 1982 Histopathology of the decubitus ulcer. Journal of the American Academy of Dermatology 6:1014–1021

Woodbury G, Houghton P E, Campbell K E, Keast D H 1999 Pressure ulcer assessment instruments: a critical appraisal. Ostomy Wound Management 45(3):42–55

FURTHER READING

Cullum N, Deeks J, Sheldon T A et al 2000 Beds, mattresses and cushions for pressure sore prevention and treatment. The Cochrane Library, issue 2. Update Software, Oxford

Nixon J 2001 The pathophysiology and aetiology of pressure ulcers. In: Morison M (ed) The prevention and treatment of pressure ulcers, 2nd edn. Mosby, Edinburgh, p 17–36

Nixon J, McGough A 2001 Principles of patient assessment: screening for pressure ulcers and potential risk. In: Morison M (ed) The prevention and treatment of pressure ulcers, 2nd edn. Mosby, Edinburgh, p 55–74

WEB-BASED SOURCES

National Pressure Ulcer Advisory Panel: www.npuap.org
European Pressure Ulcer Advisory Panel: www.epuap.org
The Cochrane Collaboration: www.cochrane.org.uk
The National Coordinating Centre for Health Technology Assessment: www.ncchta.org

CHAPTER 15

Leg ulcers

Moya J Morison and Chris Moffatt

INTRODUCTION

Leg ulceration is a common problem, affecting 1–2% of the population in the UK, US and Europe, and an even higher proportion of the population in less developed countries (Nelzen et al 1991). In the developed world, most leg ulcers are of vascular origin and the highest prevalence occurs in the very elderly. In this population the recurrence rate is high, with 20% of sufferers having more than six episodes and many ulcers failing to heal over a period of many years (Callam et al 1987). However, in tropical climates, where the major causes are trauma and infection, leg ulceration can occur at any age and can become life threatening in the absence of appropriate care.

The 1990s saw major advances in treatment and in the ways that patient care is organized in many countries. New services are emerging to bridge the gap between community and acute care, and embrace the multidisciplinary approach. A number of such services are now nurse led, and have explicit referral criteria in place for more specialist assessment and care (Ghauri et al 1998, Moffatt et al 1992). The possibility of improved health outcomes for patients and the high costs associated with long-term care have all contributed to raising the profile of leg ulceration and to the drive for audited, evidence-based practice (Bosanquet et al 1993, Morrell et al 1998).

At a personal level, research is uncovering the considerable impact of leg ulceration on quality of life for patients of all ages (Franks & Moffatt 1998, Philips et al 1994). Risk factors for delayed healing, such as ulcer chronicity and size, highlight the importance of early intervention and appropriate treatment (Margolis et al 1999). Social risk factors relating to the patient's environment and lifestyle may also contribute to delayed healing, and this is an area that requires further research (Flett et al 1994).

This chapter begins by reviewing the causes of leg ulceration, with particular emphasis on ulcers of vascular origin. Understanding the anatomy of the blood supply to the lower limb, and its related pathophysiology, are prerequisites to understanding the principles of patient assessment and treatment that follow.

CAUSES OF LEG ULCERS

A number of pathological conditions are associated with ulceration in the lower limb (Box 15.1). The most common of these aetiologies are described below, beginning with ulcers associated with chronic venous hypertension.

Venous ulcers

An understanding of the cause of venous ulceration requires an understanding of the anatomy of the venous system of the lower limb (Fig. 15.1) and the mechanics of its blood flow.

Box 15.1
Causes of leg ulcers

1. Principal causes
- Chronic venous hypertension, usually because of incompetent valves in the deep and perforating veins
- Arterial disease, for example, atherosclerotic occlusion of large vessels leading to tissue ischaemia
- Combined chronic venous hypertension and arterial disease

2. More unusual causes (2–5% in total)
- Neuropathy, for example, associated with diabetes mellitus, spina bifida, leprosy
- Vasculitis, for example, associated with rheumatoid arthritis, polyarteritis nodosum
- Malignancy, for example, squamous-cell carcinoma, melanoma, basal-cell carcinoma, Kaposi's sarcoma
- Blood disorders, for example, polycythaemia, sickle-cell disease, thalassaemia
- Infection, for example, tuberculosis, leprosy, syphilis, fungal infections
- Metabolic disorders, for example, pyoderma gangrenosum, pretibial myxoedema
- Lymphoedema
- Trauma, for example, lacerations, burns, irradiation injuries
- Iatrogenic, for example, overtight bandaging, ill-fitting plaster cast
- Self-inflicted

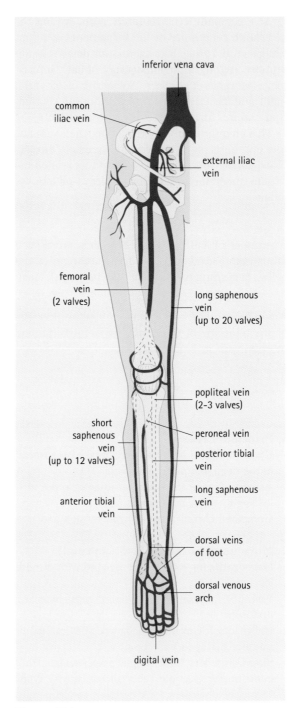

Figure 15.1
Veins of the pelvis and lower limb, illustrating the right
common iliac vein and its tributaries

Anatomy of the venous system and the mechanics of blood flow

The leg consists of three systems of veins: the deep, superficial and perforating veins. These contain valves to prevent back-flow of blood (Fig. 15.2). Venous return is aided by a combination of mechanisms, including calf muscle contraction, variations in intra-abdominal and intrathoracic pressure. Failure of the valves allows reverse flow of blood causing further damage to other valves, leading to varicose veins (Fig. 15.3). Damaged valves in the deep and perforating veins are one cause of chronic venous hypertension in the lower limb leading to venous stasis and oedema. Venous return is also facilitated by ankle movement (extension of the Achilles tendon) and by foot pumps, which are activated as the heel strikes the ground in walking. Limitation in a patient's mobility can therefore seriously affect venous function (Sochart & Hardinge 1999).

Clinical signs of chronic venous hypertension

Some of the complications arising from chronic venous hypertension, including varicose veins, staining of the skin, stasis eczema and lipodermatosclerosis are summarized in Fig. 15.4, illustrated in Fig. 15.5 and described below.

Varicose veins.   Varicose veins are a common problem, found in 10–20% of the adult population. People in occupations that involve prolonged standing in warm conditions, such as nurses, teachers and warehousemen, are particularly at risk (Evans et al 1997).

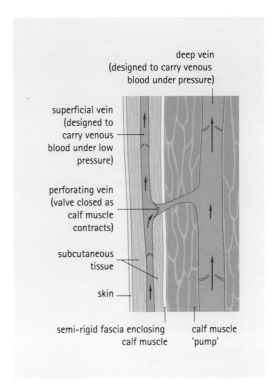

Figure 15.2
Healthy, intact valves prevent backflow of blood from the deep to the superficial veins

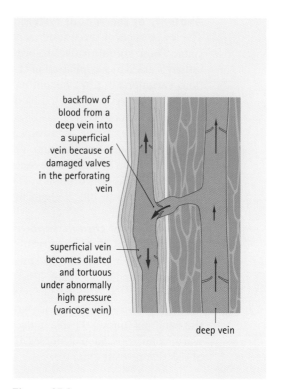

backflow of
blood from a
deep vein into
a superficial
vein because of
damaged valves
in the perforating
vein

superficial vein
becomes dilated
and tortuous
under abnormally
high pressure
(varicose vein)

deep vein

Figure 15.3
An incompetent valve in a perforating vein allows
backflow of blood from the deep to the superficial
venous system

Varicose veins are a sign of chronic venous hypertension in the lower limb, which is usually due to damage to the valves in the leg veins. The damage may be congenital or acquired. The result is that the superficial venous network is exposed to much higher pressures than normal (up to 90 mmHg instead of 30 mmHg). The superficial veins, especially the relatively thin-walled tributaries of the long and short saphenous veins, become dilated, lengthened and tortuous. About 3% of patients with varicose veins go on to develop leg ulcers but not all patients with venous ulcers have varicose veins. It is therefore not clear whether varicose veins and venous ulcers are merely associated conditions with a common aetiology, or whether varicose veins are a predisposing factor for venous ulcers.

Staining of the skin in the gaiter region. Chronic venous hypertension leads to distension of the blood capillaries and damage to the endothelium, leading to leakage of red blood cells. The breakdown products of haemoglobin cause pigmentation. This can clearly be seen in Fig. 15.5.

Ankle flare. This is distension of the tiny veins on the medial aspect of the foot. It is frequently associated with perforator vein incompetence.

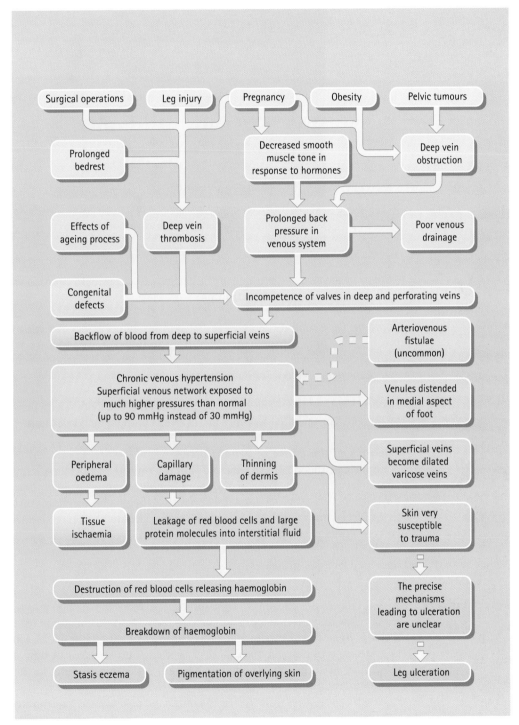

Figure 15.4
Complications arising from chronic venous hypertension (reproduced from Morison & Moffatt 1994)

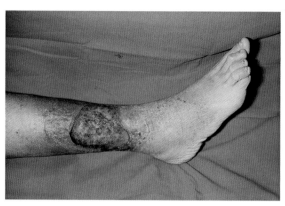

Figure 15.5
Leg ulceration in a patient with chronic venous hypertension

Atrophy of the skin.   Thinning of the dermis associated with poor blood supply makes the skin susceptible to trauma.

Eczema.   Eczematous changes to the skin are often associated with venous insufficiency and can be aggravated by a number of wound care products through irritation and allergy, as described in Chapter 10. Secondary infection can occur if the patient scratches persistently.

Lipodermatosclerosis.   This is 'woody' induration of the tissues, with fat replaced by fibrosis. The leg often assumes an inverted champagne bottle shape.

Theories of the cause of venous ulcers

A number of theories have emerged that attempt to explain the pathogenesis of venous ulceration. Four of the more popular theories are summarized in Table 15.1. It must be stressed, however, that the precise mechanisms leading to leg ulceration are still the subject of intense debate (Agren et al 2000). The current thinking suggests that reperfusion injury is the most likely mechanism, which in turn leads to neutrophil activation, free-radical production and increased levels of proteases.

Arterial ulcers   Arterial ulcers are caused by an insufficient arterial blood supply to the limb resulting in tissue ischaemia and necrosis (Fig. 15.6). Occlusion may occur in major or more distal arteries and may be chronic or acute (Box 15.2). Clinically, the skin surrounding an arterial ulcer is often shiny and loss of hair, adipose tissue and sweat glands is common. There is no brown staining in the gaiter region unless chronic venous hypertension is also present (Fig. 15.7).

   Atherosclerosis is by far the most common cause and is the deposition and accumulation of fatty material in the walls of arteries to form plaques. The plaques cause narrowing of the lumen of the vessels, causing increased resistance to blood flow. The plaques fissure and haemorrhage leading to thrombosis, embolization and consequent ischaemia. Other risk factors that can influence the severity of the atherosclerosis include: being male, hypertension,

Table 15.1
Four theories of the cause of venous ulcers

The fibrin cuff theory	White-cell trapping theory	Mechanical theory	The 'trap' growth factor theory
Layers of fibrin laid down as cuffs around the capillary wall cause a diffusion barrier to oxygen and nutrients, leading to trophic skin changes	Accumulation and activation of white cells in the microcirculation of patients with venous hypertension. Production of toxic metabolites leads to tissue breakdown	Ulceration results from mechanical stress on the patient's limb. High pressure in the capillary bed leads to oedema, which in turn raises tissue pressure resulting in stretching of the skin. Ulceration is thought to result from tissue ischaemia	Leakage of fibrinogen and protein bound growth factors. The growth factors are trapped in the fibrin cuff, preventing their use in normal epidermal tissue repair

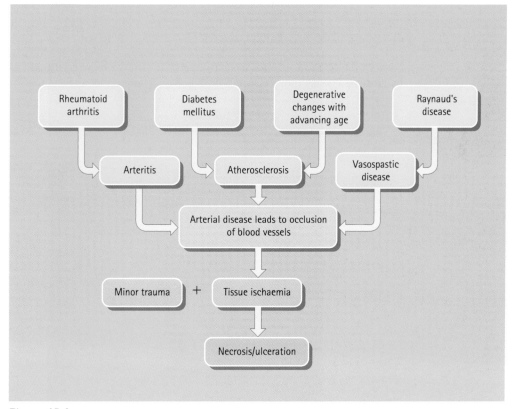

Figure 15.6
Diseases and disorders associated with arterial ulcers: a tentative model (reproduced from Morison & Moffatt 1994)

Box 15.2 *Causes of* *ischaemia in* *the leg*	• Atherosclererosis • Arterial embolism • Vasospastic disease, for example, Raynaud's • Trauma, for example, open or closed injuries, such as leg fractures or dislocation • Cold, for example, frostbite or immersion

hyperlipidaemia, diabetes mellitus and smoking. Diabetes and smoking are most strongly linked with ischaemia in the legs (Fowkes & Callam 1994). Combinations of risk factors, rather than one isolated risk factor, seem to be particularly hazardous. The most common sites for atherosclerosis in the lower limb are the lower superficial femoral artery (60%) and the aortoiliac segments (30%), with multiple segment involvement occurring in about 7% of cases (Orr & McAvoy 1987). The degree of ischaemia and the symptoms experienced depend not only on the site of the occlusion but also on the presence or absence of an effective collateral circulation.

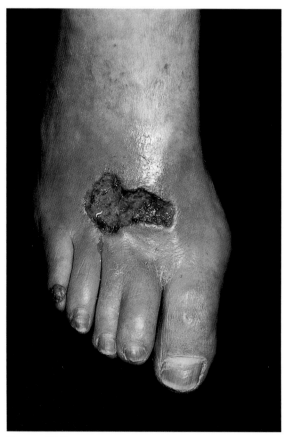

Figure 15.7
Leg ulceration in a patient with advanced arterial disease

Acute ischaemia due to arterial embolism is potentially the most damaging because the body has not had the time to develop a collateral circulation to compensate. Where an occlusion has developed over a prolonged period of time it may cause no noticeable effects for the individual. At rest, an individual may be able to tolerate up to 70% occlusion of an artery in the lower limb without being aware of any ill effects. On exercise, the increased demands for oxygen in the muscle cannot be met, causing intermittent claudication. In patients with ischaemic pain at rest, the blood vessel is likely to be 90% occluded, indicating a severely compromised arterial circulation.

Critical ischaemia is associated with persistently recurring rest pain requiring regular analgesia, with an ankle systolic pressure ≤ 50 mmHg or toe systolic pressure of ≤ 30 mmHg or ulceration or gangrene of the foot or toes. The foot ulcer of a patient presenting with critical ischaemia is illustrated in Fig. 15.8.

Rheumatoid arthritis and vasculitic ulcers

Leg ulceration is common in patients with rheumatoid arthritis, with up to 10% of patients developing an ulcer at some stage (Pun et al 1990) (Fig. 15.9). Prolonged use of steroids and susceptibility to trauma often leads to delayed healing in these patients. Vasculitic ulcers may be associated with venous insufficiency, trauma 'including pressure', arterial insufficiency and with other connective tissue disorders such as polyarteritis nodosa and systemic lupus erythematosus. The ulcers are often small, multiple and extremely painful. Healing of these ulcers is likely to be slow and is very much affected by the course of the underlying disease (McRorie et al 1998).

Diabetic ulcers

Ulceration of the lower limb, especially the foot, is a common complication for patients with diabetes mellitus (Bowker & Pfeifer 2001). Delayed wound healing and increased vulnerability to infection are likely. Gangrene may develop and there is a high risk of the need for lower limb amputation. However, it has been suggested that 50–75% of amputations are preventable.

The two most common causes of foot ulceration are peripheral neuropathy and peripheral vascular disease. They frequently occur in combination and are complicated by infection. Risk factors for foot ulceration are: previous foot

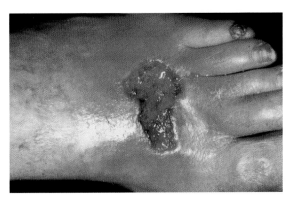

Figure 15.8
Critical ischaemia in an arterial ulcer

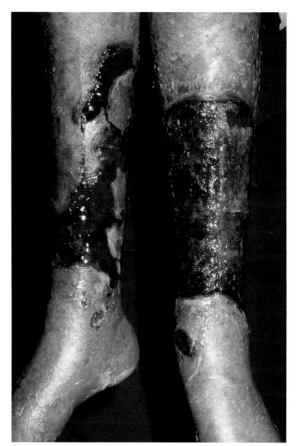

Figure 15.9
Leg ulceration in a patient with severe rheumatoid
arthritis

ulceration or gangrene, increasing age, peripheral vascular disease, male gender, neuropathy, structural deformity of the foot, nephropathy, retinopathy, living alone and duration of the diabetes.

Angiopathy in the diabetic patient

In non-diabetics, arterial occlusion or stenosis is commonly found in the iliac and femoral arteries, while in the diabetic occlusion usually occurs more distally, affecting the tibial, peroneal and distal arteries. Occlusion is likely to be multi-segmental, bilateral and to occur more rapidly and at an earlier stage than in the non-diabetic. Medial calcinosis occurs in the medial lining of the artery. This can result in difficulties in interpreting non-invasive investigation with Doppler ultrasound. Risk factors for the disease include increasing age, duration of diabetes, smoking, hypertension and hypercholesterolaemia. Microcirculatory damage in the diabetic occurs frequently, causing damage to the retina, renal glomeruli and digits of the lower limb. Microcirculatory damage occurs more frequently if glycaemic control is poor.

Neuropathy in the diabetic patient

Three main types of peripheral neuropathy occur: sensory, motor and autonomic.

Sensory neuropathy.   This is characterized by reduced or absent pain sensation in the feet which can result in unnoticed mechanical, thermal or chemical trauma.

Motor neuropathy.   This results in foot deformity due to atrophy of the small muscles of the foot causing clawing of the toes, and prominent metatarsal heads. A changed gait and repeated prolonged pressure can cause a build up of callus leading to ulceration on the sole of the foot, especially under the first metatarsal head (Fig. 15.10) and over enlarged bunions and bony prominences of the toes (Fig. 15.11).

Autonomic neuropathy.   This causes alteration in blood flow. The foot is dry, with lack of sweating. The skin cracks and develops fissures allowing entry of fungi and bacteria. Deep perforating ulceration develops below the calluses, leading to infection and abscess formation. The callus may mask the extent of the underlying ulceration. Infection and osteomyelitis are common complications that need prompt and aggressive treatment with debridement and systemic antibiotics.

Other causes of ulceration in the patient with diabetes

Diabetic patients can, of course, develop ulcers due to other pathologies, such as chronic venous hypertension (Nelzen et al 1993). It is crucial to determine the underlying cause of the ulceration for each individual. The role of

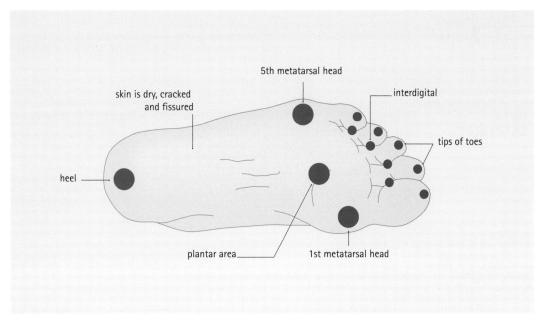

Figure 15.10
Areas of callus formation and neuropathic ulceration beneath calluses.

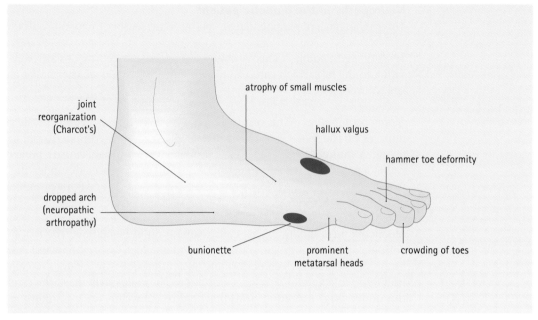

Figure 15.11
The neuropathic foot

prevention is particularly important in the diabetic as tissue damage may have devas-tating consequences.

More unusual causes of leg ulcers

Some of the more unusual causes of leg ulcers are summarized in Table 15.2. In developed countries approximately 2–5% of leg ulcers are due to these more uncommon causes, but in the tropics the incidence of ulceration due to trauma and infection is much higher.

PATIENT ASSESSMENT

When a patient presents for the first time with a leg ulcer, a general patient assessment is required to determine:

- the immediate cause of the ulcer
- any underlying pathology in the lower limb
- any local problems at the wound site, which may delay healing
- other more general medical conditions, which may delay healing
- the patient's social circumstances and the optimum setting for care.

Assessing the immediate cause of the ulcer and any underlying pathology

It is important to determine the immediate cause of the ulcer to facilitate the development of a plan with the patient to prevent recurrence. It is of para-mount importance to go on to determine any underlying pathology.

Assessment of the patient's clinical signs and symptoms, past medical history and some simple investigations normally give sufficient information to deter-mine if an ulcer is due to:

Table 15.2
More unusual causes of leg ulceration

Cause	Description
Malignant ulcers	
Squamous cell carcinomas	Can be seen as a primary carcinoma or with an ulcer that undergoes malignant change (Marjolin's ulcer)
Basal cell carcinoma	Usually found on the face but may occur on the leg. Lesion usually presents as a scab, which when knocked, bleeds profusely
Melanomas	Currently on the increase, probably due to exposure to ultraviolet sunlight. These tumours metastasize rapidly. Ulceration of the lesion is indicative of an advanced stage of malignancy
Kaposi's sarcoma, lymphangiosarcoma and bone tumour	Seen often in patients with HIV (AIDS). The lesions can mimic the presentation of a melanoma or of a venous ulcer
Blood disorders	
Sickle-cell disease	Small, perforating ulcers on the lower limb frequently follow a sickle-cell crisis. Frequently wrongly described as arterial in origin, they develop because of thrombosis occurring in the veins following sickling. Treatment is therefore compression therapy
Thalassaemia	Small painful ulcers, most commonly in teenagers and young adults
Polycythaemia	Seen in older people, usually occurring as atypical ulcers on the foot
Macroglobulinaemias	Rare blood disorders in which ulceration presents as one of many symptoms. Ulceration occurs due to damage in the microcirculation following the accumulation of large protein molecules
Infection	
Tuberculosis	Currently on the increase. Skin ulceration may present alone but often with chest involvement. The ulcer base is usually grey–pink with irregular, bluish friable edges
Syphilis	Rare cause of ulceration today, but still occurs occasionally. Often presenting in the tertiary stage of the disease with accompanying osteomyelitis. Tends to occur high on the calf or outer aspect of the lower leg
Leprosy	Progressive destruction of digits and ulceration with associated neuropathy, ulcers usually occur on plantar surface
Fungal infection	Occurs in tropical areas associated with malnutrition, poor hygiene and poverty
Metabolic disorders	
Pyoderma gangrenosum	Often accompanies systemic disorders such as ulcerative colitis, Crohn's disease, rheumatoid arthritis or myeloma
Pretibial myxoedema	Rare type of ulceration occurring in patients with myxoedema
Necrobiosis lipodica	Occurs predominantly in patients with diabetes mellitus. Pigmented areas with ulceration in the gaiter region involving secondary infection of the dermis, which becomes progressively necrotic

continued

Table 15.2—cont'd
More unusual causes of leg ulceration

Cause	Description
Lymphoedema	1. Primary lymphoedema due to congenital absence of lymphatic vessels, rarely presenting with ulceration 2. Secondary lymphoedema accompanying venous disease 3. Parasitic elephantiasis caused by filiasis causing lymphatic destruction
Iatrogenic	Compression-induced ulceration where there is arterial insufficiency, or overtight bandaging over a bony prominence where compression is indicated
Self-inflicted ulceration	Deliberate attempts to create or sustain ulceration Possible indicators include: • ulceration in unusual sites • no other pathology • immediate improvement when limb is immobilized and protected from damage Evidence of tampering with dressings or bandages is *not*, in itself, evidence of self-inflicted injury. It may be a very understandable but unwise response to a dermatological problem

- chronic venous hypertension
- arterial disease
- a combination of chronic venous hypertension and arterial disease.

The differential diagnosis of the more unusual causes of ulceration is more complex and beyond the scope of this chapter.

> Specialist assessment is particularly important for patients with diabetes mellitus or suspected arterial disease as the consequences of mismanagement can be catastrophic.

Clinical signs and symptoms

Clinical signs and symptoms of venous and arterial disorders are summarized in Boxes 15.3 and 15.4. Interpretation of the symptoms of vascular disease requires considerable clinical experience. Problems causing pain with walking, such as arthritis, must be differentiated from arterial insufficiency, with associated intermittent claudication. It is important to note that, while intermittent claudication most commonly occurs as pain in the calf, high vascular obstruction can cause pain in the buttocks and thighs and may be accompanied by impotence.

Rest pain usually indicates at least two significant arterial stenoses or occlusions in series. It decreases with dependency of the lower limb and is made worse by heat, elevation and exercise. In the course of peripheral vascular disease, nocturnal, ischaemic pain usually precedes rest pain. It occurs at night during sleep when peripheral perfusion is reduced. The person gains relief by dangling

Box 15.3
Venous problems:
clinical signs and
symptoms

1. **Prominent superficial leg veins or symptoms of varicose veins, such as:**
   - Aching or heaviness in legs, generalized or localized
   - Mild ankle swelling
   - Itching over varices
   - Symptoms caused by thrombophlebitis, localized pain, tenderness and redness (gentle exercise such as walking round the room or repeated heel raising helps to show distension of the veins)

2. **Ankle flare.** Distension of the tiny veins on the medial aspect of the foot below the malleolus

3. **Pathological changes to the skin and tissues surrounding the ulcer, including:**
   - Pigmentation. 'Staining' of the skin around the ulcer
   - Lipodermatosclerosis. Hardening of dermis and underlying subcutaneous fat, which may feel 'woody'
   - Stasis eczema
   - Atrophe blanche. Ivory white skin stippled with red 'dots' of dilated capillary loops

4. **Site of ulcer.** Frequently near the medial malleolus, sometimes near the lateral malleolus but can be anywhere on the leg

the feet over the edge of the bed. In diabetic patients, severe pain in the legs at night can be due to diabetic neuropathy or vascular insufficiency, or both (Vowden & Vowden 1997).

The signs and symptoms of acute arterial occlusion are given in Box 15.5. Irreversible damage to skeletal muscle and peripheral nerves occurs within 4–6 h of severe ischaemia, in the absence of an adequate collateral circulation.

Patients known to have severe peripheral vascular disease must be warned to seek immediate medical help should they develop sudden extreme pain in the leg.

For the diabetic patient, peripheral neuropathy is the most significant cause of ulceration. The neuropathy may be sensory, motor or autonomic, as described above. The signs and symptoms of diabetic neuropathy are summarized in Box 15.6.

Diabetic neuropathy is frequently bilateral and tends to be symmetrical. Patients are inclined to underreport symptoms of reduced sensation (hypoaesthesia), yet knowledge of such symptoms is crucially important for planning appropriate care and attempting to prevent recurrence of ulceration.

It is important to note that there are other causes of peripheral neuropathy. These include alcoholism, collagen disorders, pernicious anaemia, malignancy affecting the spinal cord and uraemia.

Box 15.4
Arterial problems:
clinical signs and
symptoms

1. Whole leg/foot

Symptoms:

- Intermittent claudication: cramp-like pain in the muscles of the leg, brought on by walking a certain distance (depending partly on speed, gradient and patient's weight). The patient gains relief by standing still to rest the ischaemic calf muscles
- Ischaemic rest pain: intractable constant ache felt in the foot, typically in the toes or heels. Usually relieved by dependency: hanging the leg over the bed or sleeping upright in a chair

Signs (many are suggestive but not specific to ischaemia):

- Coldness of the foot
- Loss of hair
- Atrophic, shiny skin
- Muscle wasting in calf or thigh
- Trophic changes in nails
- Poor tissue perfusion, for example, colour takes more than 3 seconds to return after blanching of toenail bed by applying direct pressure
- Colour changes: foot/toes dusky pink when dependent, turning pale when raised above the heart
- Gangrene of toes
- Loss of pedal pulses

2. Site of ulcer

- Usually on the foot or lateral aspect of the leg but may occur anywhere on the limb, including near the medial malleolus, which is the most common site for venous ulcers

Box 15.5
Clinical signs and
symptoms of acute
arterial occlusion
in the lower limb

- Pain of sudden onset and severe intensity
- Pallor
- Paraesthesia (numbness)
- Pulselessness (absence of pulses below the occlusion)
- Paralysis (sudden weakness in the limb)
- Polar (a cold extremity)

The importance of specialist vascular assessment for patients thought to have a significant degree of peripheral arterial disease, and for patients with diabetes mellitus, cannot be overemphasized.

Past medical history

The factors in a patient's past medical history that might throw some light on the underlying aetiology are summarized in Box 15.7. Chronic venous hypertension is suggested by a history of varicose veins or thrombotic episodes during surgery or pregnancy. A history of stroke, transient ischaemic attacks, angina

Box 15.6
Clinical signs and symptoms of neuropathy in the diabetic foot and leg

1. Foot deformity (e.g. hammer toes), Charcot's foot with collapse of the metatarsal joints giving a 'club foot' appearance
2. Excessive callus formation over bony pressure points, for example, under the metatarsal heads and the plantar surface of the foot
3. Altered sensation (paraesthesia)
   - Hyperaesthesia. Excessive sensitivity of the feet which may be so great that the individual cannot bear the slightest touch. The pain may be constant and is often more severe at night, or
   - Hypoaesthesia. Diminished sensitivity to pain, vibration, temperature or position. The foot may feel 'dead' or the individual may report unusual sensations when walking, for example, likening it to walking on cushions
4. Reduced or absent sweating, often accompanied by dry skin with cracks and fissures

Box 15.7
Medical history: indicators of possible venous or arterial problems

1. Indicators of possible venous problems
- Previous thrombogenic events
  Has the patient ever suffered from one or more of the following?
  - Deep vein thrombosis
  - Thrombophlebitis
  - Leg or foot fracture in the affected limb
- Varicose veins
  - Does the patient have prominent superficial leg veins, with signs of valve incompetence?
  - Has the patient ever had any varicose vein surgery or sclerotherapy in the affected leg?

2. Indicators of possible arterial problems
- Generalized arterial disease
- Are there any indicators of arterial disease such as:
  - Previous myocardial infarction
  - Angina
  - Transient ischaemic attacks
  - Intermittent claudication
  - Cerebrovascular accident

or myocardial infarction increases the probability of there being arterial impairment in the lower limb, and a history of intermittent claudication is almost invariably associated with poor peripheral perfusion.

Simple vascular assessment tests
A number of simple tests can yield very useful information.

Palpation of foot pulses.   In the past, the presence of palpable foot pulses has been taken as a sign of unimpaired arterial circulation in the lower limb and the absence of pulses as indicative of arterial impairment. This is not an entirely fail-safe test, depending as it does on the clinical skills of the assessor.

It is important to note that the dorsalis pedis pulse is congenitally absent in up to 12% of individuals; if the dorsalis pedis pulse is not felt, it is important to palpate the posterior tibial pulse. Oedema is a common problem in patients with ulcers, and this can make pulses hard to feel.

There are a number of other clinical situations where the presence of pedal pulses can give a false impression of a good peripheral arterial circulation. Patients with intermittent claudication may have palpable foot pulses at rest but, following a brisk walk, the pulses disappear. Further investigations are required to determine the severity of the underlying disease. Patients with diabetes mellitus may have bounding pedal pulses but this does not rule-out the possibility of a severely compromised blood supply more distally to the toes. Palpable pulses are usually present in patients with small vessel disease unless there is coexisting and severe atherosclerosis.

Palpation of pedal pulses remains a subjective test. The use of Doppler ultrasound to record a resting pressure index, in conjunction with a comprehensive assessment that takes account of the patient's signs, symptoms and medical history can provide objective evidence of the arterial status of the patient.

The resting pressure index (RPI).   A simple vascular assessment technique that can be readily carried out following training, is the resting pressure index (RPI). This is sometimes referred to as the ankle/brachial pressure index (ABPI). It involves determining the ratio of the ankle to the brachial systolic pressure with the aid of a simple, hand-held, battery-operated Doppler ultrasound probe in place of a stethoscope.

$$\text{Resting pressure index (RPI)} = \frac{\text{ankle systolic pressure}}{\text{brachial systolic pressure}}$$

The procedure for recording the resting pressure index is described in Box 15.8.

To overcome the effects of previous exercise on blood pressure, the patient should lie flat for 15–20 min, during which time the patient's history can be

Box 15.8 ***Procedure for recording the resting pressure index (RPI)***	1. Ensure that the patient has been lying flat for 15–20 min and is comfortable and relaxed. 2. Place the cuff around the arm and apply ultrasound gel over the brachial pulses. Hold the Doppler probe until a good signal is obtained. Inflate the cuff until the signal disappears and gradually lower pressure until the signal returns (this is the brachial systolic reading). Repeat this procedure using the other arm, and take the higher of the two readings to calculate the RPI. 3. Examine the foot and attempt to palpate the posterior tibial and dorsalis pedis pulses. 4. Secure sphygmomanometer cuff just above the ankle, covering any ulcerated area with cling film or a sterile towel. Locate posterior tibial, dorsalis pedis and peroneal pulses. Record the ankle systolic pressures. Take the highest of the readings. 5. To calculate the RPI, divide ankle systolic pressure by brachial systolic pressure.

taken. Patients with dyspnoea may not be able to lie completely flat; this should be recorded. It is important to check that the cuff is an appropriate size and length for the patient's limb. It is recommended that the cuff is 40% of the limb circumference at the mid point of the limb.

To assess the ankle systolic pressure, the cuff is sited just above the malleolar area. Positioning of the cuff is important. The measurements reflect the pressure required to occlude the artery beneath the cuff, and not where the Doppler probe is held. Applying the cuff higher up the limb means that a resting pressure index is not being recorded at the ankle. While it is generally recommended that the Doppler probe be held at a 45–60° angle, it is often necessary to adjust the position if the blood vessel does not lie parallel with the skin. The appropriate ultrasound gel should be used to ensure good transmission of the signal and to prevent corrosion of the probe. A beam of ultrasound waves, emitted by a crystal in the probe, travels to the underlying blood vessels where it is reflected from red blood cells in proportion to the flow velocity of the cells. The returning signal is picked up by a second crystal in the probe.

A normal RPI in a healthy adult is usually greater than 1.0. Patients with a ratio of 0.9–0.95 probably have a mild degree of arterial disease. If the RPI is less than 0.8, there is a significant impairment of blood supply. High compression is contraindicated in patients with a RPI of less than 0.8 and further vascular assessment is required. Patients with a RPI of 0.5–0.75 frequently suffer from intermittent claudication and below 0.5 ischaemic rest pain is common.

Patients with a significantly elevated RPI above 1.5 may have underlying vascular disease such as medial calcinosis. This is found in 10–12% of patients with diabetes. Patients with severe oedema and atherosclerosis (due to calcification) may have abnormal readings and should be treated with great care. Conditions such as atrial fibrillation may make the procedure difficult and the practitioner may be unsure of the true reading. If there is any doubt about the significance of the RPI seek medical advice.

Further vascular assessment methods. Specialist vascular assessment for both arterial and venous disease may be required for patients and are beyond the scope of this chapter.

Other simple investigations

Some simple investigations which can yield valuable results are summarized in Box 15.9.

Box 15.9 ***Other simple*** ***investigations***	• Blood test to test for factors which may indicate potential arteritis or auto-immune disorders; full blood count and estimation of haemoglobin levels • Patch testing for allergens (e.g. lanolin and parabens) which are present in many commonly used wound-care products • Tissue biopsy if malignant changes are suspected • Wound swabs to identify the nature and antibiotic sensitivity of any organisms causing clinical signs of infection

More unusual ulcers

A small proportion of leg ulcers are not vascular in origin, as summarized in Table 15.2. If the wound has an unusual appearance, is in an unusual site, or fails to progress, another aetiology should be suspected and the patient should be investigated further.

Local wound assessment

After assessing the underlying cause of the ulcer, assessment of the wound itself should be undertaken (Chapter 5). This will influence the method of wound cleansing, and the most appropriate primary wound contact dressing (Chapter 8).

The reasons for pain at the wound site should be very carefully assessed as many are easily correctable, and correction can significantly improve the quality of the patient's life (Krasner 1998) (Chapter 12).

Assessing other factors that might affect healing

When taking the patient's history and carrying out an assessment of the patient's current general physical condition, it is worth noting any other factors that could contribute to delayed wound healing such as:

- evidence of, or suspected, malnutrition
- poor mobility, of whatever cause, which may adversely affect the calf muscle pump and venous return
- decreased resistance to infection, whatever the cause
- poor social circumstances.

Assessment of the patient's psychosocial problems is also very important (Chapter 18). The patient's occupation and social circumstances should be considered when deciding on the practical arrangements for managing the ulcer and for patient education (Chapter 13).

TREATMENT OPTIONS

Thorough, systematic and accurate assessment of the patient, the identification of the underlying cause of the ulcer and any local problems at the wound site are prerequisites to planning appropriate care and to preventing avoidable delays in healing. The main management priorities are summarized in Box 15.10 and these principles are described in the context of the aetiology of the ulcer in the following sections.

Box 15.10
The *main* *treatment* *priorities when* *managing leg* *ulcers*

These are to:
- correct the underlying cause of the ulcer
- create the optimum local environment at the wound site
- improve all the wider factors that might delay healing, especially poor mobility, malnutrition and psychosocial issues
- prevent avoidable complications such as wound infection, medicament dermatitis or tissue damage due to overtight bandaging
- maintain healed tissue

Management of venous ulcers

As described above, the main cause of venous ulceration is chronic venous hypertension, with very high pressures being exerted on the superficial venous system, usually due to incompetent valves in the deep or perforating veins. The primary aims of venous ulcer management are therefore to:

- reduce blood pressure in the superficial venous system
- aid venous return of blood to the heart, by increasing the velocity of flow in the deep veins
- reduce oedema by reducing the pressure difference between the capillaries and the tissues.

The use of compression

The best way to achieve these aims is to apply graduated compression from the base of the toes to the knee. Methods of achieving graduated compression include the application to the lower limb of:

- single-layer elastic bandaging
- single-layer inelastic bandaging
- multilayer bandages
- compression stockings.

The advantages and disadvantages of these methods are summarized in Table 15.3. It is very important to understand the performance characteristics of the different bandages available. While all are aiming to apply graduated compression they do so in different ways. Some of the factors affecting the pressure that can be achieved under a bandage are indicated by La Place's law (Box 15.11). Table 15.4 shows the practical implications of this equation and how this relates to problems in bandage application. Figures 15.12 and 15.13 illustrate how to apply a bandage in a spiral or in a figure-of-eight.

It is likely that compression will remain the most important component of treatment for venous and lymphatic disorders (Cullum et al 1999). Systematic reviews of the literature have shown that high compression is more effective than low levels. There is insufficient evidence to recommend individual systems but compression applied in layers is more effective than single layer systems. Training in the application of compression bandaging is important and practitioners need to understand the scientific principles that underpin its effective use.

Box 15.11
La Place's law

Some of the factors affecting the pressure that can be achieved under a bandage are given in the following equation:

$$P \text{ is proportional to } \frac{N \times T}{C \times W}$$

where: P is the pressure exerted by the bandage, N is the number of layers of bandage, T is the bandage tension, C is the circumference of the limb, W is the bandage width.

Table 15.3
Methods of achieving
graduated compression

Type of compression	Advantages	Potential problems
Single elastic bandages	1. Pressure is sustained over time (useful for immobile patients) 2. Useful in patients with limited mobility	1. Potential risk of excessive high pressures with over extension (many bandages have symbols to help practitioners gauge correct extension) 2. High compression bandage may lack ability to conform to limb contours
Inelastic bandages	1. Bandage action enhanced with patient activity 2. Can be applied to patients with mild arterial disease – low resting pressure index 3. Cost effective	1. Bandage may slip during initial treatment to reduce oedema 2. Restricted availability in some places
Multilayer bandages	1. Requires infrequent reapplication 2. Adapted for individual limb size and shape, preventing slippage and limb trauma 3. Use of bandages in combination avoids excessive rises in sub-bandage pressure	1. Not always available on prescription in the community
Elastic compression stockings	1. Pressure profiles of stockings are tested and known 2. A range of compression profiles is available to meet individual needs 3. Much safer than inappropriately applied heavy compression bandages 4. Cosmetically acceptable 5. Useful in preventing recurrence of ulceration	1. Require proper fitting for length, ankle and calf size 2. Initial cost is high, but compares well with the cost of compression bandages over time 3. Can be difficult for patients with restricted movement to apply themselves 4. Compliance rate variable; high compression stockings often poorly tolerated by the elderly but well liked by younger patients who are more mobile

Table 15.4
The application of
La Place's law in practice

Application	Problems relating to application
Number of layers The more layers applied, the higher the sub-bandage pressure	Excessive layers can be applied during bandage application, particularly when bandages are joined or excess bandage remains. This may form a tourniquet and prevent venous return
Bandage tension The greater the extension of the bandage the higher resulting sub-bandage pressure Bandage tension is proportional to: • the elasticity of the bandage • how much the bandage is stretched • how many times it has been washed • how long the bandage is in place	Bandages can be overextended as the bandage is being applied to the limb. Common sites for overextension are around the ankle and at midcalf. Vulnerable points on the limb, such as the tibia, malleoli and dorsum of the foot, should be protected with padding, particularly when single elastic bandages are used

Limb circumference
The pressure exerted by the bandage is inversely proportional to the circumference of the limb
	Thin limbs are at risk of excessive pressure. Bandages are designed to apply the correct pressure to a range of ankle circumferences. The manufacturer's instructions should be carefully read prior to application
	    Thin limbs must be protected with padding and the bandage not over extended
	    Extra padding around the calf will increase the gradient and reduce the risk of pressure damage
	
	Large limbs may not receive a therapeutic level of compression and a stronger elastic bandage may need to be applied. Ulcers occurring in the hollow behind the malleoli may receive inadequate compression. Local pressure can be increased by placing a foam or gauze pad over the primary dressing covering the ulcer
	
	Inverted champagne legs
	Extra padding around the gaiter region may be required to reduce the steep gradient and prevent bandage slippage

Bandage width The pressure exerted by a bandage is inversely proportional to its width	Higher pressures are obtained with narrower bandages and lower pressures with wider ones. Most bandages are a standard 10 cm in width

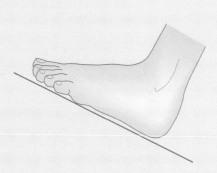

(a) Position the foot in a comfortable position, at a right angle to the leg.

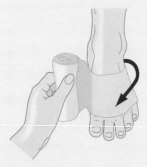

(b) Begin by making two anchoring turns around the foot. Be sure to include the base of the toes.

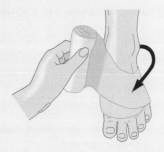

(c) Next take a high turn above the heel.

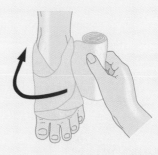

(d) Then fill the base of the foot with a low turn. From here, the bandage can be applied in a spiral as in this figure or in a figure of eight (Figure 15.13).

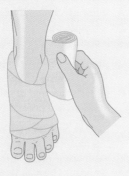

(e) Apply the bandage in a spiral, ensuring there is a 50% overlap.

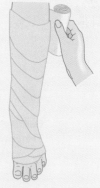

(f) Ensure the bandage is applied right up to the tibial tuberosity.

Figure 15.12
Applying a bandages in a spiral

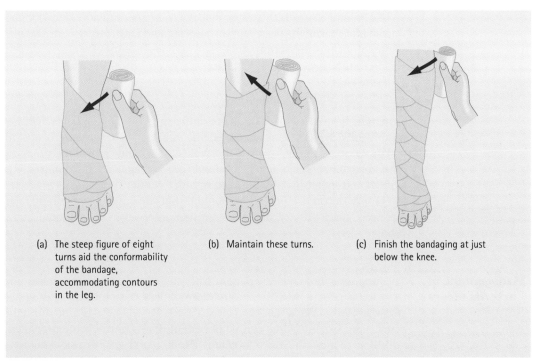

(a) The steep figure of eight turns aid the conformability of the bandage, accommodating contours in the leg.

(b) Maintain these turns.

(c) Finish the bandaging at just below the knee.

Figure 15.13
Applying a bandage in a figure-of-eight

Criteria for using reduced compression. When the underlying cause of the ulcer appears to be a combination of chronic venous hypertension and poor peripheral arterial circulation, it is the degree of arterial insufficiency that will determine whether compression can be applied. If the RPI is below 0.8 reduced compression (no more than 25 mmHg) can be applied on selected patients, according to the patient's symptoms. Patients with an RPI below 0.5 should not have compression applied.

Frequently, patients will undergo reconstructive surgery or angioplasty to correct the arterial impairment. Providing the RPI returns to 0.8 or above, compression can then be applied, but with care. These patients must be followed up regularly and their RPI checked monthly, or more frequently if any change in symptoms occurs. A Duplex scan of the graft or vessel should frequently be undertaken. Following correction of the arterial problem it may be possible to correct any venous abnormality which is amenable to surgery.

Compression hosiery and the prevention of recurrence of a venous ulcer

Compression hosiery is used to control oedema, manage varicose veins and in the prevention and treatment of venous and lymphatic disorders. They have a number of advantages over bandages, provided that they have been correctly fitted and the patient is able to apply them (see Table 15.3). Compression hosiery is graded into three classes according to the compression exerted at the ankle:

- 10–17 mmHg: light compression used to treat mild, early varicose veins

- 18–24 mmHg: medium compression, for more serious varicosities, for patients who have had acute deep vein thrombosis, and for the treatment and prevention of venous ulceration
- 25–35 mmHg: strong compression, for severe chronic venous hypertension, severe varicose veins, and for ulcer prevention and treatment in patients with very-large-diameter calves.

Generally, below-knee stockings are sufficient. However, patients with severe postphlebitic syndrome or lymphoedema may require thigh-length stockings.

The recurrence rate for leg ulceration is high. While providing hosiery is the most important aspect, the patient should be seen regularly and requires ongoing support and encouragement to comply with treatment once the ulcer has healed (Moffatt & Dorman 1995). It is essential that the patient understands why he has been given hosiery, and this can be reinforced by educational literature (Chapter 13).

Management of arterial ulcers

The prognosis for an elderly patient with an arterial ulcer is much less hopeful than for a patient with a venous ulcer, unless the problem is amenable to surgery (Wutschert & Bounameaux 1998). Vasodilators are of questionable benefit, but oxpentifylline can be of benefit. Pain control is often challenging and may require the use of opiates (Hollinworth 1995) (see Chapter 12). Effective wound management and the prevention of infection are critical, as is a reduction of risk factors such as smoking and hypertension.

> Compression bandaging should *not* be applied because severe damage to the leg can result.

Management of ulcers associated with rheumatoid arthritis

The management of a patient with rheumatoid arthritis depends on the underlying aetiology of the ulcer. If compression is required, this should be applied with great care, avoiding excessive pressure to bony prominences. The long-term use of corticosteroids causes dermal thinning and the limb must be protected from trauma. Skin grafts are frequently unsuccessful in these patients and often only palliative care can be offered. Particular attention should be paid to keeping the skin supple with emollients, maintaining mobility and reducing pain. Malnutrition is a frequent problem in these patients, as is an increased risk of infection.

Management of the diabetic foot

The long-term management of diabetic patients, and the prevention of complications, is challenging. It requires a coordinated, multidisciplinary team approach and informed patient cooperation (Edmonds & Foster 2000). As described above, diabetic foot ulcers usually result from the triad of:

- peripheral neuropathy (the insensate foot)
- peripheral vascular insufficiency (ischaemia)
- infection.

Management of diabetic foot ulcers requires aggressive treatment. In the short term, this involves:

- radical local debridement, leaving only healthy tissue
- systemic antibiotic therapy to combat any infection, following antibiotic sensitivity testing (Schmidt et al 2000)
- diabetic control, which, among other effects, optimizes efficiency of the immune system
- non-weight bearing for plantar ulcers.

Appropriate wound dressing selection, as discussed in Chapter 8, is important, but this is merely an adjunct to the above therapies. If an ulcer is refractory to all treatment, the physician may request an X-ray or bone scan to exclude the possibilities of osteomyelitis, or a retained foreign body that the patient is unaware of.

Feet should be kept dry. Soaking the feet causes maceration between the toes and increases the risk of infection. Attention should also be given to rehydrating dry skin around the ulcer and over the lower leg with emollients.

For some patients, it is possible to improve the peripheral circulation through vascular bypass surgery, percutaneous angioplasty, laser treatment and the use of haemorrheologic agents, such as oxpentifyllin, which improves red cell flexibility and blood flow. The combination of endovascular revascularization, growth factor therapy and comprehensive wound-care protocols can lead to very high limb-salvage rates in specialist centres. However, prevention is infinitely preferable to cure. Some risk factors for peripheral vascular disease in diabetic patients are not treatable, such as age and the duration of the diabetes, but many risk factors are amenable to change, such as smoking, hypertension, hyperlipidaemia, hyperglycaemia and obesity, and many long-term complications can be significantly reduced when the patient takes responsibility for self care and has a positive attitude towards health promotion (Chapter 13). Patient education is, in fact, the key to preventing foot ulceration. Patients' feet should be inspected at every routine outpatient visit. They should be encouraged to report foot problems as soon as they occur, however minor. The chiropodist should trim the patient's toe nails and treat calluses and other local foot problems.

Patients should be assessed for the need for special footwear to reduce pressure over bony prominences. Extra-depth shoes can be designed to accommodate clawed toes, and insoles can be made to reduce plantar pressures. Total contact casting may be required for the management of diabetic neuropathic ulcers. Lightweight walking casts are also available in some centres.

Diabetic patients can develop ulcers due to chronic venous hypertension in the absence of any history, clinical signs or symptoms of peripheral vascular disease or peripheral neuropathy. Compression should, however, always be applied with caution and under strict medical supervision.

Creating the optimum local environment for healing

There is no doubt that correcting the underlying cause of an ulcer, where possible, is the first priority of leg ulcer management. However, it is also important to select an appropriate dressing in relation to any local problems at the wound site (see Chapter 8).

Correcting more general causes of delayed wound healing

There are many factors that contribute to delayed healing and which should be addressed in any care plan (Fig. 5.3). Four factors, of particular relevance to leg ulcer patients are: restricted mobility, oedema in the limb, malnutrition and psy-chosocial problems.

Restricted mobility

Reduced mobility in general, and reduced ankle function in particular, are significant factors in delaying venous ulcer healing (Helliwell & Cheesbrough 1994). Patients should be encouraged to maximize their mobility within the limits of their capability and, if they are unable to walk, to carry out ankle extension, flexion and rotation exercises every hour. The physiotherapist can play an important role in increasing patient mobility.

Peripheral oedema

There are many causes of peripheral oedema, including cardiac failure, liver disease, venous and lymphatic disease and malnutrition. Peripheral oedema in a dependent limb can also be encountered in a patient with hemiparesis, following a cerebrovascular accident.

> Identification of the *cause* of the oedema is imperative, because this will determine treatment. In many cases, reducing the oedema by compression is contraindicated.

Peripheral oedema in the lower limb delays healing by increasing the diffusion distance between blood capillaries and the tissues that they serve. The tissues become starved of oxygen and nutrients and metabolic waste products build up.

Oedema can be improved by exercise and leg elevation. Patients with venous ulceration should be encouraged to sit with their legs elevated above the level of their hips and to raise the end of their beds by 23 cm (9 inches) with blocks. However, care must be taken in patients with severe ischaemia and dependency oedema. High elevation will cause severe pain and further compromise the circulation. While severe oedema can be reduced by bed rest and elevation this is rarely a sensible option, leading as it does to other complications such as stiffened joints, deep vein thrombosis and chest infections.

> Oedema due to severe heart failure can occur suddenly. Compression should never be used to reduce this type of oedema because this can exacerbate the condition.

Malnutrition

As with all wounds, malnutrition can lead to delayed wound healing. Malnutrition is a common problem for the elderly for many reasons, including poverty, difficulty in getting to the shops or preparing food, loss of interest in diet when living alone, ill-fitting dentures or specific gastrointestinal disorders. Obese patients can equally be at risk as undernourished patients. Obesity will also contribute to poor ulcer healing through immobility and poor venous return. The role of nutrition in wound healing is discussed extensively in Chapter 11.

Psychosocial issues

Many patients with leg ulcers are elderly, poor and alone. Recent research has shown that social conditions can play a role in delaying healing (Franks et al 1995) (see Chapter 18).

CONCLUSION

The 1990s saw the development of many new treatments and initiatives. It is now recognized that significant improvements in healing can be achieved when research-based methods of assessment and treatment are used. There is, however, no room for complacency. Many questions remain unanswered, such as the underlying pathology of those leg ulcers that fail to heal despite best practice (Salaman & Harding 1995). Interest and excitement in new developments, such as the use of growth factors, has been tempered with caution as the complexity of the situation emerges. Research into the pathogenesis of venous ulceration continues to bring with it the hope that a drug therapy will be developed that breaks the cycle of tissue destruction.

REFERENCES

Agren M S, Eaglstein W H, Ferguson M et al 2000 Causes and effects of the chronic inflammation in venous leg ulcers. Acta Derm Venereol Suppl 210:3–17

Bosanquet N, Franks P J, Moffatt C J 1993 Community leg ulcer clinics: cost effectiveness. Health Trends 25(4):145

Bowker J H, Pfeifer M A (eds) 2001 Levin and O'Neal's the diabetic foot, 6th edn. Mosby, St Louis

Callam M J, Harper D R, Dale J J, Ruckley C V 1987 Chronic ulcer of the leg: clinical history. British Medical Journal 294:1389–1391

Cullum N, Nelson E A, Fletcher A W, Sheldon T A 1999 Compression bandages and stockings for leg ulcers. Systematic review. Cochrane Wounds Group. Cochrane database of systematic reviews issue 4. Update Software, Oxford

Edmonds M, Foster A V M 2000 Managing the diabetic foot. Blackwell Science, Oxford

Evans C J, Fowkes F G R, Ruckley C V et al 1997 Edinburgh vein study: methods and response in a survey of venous disease in the general population. Phlebology 12:127–135

Flett R, Harcourt B, Alpass F 1994 Psychosocial aspects of chronic lower leg ulceration in the elderly. Western Journal of Nursing Research 16(2):183–192

Fowkes F G R, Callam M J 1994 Is arterial disease a risk factor for chronic leg ulceration? Phlebology 9:170

Franks P J, Moffatt C J 1998 Who suffers most from leg ulceration? Journal of Wound Care 7(8):383–385

Franks P J, Bosanquet N, Connolly M et al 1995 Venous ulcer healing: effect of socio-economic factors in London. Journal of Epidemiology and Community Health 49:385–388

Ghauri A S, Nyamekye I, Grabs A J et al 1998 Influence of a specialised leg ulcer service and venous surgery on the outcome of venous leg ulcers. European Journal of Vascular and Endovascular Surgery 16(3):238–244

Hellewell P S, Cheesbrough M J 1994 Arthropathica ulcerosa: a study of reduced ankle movement in association with chronic leg ulceration. Journal of Rheumatology 21(8):1512–1514

Hollinworth H 1995 Nursing assessment and management of pain at wound dressing changes. Journal of Wound Care 4(2):77–83

Krasner D 1998 Painful venous ulcers: themes and stories about their impact on quality of life. Ostomy/Wound Management 44(9):38–49

McRorie E R, Ruckley C V, Nuki G 1998 The relevance of large-vessel vascular disease and restricted ankle movement to the aetiology of leg ulceration in rheumatoid arthritis. British Journal of Rheumatology 37(12):1295–1298

Margolis D J, Berlin J A, Strom B L 1999 Risk factors associated with the failure of a venous leg ulcer to heal. Archives of Dermatology 135(8):920–926

Moffatt C J, Dorman M C 1995 Recurrence of leg ulcers within a community ulcer service. Journal of Wound Care 4(2): 57–61

Moffatt C J, Franks P J, Oldroyd M et al 1992 Community clinics for leg ulcers and impact on healing. British Medical Journal 305:1389–1392

Morrell C J, Walters S J, Dixon S et al 1998 Cost effectiveness of community leg ulcer clinics: randomised controlled trial. British Medical Journal 316: 1487–1491

Nelzen O, Bergqvist D, Lindhagen A, Hallbook D 1991 Chronic leg ulcers – an underestimated problem in primary health care among elderly patients. Journal of Epidemiology and Community Health 45:184–187

Nelzen O, Berqvist D, Lindhagen A 1993 High prevalence of diabetes in chronic leg ulcer patients: a cross-sectional population study. Diabetic Medicine 10:345–350

Orr M M, McAvoy B R 1987 The ischaemic leg. In: Fry J, Berry H E (eds) Surgical problems in clinical practice. Edward Arnold, London, p 123–135

Philips T, Stanton B, Provan A, Lew R 1994 A study of impact of leg ulcers on quality of life: financial, social and psychologic implications. Journal of the American Academy of Dermatology 31(1):49–53

Pun Y L W, Barraclough D R E, Muirdeu K D 1990 Leg ulcers in rheumatoid arthritis. Medical Journal of Australia 153(10):585–587

Salaman R, Harding K 1995 The aetiology and healing rates of chronic leg ulcers. Journal of Wound Care 4(7):320–323

Schmidt K, Debus E S, St Jessberger E et al 2000 Bacterial population of chronic crural ulcers: is there a difference between the diabetic, the venous, and the arterial ulcer? Vasa 29(1):62–70

Sochart D H, Harding K 1999 The relationship of foot and ankle movements to venous return in the lower limb. Journal of Bone and Joint Surgery – British Volume 81(4):700–704

Vowden K R, Vowden P 1997 Peripheral arterial disease. Journal of Wound Care 5(1):23–26

Wutschert R, Bounameaux H 1998 Predicting healing of arterial leg ulcers by means of segmental systolic pressure measurements. Vasa 27(4):224–228

Other chronic wounds

16

Tami de Araujo and Robert S Kirsner

CHAPTER CONTENTS

INTRODUCTION

Chronic wounds or ulcers are most commonly due to prolonged pressure (pressure ulcers), venous insufficiency (venous leg ulcers), complications of long-standing diabetes mellitus (diabetic foot ulcers) or poor vascular supply (arterial ulcers).

Less frequently encountered, and unfortunately also less well understood, are wounds due to uncommon aetiologies, termed atypical wounds. As a group, their prevalence has not been well studied but it is estimated of the over 500 000 leg ulcers in the US, 10% may be due to unusual causes (Philips & Dover 1991). Atypical wounds can be caused by infections, external or traumatic causes, metabolic disorders, genetic diseases, neoplasms or inflammatory processes (Falabella & Falanga 1998).

DEFINITION AND EVALUATION OF ATYPICAL WOUNDS

It is of paramount importance to recognize that a wound is indeed atypical so that appropriate measures can be undertaken to render a diagnosis and provide appropriate therapy. A wound should be evaluated for an atypical aetiology if it:

- is present in an unusual distribution
- has an atypical appearance
- does not respond to conventional therapy.

For example, a wound on the dorsum of the foot is an atypical location for a pressure, or venous, arterial, or diabetic ulcer, and should raise the consideration of an unusual cause. A wound on the medial aspect of the leg in a typical location for a venous ulcer would be considered atypical if it extended deep to the tendon, an appearance atypical for venous ulcers. Finally, all wounds that are not healing after 3–6 months of appropriate treatment should raise the consideration of an atypical cause, even if the distribution and clinical appearance are classic for a common chronic wound.

Once a wound is deemed atypical, a tissue sample of the wound is critical. This is to include histology evaluation with special stains, tissue culture (for infectious causes) and immunofluorescence testing (for inflammatory or immune based causes). The reason tissue samples are mandatory is because many of the unusual causes of wounds can resemble each other clinically (Fig. 16.1).

AETIOLOGIES OF ATYPICAL WOUNDS

Some of the most commonly encountered aetiologies for an atypical wound are presented in Table 16.1. It is important to note that this list is not all-inclusive. However, a thorough medical history, including epidemiological exposure, family history, personal habits, concomitant systemic diseases and an attentive physical examination in combination with histological evaluation and laboratory testing will provide critical information necessary for a correct diagnosis of an atypical wound.

Inflammatory causes

Among the most interesting and probably more common causes of atypical wounds are the inflammatory ulcers. Although a variety of inflammatory and immunological diseases affect the skin, two causes of inflammatory ulcers that are relatively more common are vasculitis and pyoderma gangrenosum.

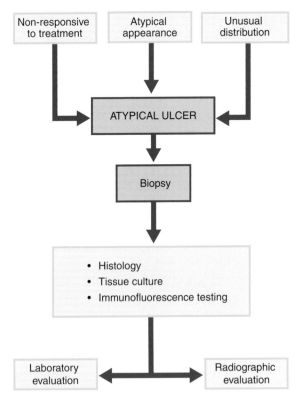

Figure 16.1
Diagnosis and evaluation of an atypical wound

Table 16.1
Sample of aetiological
agents of atypical wounds

Aetiology	Examples
Inflammatory	Vasculitis, pyoderma gangrenosum, collagen vascular disease
Infection	Atypical mycobacteria, deep fungal infections, Hansen's disease
Vasculopathies	Cryoglobulinaemia, cryofibrinogenaemia, antiphospholipid antibody syndrome
Metabolic and genetic	Calciphylaxis, sickle-cell anaemia, epidermolysis bullosa
Malignancies	Squamous cell carcinoma, basal cell carcinoma, lymphoma, Kaposi's sarcoma
External	Trauma, burns, stings, radiation

Vasculitis

Vasculitis is characterized by inflammation and necrosis of blood vessels, which can ultimately result in end-organ damage (Lotti et al 1998). Although often idiopathic, vasculitis is a reaction pattern often triggered by, among other causes, underlying infections, malignancy and medications, as well as connective tissue diseases (Table 16.2). Clinical presentation can vary depending upon the size of the underlying vessel affected. For example, lesions may include a reticulated erythema due to disease of the superficial cutaneous plexus or may present as widespread purpura, necrosis and ulceration due to disease in larger, deeper vessels. Patients may also have similar involvement of different end organs (kidney, lung, central nervous system, gastrointestinal tract, etc.) (Gibson 1990).

Circulating immune (antibody–antigen) complexes, which deposit in blood vessel walls, are the cause of vasculitis (Jennette & Falk 1997). Diagnostic tests for vasculitis are given in Table 16.3. Tissue biopsies will confirm the presence of vasculitis and biopsies of perilesional skin can detect the type of immunoglobulin involved in the process, if performed early on. Biopsies taken

Table 16.2
Various aetiologies of
vasculitis

Aetiology	Examples
Infections	Streptococci, *Mycobacterium tuberculosis*, staphylococci, *Mycobacterium leprae*, hepatitis virus A–C, herpes virus infection, influenza virus infection, *Candida*, *Plasmodium*, *Schistosomiasis*
Medications	Penicillin, sulfonamides, tamoxifen, streptomycin, oral contraceptives, thiazides
Chemicals	Insecticides, petroleum products
Food	Milk, gluten
Connective tissue and other inflammatory diseases	Systemic lupus erythematosus, dermatomyositis, Sjogren's syndrome, rheumatoid arthritis, Behçet's syndrome, cryoglobulinaemia, scleroderma, primary biliary cirrhosis, HIV
Malignancies	Lymphomas, leukaemias, multiple myeloma

Table 16.3
Diagnostic tests for
vasculitis

Purpose of test	Examples of tests
To determine aetiology	Antineutrophilic cytoplasmic antibody, rheumatoid factor, antinuclear antibody, hepatitis A, B, C profile, complete blood count, anti-Streptolysin O titre, cryoglobulin level, serum protein electrophoresis, chest radiograph, PPD, throat culture, tissue culture
To determine extent of disease	Urinalysis, stool guaiac, chest radiograph, renal function tests, liver function tests, complete blood count

later might fail to reveal immunoreactants because inflammatory cells and their byproducts will degrade immunoglobulins. Tissue culture can help by determining if the vasculitis is due to an infectious process. Once a diagnosis is confirmed histologically, evaluation of other organ systems and attempt to determine the eliciting factor is mandated.

If identified, and if possible, the causative agent should be addressed. Additionally, treatment of the vasculitis is based on the extent of the disease (Table 16.4). Mild disease, limited to the skin, can be treated with only supportive care (e.g. leg elevation, dressings). Treatments with limited side-effect profile, such as colchicine, dapsone, antihistamines, and/or non-steroidal anti-inflammatory agents can also be used. If skin disease is extensive or if systemic involvement is present, more aggressive treatment, including systemic steroids, other anti-inflammatory agents or immunosuppressants and other potential agents, might be needed (Scott & Watts 2000).

Pyoderma gangrenosum

Pyoderma gangrenosum (PG) is characterized by the appearance of one or many chronic ulcerations with violaceous undermined borders (Von Den Driesch 1997). The term 'pyoderma gangrenosum' is a misnomer, as it is neither infectious nor gangrenous, rather it is an inflammatory process of unknown aetiology, leading to painful skin ulcers. PG affects mainly adults and its usual course is that of recurring destructive ulcers, which begin as pustules and resolve with cribriform scars. Several clinical variants of PG have been described, including ulcerative, pustular, bullous, vegetative and peristomal types (Table 16.5). Because a diagnostic test to confirm PG does not exist, and a number of other conditions can resemble it clinically, the diagnosis of PG relies on the clinical presentation and exclusion of other causes. When a diagnosis of

Table 16.4
Treatment options for
vasculitis

Degree of disease	Treatment options
Mild disease	Leg elevation, compression dressings, antihistamines, NSAIDs, anti-inflammatory antibiotics, topical steroids, support stockings, dapsone, colchicine, potassium iodide, others
Extensive or systemic disease	Dapsone, systemic steroids, stanozolol, cyclophosphamide, methotrexate, azathioprine, cyclosporin, plasmapheresis, mycophenolate mofetil, tacrolimus, other anti-inflammatory and/or immunosuppressant drugs

Table 16.5
Pyoderma gangrenosum
(PG) – types and
characteristics

Type	Clinical description	Histopathology	Associated systemic diseases
Ulcerative	One or many small pustules with inflammatory halo typically on the lower extremities or trunk. These rapidly enlarge into painful ulcers with violaceous, inflamed, undermined borders	Subcorneal collections of neutrophils in inflamed skin; endothelial cell swelling; fibrin deposition in dermal vessel walls; thrombosis	Inflammatory bowel disease, seronegative monoarthritis, rheumatoid arthritis, Felty syndrome, osteoarthritis, sacroiliitis, monoclonal gammopathy, malignancy
Pustular	One or many painful pustules with halo of erythema on lower extremities and upper trunk; associated with fever and arthralgias	Subcorneal pustules with perifollicular` neutrophilic infiltrate; dense dermal neutrophilic infiltrates; subepidermal oedema	Inflammatory bowel disease, jejunoileal bypass, polycythemia rubra vera, hepatobiliary disease
Bullous	Painful superficial bullae with inflamed borders, which can develop into superficial ulcers; less deep destruction than ulcerative type	Subepidermal bullae with intraepidermal and dermal neutrophilic infiltrate	Leukaemia, myelodysplasia, inflammatory bowel disease
Vegetative	Limited, solitary, exophytic superficial ulcers; rapid response to treatment; sinus tracts formation may occur	Pseudoepitheliomatous hyperplasia; dermal neutrophilic abscesses; sinus tracts; palisading granulomatous reaction	No systemic diseases
Peristomal	Painful pink–purple papules develop into ulcers with violaceous undermined borders; multiple fistulous tracts; may cause leakage of stoma bag	Neutrophilic collections with granulation tissue; mixed dermal inflammatory infiltrate (neutrophils, lymphocytes, histiocytes)	Inflammatory bowel disease, abdominal malignancies, monoclonal gammopathy, connective tissue disease

PG is rendered it is important for the clinician to search for underlying diseases because PG is associated with other conditions in up to 75% of patients (Table 16.6) (Callen 1998).

The mechanism by which PG lesions develop is unknown, although it is believed that pathergy – defined as development of lesions in areas of trauma – plays a role. In susceptible people even minimal trauma to the skin can result in the production of PG lesions, such as pustules and/or ulcers.

Curative treatment does not appear to exist and the course waxes and wanes; however, corticosteroids are invariably helpful for the treatment of pyoderma gangrenosum (Powell & Collins 2000). For limited or mild disease, topical or intralesional steroids can be utilized. For more severe or widespread disease, systemic steroids can be used, although their side-effects limit their long-term use. A variety of systemic therapies can be used, including antibiotics with anti-inflammatory properties; systemic steroids, immunosuppressant or anti-inflammatory agents can also be useful, for example, cyclosporine appears quite effective in treating PG. A randomized study evaluating the efficacy of different treatment modalities for PG has not been done.

Infectious causes

Infectious causes of atypical wounds can be due to a variety of different organisms, some of which are not commonly encountered in the UK, Europe or United States. For example, atypical mycobacteria (other than leprosy and tuberculosis) and fungi (other than dermatophytes and candida) infections are occasionally detected upon diagnostic testing. Infection caused by *Vibrio vulnificus* can be responsible for lower leg ulcers in areas of warm, salt water.

Atypical mycobacterial infection

Atypical mycobacteria are ubiquitous in the environment and were not generally viewed as human pathogens until the 1950s, when several cases of disease caused by these organisms were reported (Groves 1995).

Cutaneous infection usually results from exogenous inoculation and predisposing factors are history of preceding trauma, immunosuppression or chronic disease. While *Mycobacterium marinum* is the most common agent of skin infection by atypical mycobacteria, many others have been reported in recent decades (Hautmann & Lotti 1994).

Table 16.6
Associated systemic diseases and differential diagnosis of pyoderma gangrenosum (PG)

Systemic diseases	Differential diagnosis
Inflammatory bowel disease	Ulcerative colitis, regional enteritis, Crohn's disease
Arthritis	Seronegative arthritis, rheumatoid arthritis, osteoarthritis, psoriatic arthritis
Haematological abnormalities	Myeloid leukaemia, hairy cell leukaemia, myelofibrosis, myeloid metaplasia, IgA monoclonal gammopathy, polycythaemia rubra vera, paroxysmal nocturnal haemoglobinuria, myeloma, lymphoma
Hepatic abnormalities	Active hepatitis, hepatitis C infection, biliary cirrhosis
Immunological abnormalities	SLE, complement deficiency, hypogammaglobulinaemia, hyperimmunoglobulin E syndrome, AIDS

The cutaneous lesions vary depending on the causative agent and can present as granulomas, small superficial ulcers, sinus tracts and/or large ulcerated lesions localized in exposed areas. Histologically, these infections present as granulomas and/or abscesses that are hard to distinguish from those of leprosy and cutaneous tuberculosis. Diagnosis will invariably depend on tissue culture or more recent techniques, such as polymerase chain reaction (PCR) and/or gene rearrangement studies.

The appropriate therapy will depend on the causative agent because susceptibility to antibiotics varies. In some cases, simple excision of the cutaneous lesions or a combination of excision and chemotherapy often is most beneficial to the patient.

Deep fungal infections

Deep fungal infections of the skin can be divided into subcutaneous and systemic mycoses. The subcutaneous mycoses result from traumatic implantation of the aetiologic agent into the subcutaneous tissue, development of localized disease and eventual lymphatic spread. In rare instances, haematogenous dissemination can occur, especially in immunocompromised hosts. As can occur with sporotrichosis or chromomycosis, ulcers from deep fungal infections are found worldwide and can present in a wide variety of clinical pictures (Kauffman 1999, Rivitti & Aoki 1999).

Systemic mycoses are the result of systemic penetration of pathogenic fungi, the lungs being the most common port of entry. They are restricted to the geographic areas where the fungi occur, especially tropical countries such as Central and South America. Therefore, careful history-taking is critical. After an initial pulmonary infection, the fungi can spread haematogenously or via lymphatic vessels to other organs, including the skin. A decrease in immunity will lead to expression of the fungal infection, as is commonly observed in HIV-infected patients.

Vasculopathies   A heterogeneous group of disorders is classified under this category. Vasculopathy is characterized by occlusion of small vessels within the skin due to thrombi or emboli which leads to tissue hypoxia and the clinical manifestations of purpura, livedo reticularis and painful ulcers (Fig. 16.2). Cryofibrinogenaemia, monoclonal cryoglobulinaemia and antiphospholipid antibody syndrome are among the vasculopathy causes that commonly present as atypical skin ulcerations of the lower extremities.

Cryofibrinogenaemia

Cryofibrinogen is a circulating complex of fibrin, fibrinogen and fibronectin along with albumin, cold-insoluble globulin and factor VIII, which is soluble at 37°C but forms a cryoprecipitate at 4°C. Additionally, this complex can be made to clot with thrombin.

Cryofibrinogenaemia occurs as a primary (idiopathic) disorder or in association with underlying diseases, such as infectious processes, malignancy, collagen vascular disease or thromboembolic disease. The clinical picture is of painful cutaneous ulcerations located on the leg and foot, usually unresponsive to treatment (Fig. 16.2). Other cutaneous findings include livedo reticularis (a net-like erythema), purpura, ecchymoses and gangrene. Presumably the

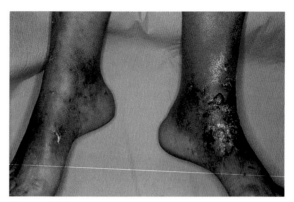

Figure 16.2
Painful punctate ulcers on the feet and legs secondary to
cryofibrinogenaemia

pathogenesis of these lesions is related to the in vivo occlusion of small blood vessels initiated in the distal extremities by the abnormal precipitate. This hypothesis is corroborated by the pathology findings of cryofibrinogenaemia, which is thrombi within superficial dermal vessels. The mechanism through which cryofibrinogen is produced is not well understood.

Treatment is symptomatic or, in secondary disease, directed to the underlying cause (Falanga et al 1991). Agents that lyse fibrin thrombi are of help. Stanazolol, streptokinase and streptodornase have been used with variable success.

Cryoglobulinaemia

Cryoglobulinaemia occurs as a consequence of deposition of cryoglobulins leading to thrombi formation in medium and small vessel walls (Piette 1990). Three types of cryoglobulins have been identified. Type I or monoclonal cryoglobulinaemia can be seen in patients with malignant diseases such as myeloma, or benign lymphoproliferative conditions such as Waldenstrom's macroglobulinaemia. This classically leads to thrombotic phenomena but can clinically resemble vasculitis (Fig. 16.3). Type II, or mixed, cryoglobulinaemia combines

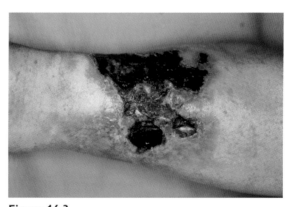

Figure 16.3
Necrotic plaque with surrounding erythema secondary to
monoclonal cryoglobulinaemia

polyclonal and a monoclonal immunoglobulin. This type of cryoglobulinaemia is less often seen in association with malignancies and is more often associated with infectious or inflammatory diseases. Type II is most commonly associated with hepatitis C infection and the monoclonal component is IgM kappa. Type III comprises only polyclonal immunoglobulin. Both type II and type III cryoglobulinaemia cause vasculitis, which can lead to skin ulcers (Rallis et al 1995). Other skin manifestations include acral cyanosis, Raynaud's phenomenon, livedo reticularis, altered pigmentation of involved skin and palpable purpura, which can progress to blistering and frank ulceration. Some patients have systemic manifestations, such as arthritis, peripheral neuropathy and glomerulonephritis.

Diagnosis is based on skin biopsies that show either vasculopathy or vasculitis and subsequent detection of cryoglobulin by electrophoresis.

Treatment should be directed to the underlying cause when associated with hepatitis C. Interferon alpha-2b can be used and might result in resolution of the associated cryoglobulinaemia. Plasmapheresis alone or in combination with prednisone or immunosuppressive drugs (cyclosphophamide/chlorambucil) has also been used.

Metabolic and genetic disorders

Metabolic diseases are uncommon causes of chronic wounds. One condition, called calciphylaxis, is seen not uncommonly in a subset of patients on chronic haemodialysis who develop secondary hyperparathyroidism (Smiley et al 2000). This causes deposition of calcium within soft tissue and the vasculature and eventually tissue death. Genetic disease can affect wound healing in a variety of ways that result in chronic wounds. Sickle-cell disease is a genetically transmitted haemoglobinopathy characterized by an alteration in the shape of the erythrocytes in the presence of low oxygen tension, leading to cell lysis (and consequent anaemia) and vascular occlusion phenomena.

Calciphylaxis

Calciphylaxis is a rare, often fatal, condition characterized clinically by progressive cutaneous necrosis, which frequently occurs in patients with end-stage renal disease (ESRD). Many eliciting factors have been suggested but the most common linking phenomenon is the development of secondary hyperparathyroidism in these patients (Roe et al 1994, Smiley et al 2000). The secondary hyperparathyroidism leads to an elevated calcium–phosphate product and development of vascular, cutaneous and subcutaneous calcification, resulting in tissue death (Fig. 16.4). Calciphylaxis typically develops after beginning dialysis and is seen in approximately 1% of patients with chronic renal failure and 4.1% of patients receiving haemodialysis (Weiss et al 1999). The prognosis for patients who develop calciphylaxis is grim, with an estimated 5-year survival of less than 50% (Budisavjevic et al 1996).

Sickle-cell disease

Lower leg ulcers are the most common cutaneous complication and a major cause of morbidity in sickle-cell disease (SCD) (Fig. 16.5). It is estimated that 25% of patients with SCD in the United States will develop leg ulcers during their lifetime (Koshy et al 1989). Risk factors appear to be older age (50 years or older), haemoglobin levels less than 6 g/dL and the presence of HLA-B35

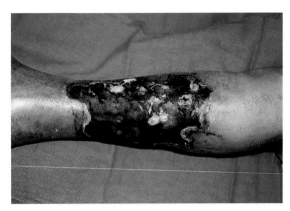

Figure 16.4
Necrotic plaque with livedo reticularis in a patient with
end-stage renal disease who is on dialysis and has
calciphylaxis

and Cw4. Once a patient has experienced a leg ulcer they are likely to have
another, and the strongest predictor of risk for new leg ulceration is a history of
previous leg ulcers.

The cause of leg ulceration in SCD is incompletely understood. The location
and characteristics of the ulcers are similar to those seen in patients with
vascular disease, diabetes and trophic ulcers. Reduction in local blood supply
appears to be common to all of these disorders, and infarction may be the
primary cause.

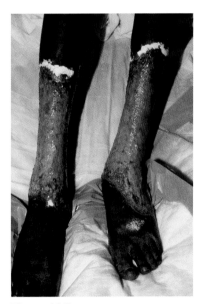

Figure 16.5
Bilateral circumferential low
extremities ulcers due to sickle-cell
anaemia

Secondary infection is a major concern as is pain. *Staphylococcus aureus* and *Pseudomonas aeruginosa* are the most consistently cultured pathogens (Koshy et al 1989). Pain is often severe and unremitting, causing significant disability.

Treatment of established ulcers includes debridement, control of oedema, pain and infections, skin grafting and use of systemic antibiotics and blood transfusions. Hydroxyurea might be of additional benefit.

Malignancies

Malignancies can either present as wounds or develop from wounds. Cancers such as non-melanoma skin cancers, lymphomas and/or sarcomas can ulcerate as they outgrow their blood supply. Alternatively, chronic wounds can develop into a malignancy, most commonly squamous cell carcinoma. This phenomenon, termed 'Marjolin's ulcer' (after the author who first described cells from an edge of a chronic wound undergoing malignant change) can be seen in up to 2% of chronic wounds (Chang et al 1998). A similar phenomenon can also occur in scars, burn wounds, sinus tracts, chronic osteomyelitis and even vaccination sites.

The precise mechanism of malignant degeneration in chronic wounds is not known and several theories have been proposed. For example, Virchow postulated that chronic irritation is a factor leading to initiation of a carcinoma. Chronic local infection or irritation, delayed healing and a prolonged latent period (20 to 30 years) often precede the development of malignancy. Neoplasia is seen with less frequency in scars that have been excised and resurfaced with a graft or flap, lending support to the chronic irritation theory. Other theories postulate that diminished blood supply and atrophic cutaneous adnexae and epidermis may render the scar less able to withstand the damaging effects of actinic radiation (Fishman & Parker 1991). Still others suggest that decreased vascularity and a weakened epithelium that are unable to withstand the effects of carcinogens, or alternatively immunosuppression produced by the relatively avascular scar tissue that predisposes the area to malignant degeneration, are responsible (Lautenschlager & Eichman 1999, Natarajan et al 2000). In addition to squamous cell carcinoma, basal cell carcinomas and other neoplasms such as Kaposi's sarcoma and lymphoma have also been found in chronic wounds.

Ideally, early identification of malignancy is critical. Biopsy of suspected lesions is paramount. Treatment options of biopsy-proven neoplasia include excision with margins; in some cases amputation of the affected limb may be necessary. We have reported successful treatment of malignancy arising from chronic osteomyelitis with Mohs surgery (Chang et al 1998) to ensure complete removal of the primary lesion.

External causes: spider bites, chemical burns, radiation and factitious wounds

External causes of atypical wounds include spider bites, chemical injury, chronic radiation exposure, trauma and factitial ulcers, among others. A careful history-taking will be the most valuable tool in determining the aetiological agent in ulcers caused by external factors.

Spider bites

At lease 50 spider species in the United States have been implicated in causing significant medical conditions, however, the *Loxosceles* (brown recluse or violin spider) and the *Latrodectus* (black widow) species are the most well-known to cause skin necrosis and ulcers in the Americas.

The bite of *Loxosceles reclusae* is usually painless and often goes unnoticed. In 10% of patients, there will be progression to more significant wounds (Newcomer & Young 1993). In these cases enlargement of the bite site occurs within 6 to 12 h, with associated pain and general symptoms such as fever, malaise, headaches and arthralgias. As the disease progresses, there is formation of a pustule, blister or large plaque at the bite site. These wounds can present as a deep purple plaque surrounded by a clear halo (vasoconstriction) and surrounding erythema, the so-called red, white and blue sign.

In bites occurring in areas of greater fat content such as the abdomen, buttocks and thighs, necrosis develops more frequently and, when the eschar is shed, an ulcer may result. Healing of the ulcer is generally very slow and can take up to 6 months (Smith et al 1997).

The differential diagnosis includes foreign body reaction, infections, trauma, vasculitis and pyoderma gangrenosum. Treatment consists of cooling the bite site, elevation (if possible) and analgesics. The use of systemic steroids can prevent the enlargement of the necrotic areas. Dapsone has also been recommended, at a dose of 100 mg per day in adults.

The black widow spider or *Latrodectus mutans* is easily recognized by a bright red hour-glass on the abdomen. The painless bite is followed by severe pain, swelling and tenderness at the site where the bite occurred. Systemic symptoms such as headaches and abdominal pain may follow, but they subside in 1 to 3 days. Treatment includes local ice, calcium gluconate and the administration of specific antivenom.

Chemical burns

Several chemical products are capable of producing skin wounds (Bates 2000). Cutaneous injury caused by caustic chemicals progresses continually after the initial exposure and, if not properly cared for, can produce painful ulcers that are difficult to heal. The lesions caused by alkalis are usually more severe than those caused by acids. However, the severity of the burn is determined by the mode of action and concentration of the chemical, and duration of contact before treatment is initiated.

Prolonged irrigation with water for 30 min or more is the most important initial treatment, followed by standard burn care.

Certain chemicals possess unique properties that require special additional therapy, such as hydrofluoric acid (the use of 25% magnesium sulfate), chromic acid (excision of the affected area) and phenol (the use of polyethylene glycol mixed with alcohol 2:1).

Radiation dermatitis

After exposure to ionizing radiation exceeding 10 Gy, local skin reactions characterized by mild erythema, oedema and pruritus may occur (Caccialanza et al 1999). This acute radiation dermatitis usually begins 2 to 7 days after exposure, peaks within 2 weeks and gradually subsides. With exposure to higher doses, intense erythema with vesiculation, erosion and superficial ulceration may ensue. Post-inflammatory pigmentary abnormalities, telangiectasia and atrophy are common. Excision of the affected area and hyperbaric oxygen have been suggested as possible treatment options.

Factitial dermatitis

The term factitial dermatitis denotes a self-imposed injury (Fig. 16.6). The clinical appearance of these ulcers is usually particular, with sharp or linear edges in an area of easy access such as the extremities, abdomen and anterior chest.

Treatment includes evaluation and treatment of underlying psychological diseases and limitation of accessibility to the wound, such as placing a dressing or cast over the wound.

CONCLUSION

Whenever possible, treating the underlying cause is the initial step in caring for patients with atypical wounds. Therefore, the appropriate use of anti-infective agents for infectious ulcers, surgical removal of malignancies and anti-inflammatory agents for inflammatory ulcers are indicated. In addition, the use of a moist pro-healing environment, the use of compression dressings (in the absence of arterial insufficiency) for leg lesions, offloading areas at risk for prolonged pressure and maximizing patients' nutritional status are essential.

Despite these measures, healing is often slow in patients with atypical wounds. Prolonged healing leads to increased morbidity, a decrease in patients' quality of life as well as an increase in both direct and indirect costs of care. Therefore adjunctive therapies are often employed aimed at both increasing the number of patients who will heal (effectiveness of therapy) and the speed at which they heal (cost-effectiveness of therapy).

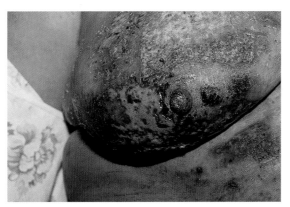

Figure 16.6
Angulated ulcer on the breast. This ulcer was created by the patient and is a factitial ulcer.

REFERENCES

Bates N 2000 Acid and alkali injury. Emergency Nurse 7(8):21–26

Budisavjevic M N, Cheek D, Ploth D W 1996 Calciphylaxis in chronic renal failure. Journal of the American Society of Nephrology 7:978–982

Caccialanza M, Piccino R, Beretta M et al 1999 Results and side effects of dermatologic radiotherapy: a retrospective study of irradiated cutaneous epithelial neoplasms. Journal of the American Academy of Dermatology 41(4):589–594

Callen J P 1998 Pyoderma gangrenosum. Lancet 351:581–585

Chang A, Spencer J M, Kirsner R S 1998 Squamous cell carcinoma arising in a nonhealing wound and osteomyelitis treated with Moh's micrographic surgery: a case study. Ostomy and Wound Management 44:26–30

Falabella A, Falanga V 1998 Uncommon causes of ulcers. Clinics in Plastic Surgery 25:467–479

Falanga V, Kirsner R S, Eaglstein W H et al 1991 Stanozolol in the treatment of leg ulcers due to cryofibrinogenemia. Lancet 338:347–348

Fishman J R A, Parker M G 1991 Malignancy and chronic wounds: Marjolin's ulcer. Journal of Burn Care and Rehabilitation 12(3):218–223

Gibson L E 1990 Cutaneous vasculitis: approach to diagnosis and systemic associations. Mayo Clinic Proceedings 65:221–229

Groves R 1995 Unusual cutaneous mycobacterial diseases. Clinics in Dermatology 13:257–263

Hautmann G, Lotti T 1994 Atypical mycobacterial infections of the skin. Clinics in Dermatology 12(4):657–667

Jennette J C, Falk R J 1997 Small-vessel vasculitis. New England Journal of Medicine 337(21):1512–1523

Kauffman C A 1999 Sporotrichosis. Clinical Infectious Diseases 29:231–237

Koshy M, Entsuah R, Koranda A et al 1989 Leg ulcers in patients with sickle cell disease. Blood 74(4):1403–1408

Lautenschlager S, Eichman A 1999 Differential diagnosis of leg ulcers. Current Problems in Dermatology 27:259–270

Lotti T, Ghersetich I, Comacchi C, Jorizzo J L 1998 Cutaneous small-vessel vasculitis. Journal of the American Academy of Dermatology 39:667–687

Natarajan S, Makhdoomi K R, Turner A R 2000 A non-healing ulcer associated with malignant lymphoma. Journal of Wound Care 9(1):45–46

Newcomer V D, Young E M Jr 1993 Unique wounds and wound emergencies. Clinics in Dermatology 11(4):715–727

Phillips T J, Dover J S 1991 Leg ulcers. Journal of the American Academy of Dermatology 25:965–987

Piette W W 1990 Hematologic associations of leg ulcers. Clinics in Dermatology 8(3–4):66–85

Powell F C, Collins S 2000 Pyoderma gangrenosum. Clinics in Dermatology 18:283–293

Rallis T M, Kadunce D P, Gerwels J W 1995 Leg ulcers and purple nail beds. Essential mixed cryoglobulinemia. Archives of Dermatology 131(3):342–343, 345–346

Rivitti E A, Aoki V 1999 Deep fungal infections in tropical countries. Clinics in Dermatology 17:171–190

Roe S M, Graham L D, Brock B B, Barker D E 1994 Calciphylaxis: early recognition and management. The American Surgeon 60:81–86

Scott D G I, Watts R A 2000 Systemic vasculitis: epidemiology, classification and environmental factors. Annals of Rheumatic Disease 59:161–163

Smiley C M, Hanlon S U, Michel D M 2000 Calciphylaxis in moderate renal insufficiency: changing disease concepts. American Journal of Nephrology 20:324–328

Smith D B, Ickstadt J, Kucera J 1997 Brown recluse spider bite: a case study. Journal of Wound, Ostomy and Continence Nursing 24(3):137–143

Von Den Driesch P 1997 Pyoderma gangrenosum: a report of 44 cases with follow-up. British Journal of Dermatology 137:1000–1005

Weiss E, Brahmatewari J, Kirsner R S, Kerdel F A 1999 Calciphylaxis in a patient with end-stage renal disease. Journal of Clinical Dermatology 2:17–18

CHAPTER

17

Trauma and wound care

William J Ennis, Wesley Valdes, Steven Salzman, Don Fishman and Patricio Meneses

CHAPTER CONTENTS

INTRODUCTION

The establishment of multidisciplinary wound clinics is a relatively recent phenomenon (Gottrup et al 2001). Wounds have been treated throughout history with a strong tradition based in the surgical services. Classically, surgeons create and manage acute wounds. Treatment regimens are frequently biased, with wound-care teams focusing on specialty dressings and wound treatment modalities, whereas surgical teams often employ mechanical debriding techniques such as wet-to-dry dressing changes and surgical debridement.

There is some evidence in the chronic wound-care literature that increasing the frequency of debridements will result in improved outcomes (Steed et al 1996). In effect, debridement places an acute inflammatory reaction within a chronic wound environment. Many have referred to this as converting a chronic wound into an acute wound. Many trauma patients have wounds that can be considered 'functionally chronic.' These wounds are in fact acute wounds that occur in compromised hosts with multiorgan failure, massive soft tissue loss, poor tissue perfusion, insensate tissue (spinal cord injury) or a combination of all of the above. Surgical incisions have an increased risk for dehiscence under these conditions. Fasciotomies are performed to release compartment pressures but the surgical wounds created can result in a chronic non-healing condition. Heavily contaminated abdominal wounds are sometimes left open to heal by secondary intention or because oedema and/or poor tissue quality precludes a tension-free wound approximation. These clinical scenarios create the need for complex, interdisciplinary wound management.

The authors have utilized many traditional chronic wound-care techniques and dressings for the treatment of acute traumatic wounds. Conversely, many surgical principles and closure techniques employed in the care of acute/ traumatic wounds are used for healing chronic wounds. The need for inter-disciplinary communication is therefore paramount. The topic of pressure-ulcer formation demonstrates an area of crossover because both younger trauma patients and elderly frail patients develop these difficult to heal wounds. A huge increase of gunshot-wound-related paraplegic and quadriplegic patients has been seen in some urban populations. These patients are at high risk of developing pressure ulcers. Treatment plans and outcome measures, however, have traditionally focused on older populations. There may be social, physiological, psychological and long-term care issues that require a new look at this problem as it relates to this new expanding demographic cohort.

In this chapter the authors, all from a 700-bed, level-one trauma centre in the US, with an active inpatient and outpatient hospital-based wound programme, as well as a dedicated 34-bed subacute wound-care unit, will review several topics. The controversial topic of wound irrigation and cleansing will be reviewed as it relates to traumatic wounds. Certain treatment options for open abdominal wounds, incisional dehiscence and fasciotomy wounds will be presented from both a surgical and wound-care team viewpoint. Lastly, the principles and management of pressure-ulcer care will be reviewed with a special emphasis on the young, spinal-cord-injured, patient population.

We hope to encourage collaboration between wound-care services and surgical teams. At a minimum, we hope to encourage sharing concepts, traditions, and biases while focusing on evidence-based collaborative solutions for our patients.

ACUTE/CHRONIC WOUNDS

The accepted definition of a chronic wound is 'a wound which has not proceeded through a timely, orderly, sequence of healing and/or fails to achieve sustained anatomic and functional integrity' (Lazarus et al 1994). The terms acute and chronic wounds do not adequately reflect the biochemical and physiological differences between healing and non-healing states. The terms acute and chronic imply a linear temporal time line for healing. Wounds can arise acutely and transform into a chronic non-healing state. Also, through the process of debridement, an 'acute' wound physiology can be re-established within a chronic wound (Falanga & Bren 2001). There are few data to describe 'normal' healing timeframes for specific wound aetiologies. Describing the 'optimal' or 'suboptimal' wound conditions that facilitate healing may represent more accurate terminology.

Wound healing is the body's attempt at restoring tissue integrity after an injury. Injured tissues heal by either regeneration or repair. Regeneration implies a complete re-establishment of the original tissue construct. A few adult human tissues (liver, epidermis, alimentary tract) are capable of this phenomenon. Recently, there has been tremendous interest in understanding the process of fetal healing (Bleacher et al 1993). Fetal healing results in scarless regeneration of tissue (Shah et al 1992). Most adult tissue heals through the process of repair with scar tissue formation as a byproduct. Scar tissue achieves the goal of re-establishing skin continuity at the price of decreased tensile strength and a loss of many specialized functions of the original tissue.

All wounds proceed through the processes of haemostasis, inflammation, proliferation and remodelling. The physiology of these phases of healing is described in Chapter 6. Surgical wounds are classically described as healing by primary intention, secondary intention or tertiary intention (delayed primary closure) (Phillips 2001). Primary intention refers to surgical closure of the wound; secondary intention implies leaving a wound open to granulate, contract and re-epithelialize; delayed primary closure describes the surgical closure of a wound that is initially left open (Bates-Jensen & Wethe 1998). Many factors affect wound healing in both acute and chronic wounds (Ennis & Meneses 2002). Duration of operation, hypothermia, pain, hypovolaemia, hypotension and poor tissue perfusion can all impact on the ability of a wound to heal. Biochemical differences have recently been described between acute and chronic wound exudates (Schultz & Mast 1998). Chronic wound fluid can decrease mitogenic activity, increase inflammation and accel-erate protease activity when compared to acute wound fluid (Staiano-Coico et al 2000). The benefit of debriding chronic wounds may be, in part, removal of this biochemically hostile environment (Falanga 2000).

Biochemical differences in wound fluid may influence future treatment protocols for both acute and chronic wounds. Because chronic wound fluid can inhibit healing, absorption and fluid management become clinically impor-tant. The presence of either acute or chronic wound fluid has implications for dressing selection and the choice of surgical closure (see Chapter 8). The metabolic impact of wound bioburden will also impact healing differently in an acute or chronic wound.

The above concepts are important because they impact on practice patterns. In an obstetrics/gynaecology practice, the majority of patients are young and healthy. It is therefore unlikely that an individual clinician would collect a large experience treating dehisced, non-healing wounds. The majority of wound complications this clinician would encounter, however, would probably respond to various topical treatments. A long history of successful outcomes can lead to the conclusion that dressing or irrigation fluid selection is clinically irrelevant. Conversely, clinical experience from a chronic wound-care centre frequently requires the use of advanced wound-care technologies to achieve adequate healing outcomes. It is possible, therefore, that a relatively uncom-plicated wound might be 'over treated' with advanced dressings or modalities based on protocols and past experience. A multidisciplinary team of providers can 'share' these concepts and experiences in an attempt to create a unified treatment approach to all wounds drawing from the expertise of these two different viewpoints.

The authors have found it useful to standardize wound care for both acute and chronic wounds using a model known as the 'least common denominator model' (Ennis & Meneses 1996). This model addresses tissue oxygenation, infection/bioburden, psychosocial issues, pressure/offloading, immune status/nutrition and wound-bed analysis for each wound encountered, irrespective of aetiology. Our data suggest that with a standard approach to all wounds, healing can be achieved without statistical differences between wound aetiologies or patient demographics (Ennis & Meneses 2000). Optimizing wound conditions at a local and systemic level is necessary for all wounds to achieve rapid, efficient, cost-effective wound closure.

WOUND CLEANSING/ IRRIGATION

Historically, cleansing and irrigation have been important components of wound care (Phillips & Davey 1997). Because of widespread acceptance that wound cleansing is necessary, there has been little interest in conducting randomized controlled trials comparing techniques and cleansing solutions. Clinicians rarely give critical thought to irrigant selection, frequency, force, or technique of irrigation. The overall function of wound cleansing is to remove necrotic tissue, exudate/slough, dressing residue as well as bacteria and their metabolic waste (Williams 1999). Swabbing, bathing and irrigation are three accepted forms of wound cleansing (Oliver 1997).

Swabbing is the least effective of the three techniques. Surface bacteria are often redistributed across the wound bed instead of being removed. The use of cotton-based products for swabbing can lead to foreign body deposition through the process of linting. Without an accurate means of measuring applied pressure during swabbing, newly formed, friable granulation tissue can be damaged. Swabbing is therefore not recommended for use in acute wounds (Towler 2001).

Bathing has some limited application in large sacral and perineal wounds but controversy exists over utilizing this technique for acute wounds. Whirlpool, a variation of bathing, uses water turbulence to remove debris and cleanse the wound. This technique can also damage healthy granulation tissue and is infrequently utilized by clinicians in wound-care centres (Williams 1999). Many departments order frequent whirlpool therapy despite the published concerns mentioned above. Whirlpool seems to have a role, however, for the treatment of 'road rash' and the elimination of loose, flaky, exudate seen in chronic lymphoedema. Whirlpool can also be useful in treating the 'pseudoeschar' that forms with long-term use of topical silvadene dressing changes.

Wound irrigation has emerged as the most useful and reproducible technique for wound cleansing. Pulse lavage, a variation of irrigation, has migrated from the operating room to the bedside in many clinical centres. Physical therapists have embraced this technology and incorporate the technique as an integral tool in their treatment armamentarium. Pulse lavage allows the clinician to prescribe a specific irrigating force (Loehne 2001). The treatment guidelines for pressure ulcers developed by the Agency for Health Care Policy and Research (AHCPR) recommended a force of 8–12 pounds per square inch for irrigation (Morse et al 1998). Pressures of 5–8 pounds per square inch, however, are adequate for wound cleansing. Irrigation fluids commonly used include sterile water, normal saline, antiseptics and antibiotic solutions. Dakin's solution (sodium hypochlorite), has been used in concentrations from 2–4 g/L (Dakin 1915). Dakin's solution was originally used for the treatment of wet gangrene in the First World War. The solution has been found to be cytotoxic to fibroblasts at concentrations of > 0.05%. Some reports imply that Dakin's solution is not safe for open wounds at any concentration while others have identified effective therapeutic concentrations (Hegers et al 1991, Kozol et al 1988). Other irrigation solutions include povidone-iodine, chlorhexidine, hydrogen peroxide and benzalkonium chloride, all of which have been used with varying degrees of success. Again, no randomized controlled trials are available to help clinicians make an evidence-based decision.

Soap solutions have also been used for wound cleansing. The formation of micelles interferes with bacterial adherence to the wound bed, facilitating their removal (Conroy et al 1999). Surfactant-impregnated sponges have been shown to atraumatically remove bacteria (Rodehever et al 1975). Bolton et al (1985) tested a large number of antiseptic agents and deduced that in vivo standards for bactericidal/cytotoxic effects are different than those used in vitro.

The goal of wound antisepsis is to maintain a low bacterial burden. A clinician's choice of a particular agent depends on both the desired spectrum of activity and duration of action. Despite this philosophy, some authors routinely state that antiseptics are only for use on intact skin and should not be used in acute or chronic wounds, while others interpret the recommendations more liberally (Bennett et al 2001, Brown & Zitelli 1993).

Riyat & Quinton (1997) found that drinking-quality tap water is useful for wound irrigation. Widespread variations in water purity, as well as living conditions, make it difficult to support the universal use of tap water for irrigation. An interesting report by Kuzan et al (1981) failed to demonstrate significant reductions in bacterial counts when comparing povidine iodine solution to normal saline. Hypertonic saline has been reported to enhance the healing of infected wounds when used as an irrigant (Junger et al 1994).

Overall, the paucity of randomized controlled trials studying wound cleansing forces clinicians to rely on clinical experience, training and local practice trends to make treatment recommendations. In actuality, most clinical decisions are conducted this way. Many chronic wound-care clinicians have taken the AHCPR guidelines as mandates and have often alienated trauma and general surgical teams by openly criticizing the use of 'cytotoxic' agents without analysing the clinical scenario and specific indication. Many of these clinicians have had years of positive clinical outcomes using these solutions. As stated previously, younger patients and those with few preinjury comorbidities may contribute to these historical positive results.

In clinical practice, infected pressure ulcers, postoperative wounds and fasciotomy wounds can be effectively treated with pulse lavage. For the first 24–72 h, antiseptic wet-to-dry dressings can be useful for a grossly infected wound. Once healthy granulation tissue appears in the wound bed, products that maintain a moist environment, require infrequent dressing changes, and enhance local immune function should be considered. Many of today's advanced wound-care dressings fill this role (Chapter 8). Wound irrigation at this point on the continuum should be non-cytotoxic with a very low irrigating pressure. Without strong evidence-based support for making clinical decisions, wound-care clinicians should be constantly asking the following questions:

- What is the goal of the cleansing?
- Is contamination/infection a concern?
- Is dressing/residue removal the goal?
- Is there any adherent slough/necrotic tissue that requires removal?

By reviewing these goals and objectives of cleansing, the irrigant solution and cleansing technique will be patient specific and positive outcomes can be achieved.

FASCIOTOMY WOUNDS

Fasciotomy is the procedure of choice for the treatment of compartment syndrome. Acute and chronic forms of compartment syndrome are well described (Mubarak et al 1989). Compartment syndrome is defined as a condition where increased interstitial pressures within a fascial compartment result in microvascular compromise and, if untreated, irreversible tissue damage (Hoover & Siefert 2000). There are many conditions that result in the development of a compartment syndrome (Tiwari et al 2002) and it has recently been described after coronary bypass surgery (Friedman et al 2002). The majority of cases treated by the authors arise secondary to traumatic injury, such as gun-shot wounds, motor vehicle accidents and crush injuries to the lower extremity.

Although compartment syndrome can occur in numerous locations, we will focus on lower extremity cases because these are the most frequently encountered by wound clinicians. Several surgical approaches are available to the surgeon for the treatment of lower extremity compartment syndrome. The fibulectomy/ fasciotomy procedure and the single incision parafibular fasciotomy are rarely used today in practice; the double incision fasciotomy is the more commonly encountered procedure. Chronic exertional compartment syndrome is a well-known clinical entity seen frequently in sports medicine. The syndrome arises secondary to repetitive, strenuous athletic activity. Surgical options for this condition include partial fasciectomy at the time of fasciotomy (Slimmon et al 2002). Endoscopic-assisted fasciotomy has been described in amputation specimens and in vitro, and represents an option in the future (Leversedge et al 2002).

The trauma service monitors a responsive patient for signs of developing compartment syndrome, including throbbing extremity pain, paraesthesias, decreasing pulses and pain with passive stretch of the involved muscle (Stack 1998). The unresponsive patient poses a clinical challenge because of the inability to monitor the clinical signs mentioned above. Compartment pressure measurements are often used to aide in the diagnosis in these settings. Concern over postoperative incisional complications can sometimes delay the decision to perform a fasciotomy. This delay in surgical decompression, however, can lead to irreversible muscle or nerve damage, wound healing problems and/or infection. Paradoxically, therefore, an initial conservative approach can yield a poor overall outcome. Guerrero et al (2002) reported a statistically significant increased limb loss in arterial trauma patients who developed compartment syndrome and in those who did not receive anticoagulation. These findings led to the suggestion of liberalizing the use of fasciotomy and anticoagulants for trauma patients with arterial injuries. Coordination of services again becomes paramount for successful outcomes. McHenry et al (2002) demonstrated a higher percentage of patients developing compartment syndrome when orthopaedic fixation occurred before revascularization, leading to a statistically increased length of stay.

French surgeons in the early eighteenth century believed that traumatic injury led to 'augmentation de volume', producing constriction of the soft tissues (Helling & Daon 1998). In the 1739 publication *Observations in surgery*, Henry Francois LeDran mentioned the use of fasciotomy and debridements to avoid 'entanglement' or choking of the tissues (Helling & Daon 1998). After the collapse of the French empire, British surgeons, led by John Hunter, began to advocate a more minimalistic approach (Helling & Daon 1998). In 1867, Joseph Lister improved the care of open fracture wounds by sterilizing them with carbolic acid (Helling & Daon 1998). Lister agreed with Hunter's non-surgical approach and advocated treating open wounds solely with antiseptics. In fact, conventional wisdom at the time implied that debridement actually worsened a pre-existing infection. A compromise position was proposed by Antoine Depage in 1914. Depage first irrigated the wound with a hypochlorite solution and then performed a delayed primary closure (Helling & Daon 1998). This technique built on the surgical concepts of the French and the antimicrobial theories of the British. Fasciotomy techniques and wound-care methods were further enhanced by Debakey in the Second World War (Debakey & Simeone 1946) and Rich et al (1970) in Vietnam, as vascular injuries became more serious with advancements in weapons.

This brief historical review helps demonstrate how surgical traditions and concepts change over time. The current wound literature has described improved healing outcomes with frequent debridements (Steed et al 1996). However, this concept was until recently frowned upon by the wound-care community. The use of bioengineered tissue, growth factors and biological dressings has driven clinicians to focus on wound-bed preparation and bioburden control (Krasner 2001). The brief use of antiseptics before and the use of topical antimicrobials after, placement of a living skin equivalent have become routine (Williamson & Sibbald 2001). These two clinical scenarios are modern examples of how treatment traditions and practices can shift radically over time.

The evaluation and treatment of an open fasciotomy wound follows the same principles described earlier for general wound care. Tissue oxygenation is assessed grossly through visual inspection and on a macrovascular level by the palpation of pulses and Doppler waveform analysis. A healthy, exposed muscle belly has a distinctive appearance, texture and colour, however, most chronic wound clinicians have no experience evaluating this muscle tissue. Wet-to-dry dressings are frequently ordered for fasciotomy wound care. This form of mechanical debridement (wet-to-dry) should only be used if there was a suboptimal initial debridement or persistent slough. After achieving a healthy bed of granulation tissue, local wound care should focus on dressing frequency, pain reduction and preparing the wound bed for closure. Communication between the wound service and trauma team is critical at this phase of care. It would be inappropriate and wasteful to utilize expensive dressings and wound closure devices if a second-look operation and/or debridement was planned.

Campbell's Operative Orthopaedics surgery textbook describes returning patients to the operating room at 72 h to re-explore the wound and remove any additional non-viable tissue (Azar & Pickering 1998). *Rockwood and Green's Fractures in Adults* textbook refers to leaving the wound open initially and attempting closure at 7–10 days (Heppenster et al 2001). Skin grafting is only utilized when persistent swelling at 7–10 days precludes direct surgical closure according to this reference. Most surgeons currently close the two-incision fasciotomy with a split-thickness skin graft medially and a delayed primary closure laterally. There is, however, wide practice variation in the management and closure techniques.

Once it has been determined that the wounds will be left open to heal by either secondary intention or delayed primary closure, then a number of chronic wound-care treatments may have application. The use of moisture-retentive dressings is a simple approach that can be overlooked by those unfamiliar with advanced chronic wound care dressings. Calcium alginate dressings perform particularly well for these exudative wounds. Dressing changes can initially be performed on a daily basis but as healing progresses the dressing interval can be increased. As granulation tissue fills the wound bed and the depth of the wound diminishes, achieving closure through skin grafting becomes relatively straightforward. Pulse lavage irrigation can be performed at dressing changes for those wounds with residual debris in the wound bed or when bacterial colonization is a concern. Recently, the use of negative pressure via the vacuum-assist closure device (VAC) has helped speed granulation tissue formation, control oedema/swelling and allow for early skin grafting (Scherer et al 2002). The VAC can assist with the removal of extravascular space oedema fluid, which allows for resuscitation of compromised microcirculation. The mechanical tension results in cellular changes, as well as allowing for fascial reapproximation at subsequent, scheduled surgeries. The use of the VAC in fasciotomy wounds is therefore beneficial (Webb 2002). The authors have now adopted a policy of placing VAC sponges at the time of initial fasciotomy with scheduled 48-h returns to the operating room for VAC dressing changes and attempts at fascial closure. The wound team evaluates the patient at the first VAC change and, along with the trauma team, decides on the most expeditious route to closure. These decisions are also based on comorbidities, medical stability, discharge planning, home environment, availability of outpatient care and the patient's personal desire. Hyperbaric oxygen has also been utilized for the treatment of compartment syndrome (Myers 2000).

In summary, the decision to perform a fasciotomy could be made with less trepidation if the chronic wound service was involved to follow the patient after the procedure. Also, trauma surgical input might allow for more expeditious wound closure than a wound team working in isolation.

OPEN ABDOMINAL WOUNDS

The management of critically injured patients has changed dramatically over the past few decades. Performing extensive surgical procedures in the face of gross physiological derangements yields morbid results even in experienced hands. This clinical reality has led to changes in the approach and treatment of the seriously injured patient.

Damage-control laparotomy

The triad of hypothermia, acidosis and coagulopathy during initial operative resuscitation efforts has been recognized as a significant cause of death in patients with traumatic injuries (Zacharias et al 1999). A staged surgical approach consisting of a brief initial laparotomy, followed by aggressive resuscitation, with a subsequent planned reoperation is the current trend (Brasel & Weigelt 2000). During the initial laparotomy the clinical endpoints include the control of bleeding and contamination. The abdominal cavity is then packed with laparotomy sponges and a temporary abdominal covering is sewn onto the surrounding skin. Gore-Tex has been used for temporary coverage while others attempt to close the skin loosely over the open fascial layer. The authors have utilized sterile plastic radiographic cassette covers to achieve the same goals. The plastic cover is readily available, cost-effective, provides for a moist environment, allows for visualization of the abdominal cavity for bowel and organ viability, and is easily removed. After subsequent aggressive resuscitation of the patient, a return to the operating room is planned for surgical re-exploration and definitive repair of any organ damage, usually in 24–48 h. Correction of hypothermia and volume repletion can reverse the acidotic state and correct any coagulopathy. One of the clinical goals for the second laparotomy includes closure of the abdominal fascia when possible. The success of this approach is well documented and the surgical community is embracing the approach. The challenge, however, continues to be patient selection, refining intraoperative techniques and expanding our understanding of the physiology of exsanguinations and reperfusion injury in resuscitation (Rotondo & Zonies 1997).

One of the negative side-effects of this approach is the accumulation of interstitial fluid (tissue oedema), which can make definitive fascial closure of the abdominal cavity technically impossible. However, eventual successful fascial closure is described in > 70% of cases treated with damage-control laparotomy, compared with 86% of patients treated in the historical standard laparotomy group (Johnson et al 2001). If closure is not possible then temporary coverage is again needed for 2–3 days. During this time, diuresis is initiated and reabsorption of tissue oedema is facilitated (Shapiro et al 2000). If surgical closure is still unachievable then long-term wound management for the open abdominal cavity becomes a necessity. Attempting closure under tension can lead to necrosis of underlying tissue, infection, bowel fistulae and abdominal compartment syndrome (discussed below).

Many techniques for the temporary management of the open abdominal wound have been described. The ideal temporary abdominal wound dressing/coverage should provide containment of the abdominal viscera, protect viscera from mechanical injury, prevent desiccation, be readily available, safe, cost-effective and promote safe closure of the abdomen at a later time (Sherck et al 1998).

Local wound care

The traditional dressing technique used for the open abdomen is the use of wet-to-dry saline packs. A healthy bed of granulation tissue will eventually form if infection can be avoided and the dressings are maintained moist throughout the day. Frequent dressing changes (i.e. every 8 h) can delay granulation tissue formation, however, and prevent wound contraction. This strategy leaves the patient with a large incisional hernia, which can be debilitating. A planned repair of the abdominal wall defect is anticipated with this technique. Often, muscle flaps and other complex reconstructions are needed to achieve closure. The use of advanced wound-care products in this clinical setting is uncommon. One reason for this lack of acceptance is cost. Open abdominal wounds can be massive and, for example, calcium alginate dressings could cost several hundred dollars per dressing change. The authors have used a thin contact layer of calcium alginate covered by slightly moistened inexpensive fluff sponges covered by a polyurethane film sheet. This dressing regimen achieves a moist wound environment and allows for a less expensive dressing protocol. The tertiary film dressing provides warmth, moisture and can help reduce dressing changes to once a day, which is helpful for granulation tissue formation and often more comfortable for the patient.

Mesh: Dexon, Gore-Tex, Composigraft

Two of the most commonly used fascial substitutes are polyglycolic acid (Dexon) and polytetrafluroethylene (Gore-Tex) mesh. These synthetic materials are sewn into the fascia and act as scaffolding for tissue repair. Pliability, resilience and permeability make them suitable options for this problem; there is no consensus as to which material achieves superior performance. Nagy et al (1999) support the use of Gore-Tex for coverage. Fewer adhesions to underlying bowel, greater wound epithelialization and lower morbidity and mortality rates were among the positive findings in this animal model. Larger sample sizes and further randomized controlled trials, however, are needed to define patient selection criteria and overall outcomes. Many biomaterials are being analysed for their ability to reduce peritoneal adhesions, fistulae formation, biological tolerance and ability to resist infection (Bellon et al 1997, Van't Riet et al 2003).

Vacuum techniques

In 1995 a group from the University of Tennessee College of Medicine published a novel method for achieving temporary abdominal closure called the 'vacuum pack' (Brock et al 1995). In this technique, a fenestrated polyethylene sheet is placed between the abdominal viscera and the anterior parietal peritoneum. Moist laparotomy towels and two closed suction drains are then applied and covered by an adhesive-backed drape. Suction is applied to the drains to create a vacuum, which facilitates drainage, provides integrity and protection for the abdominal cavity and allows for ease of re-entry. In subsequent follow-up reports this technique has been successful over 7 years on 112 patients (Barker et al 2000, Smith et al 1997). In 1997 Argenta and Morykwas (1997a, 1997b) published their technique for vacuum-assisted closure for wound closure. This technique involves using a polyurethane sponge applied to a wound bed, attached to a suction pump and then occluded with a polyurethane film dressing to create the vacuum seal. The commercially available VAC (Vacuum-assisted Closure Device, Kinetic Concepts Inc., San Antonio, TX) is now widely used for the treatment of a wide variety of complex wounds (Brown et al 2001, Genecov et al 1998, Morykwas et al 1999a, 1999b). Case reports now describe salvaging PTFE mesh using the VAC where in the past exposed mesh often resulted in mesh removal (Kercher et al 2002). Complications of VAC therapy are rare but enterocutaneous fistula development was most feared. Current literature describes the use of the VAC for the management of both perifistula skin and, paradoxically, the fistula itself (Cro et al 2002, Erdmann et al 2001, Saklani & Delicata 2002). In a report from Garner et al, 13 of 14 patients achieved fascial closure of their open abdomen with the use of VAC (Garner et al 2001). This technique utilizes the placement of the VAC device every 48 h in the operating room with serial fascial approximation until closure is achieved, in this study, an average of 10 days. The VAC has recently gained popularity for the treatment of sternal incisional dehiscence as well (Fleck et al 2002, Hardy 2002). The VAC can also be used as a 'bridge' to sternal closure; benefits include less frequent dressing changes and the return of chest wall mechanics (Song et al 2003).

ABDOMINAL COMPARTMENT SYNDROME

Abdominal compartment syndrome is another wound condition that requires cooperation between the trauma/surgical service and the wound-care department. The condition was first described in 1890 but has only been fully appreciated in the past decade. Increases in abdominal cavity pressure can lead to altered respiratory mechanics, haemodynamic instability and decreased renal function. Unrecognized, this disorder is universally fatal. Common causes include ruptured abdominal aortic aneurysm, intra-abdominal infection and abdominal trauma. The syndrome can occur in the trauma patient without a definitive intra-abdominal injury (Balogh et al 2002). Clinical symptoms include increasing abdominal girth, elevated peak airway pressures and decreasing urinary output. Because many clinical situations share these clinical findings, the diagnosis is often overlooked. Intraluminal bladder pressures provide a urometric window for detecting and monitoring intra-abdominal pressures. Bladder pressures greater than 25 mmHg in addition to clinical findings strongly suggest the diagnosis (Johna 2001). The treatment requires performing a decompressive laparotomy. A vertical midline incision relieves the pressure and allows for the restoration of organ perfusion along with improved respiratory mechanics. As with the previously mentioned damage control laparotomy patients, tissue oedema often precludes surgical closure. Similar wound problems to those mentioned above are therefore encountered, and the same techniques for treatment can be utilized.

ABDOMINAL DEHISCENCE

Dehiscence is defined as a separation within the fascial layer (Fisher et al 1999). Dehiscence most often occurs in abdominal incisions, although it can occur anywhere in the body; the incidence of abdominal dehiscence is between 0.5% and 3.0% (Pavlidis et al 2001). Many factors contribute to fascial dehiscence but technical error is the most common aetiological factor. Other contributing factors include malnutrition, hypoproteinaemia, obesity, malignancy, uraemia, diabetes, infection, immunological deficiency, increased abdominal pressures secondary to coughing and local haemorrhage (Riou et al 1992); elderly patients are also at greater risk.

The presence of a dehiscence is usually heralded by the drainage of fluid from the incision. The fluid is classically described as salmon coloured and is noted on postoperative days 4 or 5 in 85% of the cases. Fascial dehiscence is sometimes diagnosed when fascial separation is noted at the time of wound incision and drainage for a local infection. The most dramatic presentation of abdominal dehiscence is the extrusion of peritoneal contents through the defect, known as evisceration.

Treatment is dependent on presentation and the patient's underlying clinical condition. Evisceration requires immediate coverage and an urgent return to the operating room for closure. The fascial edges are debrided and a mass closure is performed. There are more clinical options for a controlled dehiscence, defined as the absence of evisceration. The patient can be returned to the operating room after medical stabilization for semi-elective mass closure. If the patient's clinical condition precludes a surgical option then local wound care and other non-operative management becomes necessary.

Large open abdominal wounds can be treated as described in the section on damage-control laparotomy. The authors use pulse lavage therapy in the treatment of dehisced abdominal wounds. This technique is particularly useful for contaminated/infected wounds and allows for continued debridement of the wound bed. In addition, electrical stimulation has been employed for the treatment of large open abdominal dehiscence wounds. This technique employs the concept of galvanotaxis and the beneficial effects have been widely published in the wound-care literature (Gardner et al 1999). Vacuum-assisted closure has also been utilized for the treatment of these large, complex wounds.

Again, cost effectiveness is a factor when selecting treatment modalities. In the US, many trauma patients do not have the financial resources to obtain expensive dressings or come to the clinic for costly modalities. This is a reflection of the socioeconomic and demographic characteristics of many trauma patients and the lack of a generalized government-sponsored health insurance plan. The hospital can achieve potential savings through the use of modern wound-care technologies by reducing hospital length of stay and the need for additional surgical procedures. Society can benefit if a patient can be returned quickly to a productive life through the use of such techniques. Several studies have demonstrated that the 'perceived' cost-effective treatment (i.e. saline gauze) turns out to be more costly when nursing time, delay in healing and complications are factored in to the economic equation (Bolton et al 1997). The most costly dressing is always the one that didn't work!

PRESSURE ULCERS

Much has been written over the past 15 years concerning the incidence, prevalence and treatment of pressure ulcers in the US. The occurrence of a pressure ulcer carries with it the perception of 'inadequate care' and many clinicians and attorneys play the blame game (Meehan & Hill 2002). Pressure, applied to tissue over time leads to microcirculatory collapse, tissue oedema and, subsequently, irreversible tissue damage. Animal models have described the amount of time and pressure required to damage tissue (Goldstein & Sanders 1998). Unfortunately, a patient's overall condition is a difficult variable to control. Tissue perfusion, nutritional status, tissue oedema, pain, sensation, infection, temperature and age are but a few confounding variables for the formation of a pressure ulcer. Recently, accreditation agencies have begun to use pressure-ulcer formation as a quality indicator (Dlugacz et al 2001). The nursing home industry has implemented comprehensive programmes to prevent pressure-ulcer formation in part secondary to increased scrutiny from survey agencies and potential litigation (Lyder et al 2002). Many clinical conferences now focus on whether pressure ulcers are all 'avoidable' or if there is an underlying basal rate that will occur despite best practice. Further confusing the issue is whether all wounds should be approached with a goal of healing (Alvarez et al 2002, Ennis 2001). The AHCPR prevention and treatment guidelines for pressure ulcers have been updated informally but no formal agency has revisited the topic since 1994; our standards of care might therefore be in need of updating.

A growing group of patients presenting to US trauma centres develop pressure ulcers and require a new approach – young, paraplegic men who have sustained gun-shot wounds to the spine are presenting, with increasing frequency, to trauma outpatient follow-up clinics with pressure ulcers. Historically, trauma services, because of the nature of their acute care, do not provide care for pressure ulcers, which are more common in chronic patient-care settings. Wound-care teams classically care for such disorders but frequently in debilitated elderly patient populations. The new group of patients contains two categories of patient.

Acute pressure ulcer patients

The first group is what the authors call the 'acute' pressure-ulcer patient, who develops a pressure ulcer within 90 days of the original injury. When a stage 3 or 4 wound develops within such a short period of time there are often educational, socioeconomic and/or financial issues that require an aggressive use of social services in addition to basic wound care. Wounds need to be assessed, staged, debrided and moist environmental products need to be utilized, as in the treatment of any pressure ulcer. However, if the patient lacks a seat cushion, adequate mattress for sleeping, the financial ability to receive treatments and home health, transportation and a home environment free of ongoing trauma, many treatment regimens will fail. It would be inappropriate to move directly to a surgical flap closure of such a patient without addressing all of the above needs. A long-term plan, which includes muscle group preservation, needs to be created. It is well known that despite the best of conditions recurrent pressure ulcers occur in up to 80% of paralysed patients (Evans et al 1994). Given the young age of these patients, the acute pressure ulcer needs to be approached within the context of a lifetime treatment plan. However, this concept must be balanced by the fact that young spinal-cord-injured patients frequently do not want to participate in a prolonged, local wound-care programme that requires numerous visits and active participation on their part. The authors have found a benefit in establishing a subacute wound programme at a local nursing home and rehabilitation centre. By cohorting like cases, patients can develop social support and learn from the experiences of their peers. After initial debridements, antibiotics when needed and local care, the patients receive 2–3 weeks of subacute wound-bed preparation prior to flap reconstruction and attempts at secondary closure. By utilizing electrical stimulation, ultraviolet light, ultrasound, vacuum closure, pulse lavage, local debridement, pressure-relieving devices and a number of synthetic and biological dressings, many patients can be healed without surgical closure. The Social Services department is also given adequate time to evaluate all other social and environmental issues that make these cases so complex. The authors have found these patients to be exceptionally challenging and, simultaneously, the most rewarding.

Chronic pressure ulcer patients

The second group of pressure ulcers patients are 'chronic', or those that occur more than 90 days after injury. Clearly, this arbitrary time line is, in actuality, a continuum, but it provides a theoretical framework for treatment protocols. Chronic pressure-ulcer patients can be approached with a more traditional wound-care focus, although Social Services involvement is still critical. Clearly, there are still major differences between patient expectations and care plans between the chronic pressure-ulcer patient and the young trauma patient. The concept of an advanced, comprehensive, subacute wound unit allows for the trauma team to discharge patients earlier with confidence that advanced wound care will continue at the next point on the continuum of care. The authors have found this results in improved compliance, follow-up and ultimately outcomes.

This topic is mentioned to raise awareness that pressure ulcers are not only a disease of the elderly and that a 'new paradigm' of care is needed when dealing with the young, paralysed patients, who seem to be making up a new and growing population for trauma and wound-care services.

REFERENCES

Alvarez O, Meehan M, Ennis W J et al 2002 Chronic wounds: palliative management for the frail population. Wounds 14(8S):5S–27S

Argenta L C, Morykwas M J 1997a Vacuum-assisted closure: a new method for wound control and treatment; clinical experience. Annals of Plastic Surgery 38(6):563–576

Argenta L C, Morykwas M J 1997b Vacuum-assisted closure: a new method of wound control and treatment; animal studies. Annals of Plastic Surgery 38(6):553–562

Azar F M, Pickering R M 1998 Traumatic disorders. In: Canale S T (ed) Campbell's operative orthopaedics, 9th edn. Mosby, St Louis, p 1405–1411

Balogh Z, McKinley B A, Kozar R A et al 2002 Secondary abdominal compartment syndrome is an elusive early complication of traumatic shock resuscitation. American Journal of Surgery 184(6):538–543

Barker D E, Kaufman H J, Smith L A et al 2000 Vacuum pack technique of temporary abdominal closure: a 7-year experience with 112 patients. Journal of Trauma 48(2):206–207

Bates-Jensen B, Wethe J 1998 Acute surgical wound management. In: Bates-Jensen B (ed) Wound care, a collaborative approach. Aspen Publishers, New York, p 219–233

Bellon J M, Contreras L A, Bujan J, Carrera-San Martin A 1997 The use of biomaterials in the repair of abdominal wall defects: a comparative study between polypropylene meshes (Marlex) and a new polythetrafluoroethylene prosthesis (dual mesh). Journal of Biomaterials Application 12(2):121–135

Bennett L L, Rosenblum R, Perlov C et al 2001 An in vivo comparison of topical agents on wound repair. Plastic and Reconstructive Surgery 108:675–683

Bleacher J C, Adolph V R, Dillon P W, Krummel T M 1993 Fetal tissue repair and wound healing. Dermatologic Clinics 11:677

Bolton L L, van Rijswick L, Schaffer F A 1997 Quality wound care equals cost-effective wound care: a clinical model. Advances in Wound Care 10(4):33–38

Bolton L, Constantine B, Kelliher B O et al 1985 Repair and antibacterial effects of topical antiseptic agents in vivo. In: Maibach H I, Lowe N J (eds), Models in dermatology, vol 2. Karger AG, Basel, p 145–158

Brasel K J, Weigelt J A 2000 Damage control in trauma surgery. Current Opinions in Critical Care 6(4):276–280

Brock W B, Barker D E. Burns R P 1995 Temporary closure of open abdominal wounds: the vacuum pack. The American Surgeon 61(1):30–35

Brown C D, Zitelli J A 1993 A review of topical agents for wounds and methods of wounding. Guidelines for wound management. Journal of Dermatology, Surgery and Oncology 19:732–737

Brown K M, Harper F V, Aston W J et al 2001 Vacuum assisted closure in the treatment of a 9-year-old child with severe and multiple dog bite injuries of the thorax. Annals of Thoracic Surgery 72(4):1409–1410

Conroy B P, Anglen J O, Simpson W A, Christensen G 1999 Comparison of Castile soap, benzalkonium chloride and bacitracin as irrigation solutions for complex contaminated orthopaedic wounds. Journal of Orthopaedic Trauma 13(5):332–337

Cro C, George K J, Irwin S T, Gardiner K R 2002 Vacuum assisted closure system in the management of enterocutaneous fistulae. Postgraduate Medicine 78(920):364–365

Dakin H D 1915 The antiseptic action of hypochlorite. British Medical Journal Dec 4th, 809–810

Debakey M E, Simeone F A 1946 Battle injuries of the arteries in World War 2. An analysis of 2,471 cases. Annals of Surgery 123:534

Dlugacz Y D, Stier L, Greenwood A 2001 Changing the system: a quality management approach to pressure injuries. Journal of Healthcare Quality 23(5):15–19

Ennis W J 2001 Healing: can we? Must we? Should we? Ostomy Wound Management 47(9):6–8

Ennis W J, Meneses P 1996 Clinical evaluation: outcomes, benchmarking, introspection, and quality improvement. Ostomy and Wound Management 42(Suppl 10A):40S–47S

Ennis W J, Meneses P 2000 Issues impacting wound healing at a local level: the stunned wound. Ostomy Wound Management 46(Suppl 1A):39S–48S

Ennis W J, Meneses P 2002 Factors impeding wound healing. In: Kloth L C, McCulloch J (eds) Wound healing alternatives in management, 3rd edn. F A Davis, Philadelphia

Erdmann D, Drye C, Heller L et al 2001 Abdominal wall defect and enterocutaneous fistula treatment with the vacuum assisted closure (V.A.C.) system. Plastic and Reconstructive Surgery 108(7):2066–2068

Evans G, DuFresne C R, Manson P N 1994 Surgical correction of pressure ulcers in an urban center: is it efficacious? Advances in Wound Care 7(1):40–46

Falanga V 2000 Classification for wound bed preparation and stimulation of chronic wounds. Wound Repair and Regeneration 8(5):347–352

Falanga V, Bren H 2001 Wound bed preparation for optimal use of advanced therapeutic products. In: Falanga V (ed) Cutaneous wound healing. Martin Dunitz, New York, p 457–468

Fisher J E, Fegelman F, Johanningman J 1999 Surgical complications. In: Schwartz S L (ed) Principles of surgery. McGraw Hill, New York, p 441–483

Fleck T M, Fleck M, Moidl R et al 2002 The vacuum assisted closure system for the treatment of deep sternal wound infections after cardiac surgery. Annals of Thoracic Surgery 74(5):1596–1600

Friedman J T, Scher L, Hall M 2002 Lower extremity compartment syndrome after coronary artery bypass. Journal of Vascular Surgery 36(5):1069–1070

Gardner S E, Frantz R A, Schmidt F L 1999 Effect of electrical stimulation on chronic wound healing: a meta analysis. Wound Repair and Regeneration 7(6):495–503

Garner G B, Ware D N, Cocanour C S et al 2001 Vacuum assisted wound closure provides early fascial reapproximation in trauma patients with open abdomens. American Journal of Surgery 182(6):630–638

Genecov D G, Schneider A M, Morykwas M J et al 1998 A controlled subatmospheric pressure dressing increases the rate of skin graft donor site reepithelialization. Annals of Plastic Surgery 40(3):219–225

Goldstein B, Sanders J 1998 Skin response to repetitive stress: a new experimental model in pig. Archives of Physical and Medical Rehabilitation 79(3):265–272

Gottrup F, Holstein P, Jorgenson B et al 2001 A new concept of a multidisciplinary wound healing center and a national expert function of wound healing. Archives of Surgery 136:765–772

Guerrero A, Gibson K, Kralovich K et al 2002 Limb loss following lower extremity arterial trauma: what can be done proactively? Injury 33(9):765

Hardy J W 2002 Treatment of open sternal wounds with the vacuum assisted closure system; a safe reliable method. Plastic and Reconstructive Surgery 109(2):710–712

Hegers J P, Sazy J A, Stenberg B D, Strock L L 1991 Bactericidal and wound healing properties of sodium hypochlorite solutions: the 1991 Linberg award. Journal of Burn Care and Rehabilitation 12:420–424

Helling T S, Daon E 1998 Advances in surgical technique. In: Flanders fields. The great war, Antoine Depage and the resurgence of debridement. Annals of Surgery 228(2):173–181

Heppenster R B, McCombs P R, DeLaurentis D A 2001 Vascular injuries and compartment syndrome. In: Rockwood and Green's fractures in adults. Lippincott, Philadelphia, p 319–352

Hoover T J, Siefert J A 2000 Soft tissue complications of orthopaedic emergencies. Emergency Medical Clinics of North America 18(1):115–139

Johna S 2001 Can we use the bladder to estimate intra-abdominal pressure? Journal of Trauma 51(6):1218

Johnson J W, Gracias V H, Schwab C W et al 2001 Evolution in damage control for exsanguinating penetrating abdominal injury. Journal of Trauma 51(2):269–271

Junger W G, Liu F C, Loomis W B, Hoyt D B 1994 Hypertonic saline solution as disinfectant. East African Medical Journal 71(2):83

Kercher K W, Sing R F, Matthews B D, Heniford B T 2002 Successful salvage of infected PTFE mesh after ventral hernia repair. Ostomy Wound Management 48(10):40–45

Kozol R A, Gillies C, Elgebaly S A 1988 Effects of sodium hypochlorite (Dakin's solution) on cells of the wound module. Archives of Surgery 123:420–423

Krasner D L 2001 How to prepare the wound bed. Ostomy Wound Management 47(4):59–61

Kuzan J O, Robson M C, Heggers J P, Ko F 1981 Comparison of silver sulfadiazine, povidone-iodine, and physiological saline in the treatment of chronic pressure ulcers. Journal of the American Geriatric Society 29(5):232–235

Lazarus G S, Cooper D M, Knighton D R et al 1994 Definitions and guidelines for assessment of wounds and evaluation of healing. Archives of Dermatology 130:489

Leversedge F J, Casey P J, Seiler J G, Xerogeanes J W 2002 Endoscopically assisted fasciotomy: description of technique and in vitro assessment of lower leg compartment decompression. American Journal of Sports Medicine 30(2):272–278

Loehne H B 2001 Pulsatile lavage with suction. In: Sussman C, Bates-Jensen B (eds) Wound Care, 2nd edn. Aspen Publishers, New York, p 643–661

Lyder C H, Shannon R, Empleo-Frazier O et al 2002 A comprehensive program to prevent pressure ulcers in long-term care: exploring costs and outcomes. Ostomy Wound Management 48(4):52–62

McHenry T P, Holcomb J B, Aoki N, Lindsey R W 2002 Fractures with major vascular injuries from gunshot wounds: implications of surgical sequence. Journal of Trauma 53(4):717–721

Meehan M, Hill W M 2002 Pressure ulcers in nursing homes: does negligence litigation exceed available evidence? Ostomy Wound Management 48(3):46–54

Morse J W, Babson T, Camasso C et al 1998 Wound infection rate and irrigation pressure of two potential new wound irrigation devices: the port and the cap. American Journal of Emergency Medicine 16:37–42

Morykwas M J, Kennedy A, Argenta J P, Argenta L C 1999a Use of subatmospheric pressure to prevent doxorubicin extravasation ulcers in a swine model. Journal of Surgical Oncology 72(1):14–17

Morykwas M J, David L R, Schneider A M et al 1999b Use of subatmospheric pressure to prevent progression of partial-thickness burns in a swine model. Journal of Burn Care and Rehabilitation 20(1, Part 1):15–21

Mubarak S J, Pedowitz R A, Hargens A R 1989 Compartment syndrome. Current Problems in Orthopaedics 3:36–40

Myers R A 2000 Hyperbaric oxygen for trauma: crush injuries, compartment syndrome, and other acute traumatic peripheral ischemias. International Clinics in Anesthesiology 38(1):139–151

Nagy K K, Perez F, Fildes J J, Barett J 1999 Optimal prosthetic for acute replacement of the abdominal wall. Journal of Trauma 47(3):529–532

Oliver L 1997 Wound cleansing. Nursing Standard 11(20):47–56

Pavlidis T E, Galatianos I N, Papaziogas B T et al 2001 Complete dehiscence of the abdominal wound and incriminating factors. European Journal of Surgery 167(5):351–354

Phillips D, Davey C 1997 Wound cleaning versus wound disinfection: a challenging dilemma. Perspectives 21(4):15–16

Phillips L G 2001 Wound healing. In: Townsend C M, Beauchamp R D, Evers B M, Maltox K L (eds) Sabiston textbook of surgery. W B Saunders, Philadelphia, p 131–143

Rich N M, Baugh J H, Hughes C W 1970 Acute arterial injuries in Vietnam: 1,000 cases. Journal of Trauma 10:539

Riou J P, Cohen J R, Johnson H Jr 1992 Factors influencing wound dehiscence. American Journal of Surgery 163(3):324–330

Riyat M S, Quinton D N 1997 Tap water as a wound cleansing agent in accident and emergency. Journal of Accident and Emergency Medicine 14:165–166

Rodeheaver G T, Smith S L, Thacker J G et al 1975 Mechanical cleansing of contaminated wounds with a surfactant. American Journal of Surgery 129:241–245

Rotondo M F, Zonies D H 1997 The damage control sequence and underlying logic. Surgical Clinics of North America 77(4):761–777

Saklani A P, Delicata R J 2002 Vacuum assisted closure system in the management of enterocutaneous fistula. Postgraduate Medicine 78(925):699

Scherer L A, Shiver S, Chang M et al 2002 The vacuum assisted closure device: a method of securing skin grafts and improving graft survival. Archives of Surgery 137(8):930–933

Schultz G S, Mast B A 1998 Molecular analysis of the environment of healing and chronic wounds: cytokines, proteases, and growth factors. Wounds 10(Suppl):1F–9F

Shah M, Foreman D M, Ferguson, M W 1992 Control of scarring in adult wounds by neutralising antibody to transforming growth factor β. Lancet 339:213

Shapiro M B, Jenkins D H, Schwab C W, Rotondo M F 2000 Damage control: collective review. Journal of Trauma 49(5):969–978

Sherck J, Seiver A, Shatney C et al 1998 Covering the "open abdomen", a better technique. The American Surgeon 64(9):854–857

Slimmon D, Bennell K, Brukner P et al 2002 Long term outcome of fasciotomy with partial fasciectomy for chronic exertional compartment syndrome of the lower leg. American Journal of Sports Medicine 30(4):581–588

Smith L A, Barker D E, Chase C W et al 1997 Vacuum pack technique of temporary abdominal closure: a 4-year experience. The American Surgeon 63(12):1107–1108

Song D H, Wu L C, Lohman R F et al 2003 Vacuum assisted closure for the treatment of sternal wounds: the bridge between debridement and definitive closure. Plastic and Reconstructive Surgery 111(1):92–97

Stack L B 1998 Compartment syndrome evaluation. In: Roberts J R, Hedges J R (eds) Clinical procedures in emergency medicine, 3rd edn. W B Saunders, Philadelphia, p 933–935

Staiano-Coico L, Higgins P J, Schwartz S B et al 2000 Wound fluids: a reflection of the state of healing. Ostomy Wound Management 46(Suppl 1A):85S–93S

Steed D L, Donohoe D, Webster M W et al 1996 Effect of extensive debridement and treatment on the healing of diabetic foot ulcers. American College of Surgeons 83:61–64

Tiwari A, Haq AI, Myint F, Hamilton G 2002 Acute compartment syndromes. British Journal of Surgery 89(4):397–412

Towler J 2001 Cleansing traumatic wounds with swabs, water or saline. Journal of Wound Care 10(6):231–234

Van't Riet M, Vos van Steenwifk PJ, Bonthuis F et al 2003 Prevention of adhesion to prosthetic mesh: comparison of different barriers using an incisional hernia model. Annals of Surgery 237(1):123–128

Webb L X 2002 New techniques in wound management: vacuum assisted wound closure. Journal of the American Academy of Orthopaedic Surgeons 10(5):303–311

Williams C 1999 Wound irrigation techniques: new steripod normal saline. British Journal of Nursing 8(2):1460–1462

Williamson D, Sibbald R G 2001 Skin substitutes. In: Krasner D L, Sibbald R G, Rodeheaver G T (eds) Chronic wound care, 3rd edn. HMP Communications, Malvern, PA, p 541–552

Zacharias S R, Offner P, Moore E E, Burch J 1999 Damage control surgery. AACN Clinical Issues 10(1):95–103

Wound management principles and resources

Professional issues

Social and psychological issues

Jane Harris and Catherine Spence

CHAPTER CONTENTS

INTRODUCTION

Wounds are rarely life threatening but they are often challenging, life-changing events. Possibly the greatest potential impact is upon the person's social and psychological well-being, two of the fundamental determinants of quality of life. Understanding and acknowledging this offers the practitioner the opportunity to create a truly person-centred and caring context that focuses on supporting individuals and their families in coping with challenge and adapting to change. Concentrating care on the physiological aspects of wound care might lead the practitioner to contribute, albeit unwittingly, to the threat to the person's quality of life.

This chapter therefore looks at this broader picture of how a wound can impact upon the social and psychological well-being of patients and those around them. It discusses variation in how individuals respond and the relevance of both the context – which includes factors such as the type of wound, existing disease, age and gender – and the coping strategies that people might access to limit the impact of the wound. Finally, the implications for practice are highlighted, based on the importance of valuing the individual and family's perspective and the role of the practitioner in supportive care.

INDIVIDUAL RESPONSES TO WOUNDS

The relationship between wound type and response of the individual and family affected has been discussed at length in the literature. Broad categories are often used to differentiate between wound types, specific effects and coping strategies. This is reflected in this section. However, it is important to remember that although generalization is useful in presenting information and aiding a general understanding of the topic, the spectrum within any one category is infinitely wide. Contextual issues are fundamental to understanding the nature of the problem for the individual and this will be discussed later.

Responses to acute wounds

Acute wounds, which are described by Dealey (1994) as wounds of sudden onset and short duration, tend to follow a timely and ordered sequence of repair and healing. They might cause minimal disruption to the individual's lifestyle and have little effect on plans for the long-term future. They may, however, have a dramatic effect, cause permanent disfigurement and loss of function and have serious psychological effects.

Responses to chronic wounds

Chronic wounds generate strong negative feelings and people not only suffer painful physiological trauma but also psychological difficulties. Their progress lacks the timely sequence of repair and healing (Neil & Barrell 1998) and they are characterized by uncertainty in terms of duration and outcome. Phillips et al (1994) reported a negative psychological impact, which included anxiety and depression, in 68% of a study sample who had chronic wounds. For some people who survive serious traumatic injury, the negative impact is transformed into what is described by Morse & O 'Brien (1995) as regrouping – choosing to move on and learning to get back into the world.

Within these two broad categories of wounds it is evident that not all responses are negative. An individual's coping style will therefore be relevant to the outcome of wound healing and adaptation to change. Some may view their wound and its implications as challenging, aiming to move forwards, and others, for a variety of reasons, cannot draw on internal resources and succumb to negative feelings and emotions.

COPING

Coping can be viewed as a process where individuals try to meet the demand placed on them, in this case the wound, with whatever resources they have available (Keeling et al 1997). However, Ritter et al (1995) emphasize that engagement in active coping processes is necessary for the demand to be met successfully. In other words, coping processes not only need to be available, they must be set in motion.

Box 18.1 illustrates a multidimensional coping inventory devised by Endler and Parker (1990), which looks at three major coping styles. Eysenck (2000) suggests that there are no simple answers in deciding which coping strategy is most effective and proposes that the nature of the stressful situation is important, for example the characteristics of the wound. Task-oriented coping is effective when the individual has the resources to deal with the wound and is able and motivated to use them. This pragmatic approach is perhaps more likely to be used for short-term acute wounds that do not have long-term consequences. In contrast, emotion-focused coping is used when the individual cannot resolve the situation. It may predominate when people live with the uncertainty and prolonged treatment associated with chronic wounds. Use of avoidance-oriented coping strategies, possibly when wounds are serious and their consequences most difficult to face, may be problematic. Family and friends feel ostracized and powerless to help. This, in turn isolates the person further. This type of coping strategy can also be difficult for the practitioner to deal with, and requires the use of a range of effective communication skills.

Apart from the nature of the stressor, age can also affect the coping style adopted. Folkman et al (cited in Eysenk 2000) suggests that older people use

Box 18.1
Multidimensional Coping Inventory
(from Endler & Parker 1990)

Task-oriented strategy
- Seeking out more information on the situation
- Viewing other courses of action and the probable outcomes
- Prioritizing and dealing with the situation directly

Emotion-oriented strategy
- Making an effort to maintain hope
- Controlling emotions
- Showing anger
- Deciding nothing can be done

Avoidance-oriented strategy
- Denying or minimizing the situation
- Suppressing stressful thoughts
- Replacing stressful thoughts with self-protective ones

more passive and emotion-focused styles in stressful situations than younger people, who tend to use more active, task- or problem-focused strategies.

Neil & Barrell (1998) used a small, qualitative study to examine the experiences of seven patients with chronic wounds. Selder's Transition Theory (1994) provided a framework for understanding patients with chronic wounds, by attempting to explain the process of restructuring reality after a period of uncertainty. This is represented in Fig. 18.1. The final stage of restructuring reality is evidently very challenging and may not always be achieved, leaving the patient in an earlier stage. This highlights the practitioner's vital role in focusing skills and available resources to prevent wounds becoming chronic. These should include accurate assessment and identification of risk factors, patient education and evidence-

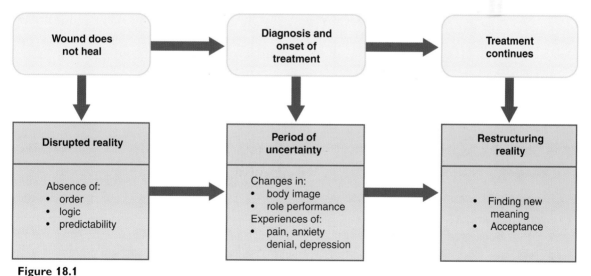

Figure 18.1
Chronic wounds: a process of restructuring reality using Selder's Transition theory (adapted from Rehabilitation Nursing, 23, 297, with permission of the Association of Rehabilitation Nurses, 4700W, Luke Avenue, Glenview, IL 60025-1485. Copyright © 1998).

based care. Support for patients and families through the transition, by helping them to understand the process and develop effective coping strategies, is essential.

Patients with acute wounds appear to have some similar but also other psychological responses. Magnan (1996) looked at the reactions of patients with acute wounds and highlighted the concept of body image as a way in which to evaluate psychological responses. Body image is a very personal concept and is closely associated with a person's self-esteem and self-worth. Both acute and chronic wounds can impact negatively on body image. Practitioners must not be tempted to make assumptions about the impact of a wound and its consequences on body image. They must recognize that it is the perception of the person themselves that is most relevant and the basis for supportive care.

The grieving process

The grieving process is believed to be a necessary adaptive response to loss. In wound care, loss may relate to a part of the body, a function or role or for some loss of attractiveness. Worden's work was based on death and bereavement and describes the grieving process in terms of four tasks. This relates well to the process of loss associated with some acute and chronic wounds and is shown in Fig. 18.2. Its application in wound care is most useful when the loss or change is permanent or of fixed duration and the person and family require to go through a process of readjustment. Where uncertainty of outcome exists, for example in some chronic wounds its application may be limited.

The grieving process demonstrates that changes in the person's physical and psychological circumstances may result in many emotions, often characterized by anxiety. The person strives to resolve anxiety by using a variety of psychological defence mechanisms (Eysenck 2000). These mechanisms are for the main part unconscious because we are not aware of employing them. The four most commonly observed defence mechanisms were identified by Magnan (1996) and are shown in Box 18.2. A person may use denial when a wound is large, unpleasant and disfiguring. Trauma wounds, which may require frequent dressing changes resulting in pain and continual reminders, may result in increasing anxiety and the turning inwards seen as regressive behaviour.

Box 18.2
Defence mechanisms
(Magnan 1996)

- Denial
- Repression (unconscious forgetting)
- Suppression (conscious forgetting)
- Regression (returning to an earlier developmental stage)

The individual context

The impact of the wound on the social and psychological well-being of the individual and the family clearly varies in extent and severity. For example, some people who live with a chronic venous leg ulcer experience minimal negative social and psychological consequences, while others become depressed, anxious and withdraw from social contact. This suggests that the interaction between the wound and its impact on the individual and their family is complex. Contextual factors profoundly influence the nature and extent of the

Task 1 To accept the reality of the loss.

People with either chronic or acute wounds must come to terms with what has happened to them and that a return to what was before is either unlikely, uncertain or impossible.

Task 2 To work through the pain of the physical or emotional loss or change.

This may be difficult when the outcome is uncertain. Failure to go through this process and recognize feelings may cut people off and lead to depression (Bowlby 1980).

Task 3 To adjust to a changed environment

This means different things to different people, including changed relationships and different roles the patient may have to play. It also involves adjusting to their own sense of self. For some this may be difficult, as they may see themselves as helpless and incapable. Some people may need help to recognize their strengths to move on.

Task 4 To get on with life

This task involves the person relocating the trauma of the wound in their emotional lives, which will enable them to go on with life. This may be a difficult task to achieve as they believe that life has stopped as a result of the trauma.

Figure 18.2
Four tasks associated with grieving. (Based on Worden 1991.)

impact. A summary of contextual factors is given in Fig. 18.3. Some of these factors are positive, for example, effective family support, while others, such as serious underlying disease, are negative. However, the context alone is not responsible for the final outcome. It is the deployment of effective coping strategies that makes the difference by restricting the influence of the negative factors and using the positive factors to minimize the impact of the wound. This is illustrated in Fig. 18.4.

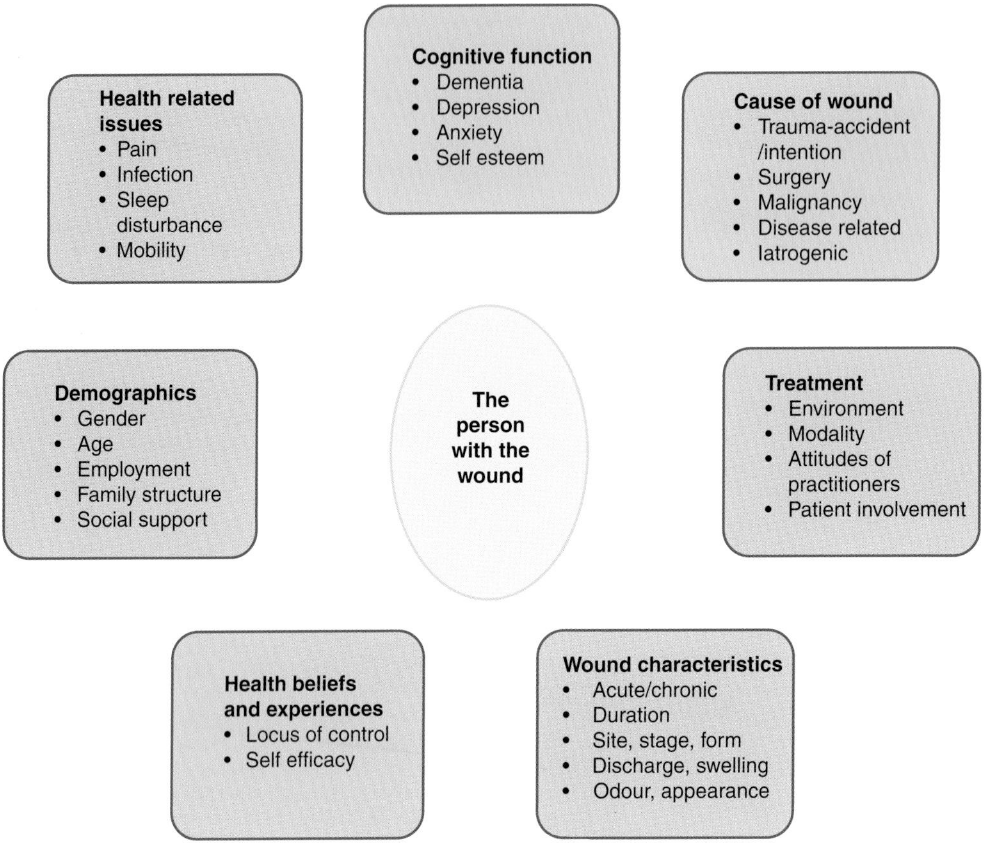

Cognitive function
- Dementia
- Depression
- Anxiety
- Self esteem

Health related issues
- Pain
- Infection
- Sleep disturbance
- Mobility

Cause of wound
- Trauma-accident /intention
- Surgery
- Malignancy
- Disease related
- Iatrogenic

Demographics
- Gender
- Age
- Employment
- Family structure
- Social support

The person with the wound

Treatment
- Environment
- Modality
- Attitudes of practitioners
- Patient involvement

Health beliefs and experiences
- Locus of control
- Self efficacy

Wound characteristics
- Acute/chronic
- Duration
- Site, stage, form
- Discharge, swelling
- Odour, appearance

Figure 18.3
The context

Box 18.3
The demands of wound care

A study by Phillips (1994) identified a strong correlation between the time spent on leg-ulcer care and feelings of anger and resentment. This could also apply to other wound types, and whether individuals receive professional care or self care. An opportunity cost is implied as time spent on wound care could be used for other activities, such as attending school, working or engaging in social activities. This cost may be greater if treatment involves hospitalization or clinic attendance. Some people may find home-based professional care intrusive, and resent interference in family routines and activities.

THE IMPACT OF WOUNDS

The psychological effects of wounds have already been discussed and include anxiety, depression, changes in body image and self-esteem. Boxes 18.3 to 18.7 contain examples of social implications, such as lifestyle changes, which may be problematic in their own right but might also be the source of or contribute to negative psychological responses.

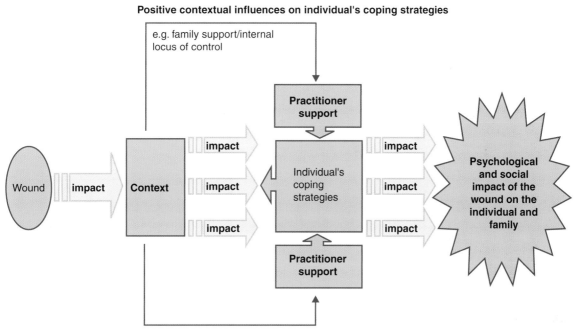

Figure 18.4
The impact of the wound on social and psychological well-being

Box 18.4 *Financial* *implications*	The wound or its consequences may affect the person's capacity to work, necessitate a change in the type of employment, or cause days off due to illness or treatment. A financial strain imposed by loss of earnings can not only cause practical problems but can also have serious psychological implications such as reduced self-esteem and depression. Those who pay for treatment and prescriptions will incur an additional financial cost and it may be necessary for some to purchase equipment to ease discomfort and assist with activities of daily living.

Box 18.5 *Challenges to* *the family*	A family member with a wound poses challenges that threaten the integrity of the family and have the potential to change familiar roles and routines. These include coping with negative psychological feelings associated with changes in the person's appearance and role within the family, taking on a carer role and becoming involved in treatment and supporting the person's own coping mechanisms. The image of the home and living arrangements may be altered to accommodate the person's needs and level of mobility. This may be difficult for others to live with and may discourage social events usually held at home.

Box 18.6
Independence and mobility

The effects of the wound may limit mobility and the person's ability to perform all the usual personal and everyday tasks associated with their role in life. These may include going to work or school, driving, engaging in sport, social and leisure pursuits, attending a place of worship, playing with children or grandchildren, shopping and other activities. Dependence on others may be the only way to engage in these activities and for those who have difficulty coming to terms with this, social and spiritual isolation may result along with feelings of resentment and depression.

Box 18.7
Social interaction

People may be reluctant to socialize with others because they have altered body image due to disfigurement, which is not only caused by the smell or sight of the wound but also by the dressing. They are afraid of friends' reactions, they feel depressed and out of touch or they cannot access the meeting place due to mobility problems. A loss of confidence may make them reluctant to meet new people and take up new activities which accommodate their changed circumstances.

Previous research has indicated that health beliefs, cognitive responses and social support can strongly influence individual responses to ill health and treatment (Bandura 1982, Cox 1986, Rosenstock 1991). Three theoretical concepts that relate to health beliefs are particularly relevant to how people respond to wounds and subsequently wound care. These are described in Table 18.1. They have been used to help explain health behaviour and can be applied to wound care in terms of prevention, recurrence and concordance with ongoing treatment.

Health beliefs

The Health Belief Model (Becker 1974) is more complex than Table 18.2 suggests. A number of factors modify the person's perception of the severity of the wound and the benefits of the treatment. These include age, gender, ethnicity, social status, knowledge of the wound and its likely outcome, and advice from others such as family members. Rotter's theory of the locus of control from 1966 offers an explanation for the distinction between the active and passive patient. Seligman (1975) described 'learned helplessness' – in which the person with an external locus of control is unable to take control, and is not given the support to do so – as a characteristic of depression. It could be suggested that someone with an internal locus of control could experience frustration, demotivation and depression, when care is imposed without informed choice and negotiation. It has been found that people with a strong sense of self-efficacy respond to stressful situations with fewer negative psychological and physical effects than those with a weaker sense of self-efficacy (Bandura et al 1985).

Cognitive responses and social support

Many chronic wounds develop as a result of pre-existing illness or disability and at a time in people's lives when they are least equipped to cope either physically or psychologically. This is particularly the case for older people, in whom there

Table 18.1
Health beliefs and their
implications for wound
care

Concept	Characteristics	Implications
Health belief model (Becker 1974)	People's motivation to act or behave in a particular way, e.g. comply with treatment, is based on their perception of: • the severity of the problem • the benefits of the action	The likelihood of the treatment reducing the severity of the wound/healing the wound is judged by: • estimating the accuracy of the diagnosis • past experience of the treatment • effectiveness of treatments in general
Internal locus of control (Rotter 1966)	People believe that they have control and influence over events in their lives	An internal locus of control suggests they would: • require information and explanation of their wound and treatment options • adopt a positive and proactive approach to decision making • be active in their treatment
External locus of control (Rotter 1966)	People believe that their life events are controlled either by fate or the actions of others and that they have no control over them themselves	An external locus of control suggests they would: • be more likely to have negative expectations of the outcome of treatment • rely on the judgement and actions of others • be reluctant to be involved themselves
Self-efficacy (Bandura et al 1985)	People will try something if they are motivated and have positive expectations of the outcome	People are more likely to comply with treatment if: • they have observed successful outcomes for others in similar circumstances • they feel that circumstances are favourable

is an increased incidence of leg ulcers and pressure ulcers. Franks & Moffatt (1999) assert that the impact of ulceration may be less for an older person than it would be for someone younger, as older people's expectations of health are lower. However, life may be characterized by multiple losses, including of cognitive and physical function, bereavement and social support networks. Older people are also more likely to be affected by dementia and problems associated with depression, anxiety and mood disturbance. The impact of a wound may therefore be severe and, with coping mechanisms difficult to mobilize, withdrawal and social isolation may result. Several authors have identified the positive effects of social support on compliance and the negative effects of social isolation. Edwards (1999) suggests that patients living in social isolation often do not comply with treatment because they fear losing the social network between themselves and the nurse when their wound heals. Families are often in a position to provide essential support for the person with the wound but it cannot be assumed that they will be able to do so. They will be as unprepared for traumatic injury as the patient and the stresses caused challenge effective family functioning. Research has shown that the stress experienced by spouses of cardiac patients can be greater than the stress experienced by the patient and include anxiety, depression and psychosomatic symptoms that continue for up to a year after the traumatic event (Miller & Wikoff 1989).

IMPLICATIONS FOR PRACTICE

- The nurse is accountable for offering the most individually tailored and effective care possible to the patient with a wound. This relies on accurate assessment that recognizes the contribution of social and psychological well-being not only to positive wound care outcomes but also as a vital determinant of the patient's quality of life in general. Assessment methods must therefore reflect this and care should be based on an appropriate model that values the patient's perspective and offers support and empowerment throughout the care process. The Davies and Oberle model of supportive care (Davies & Oberle 1990) is a good example and is recommended reading.
- Wound care should itself be aimed at minimizing 'costs' to patients in terms of time, opportunity costs, financial and emotional costs. Shorter, simpler modalities will reduce the burden of care and enable self-treatment and family involvement. This must be balanced with quality evidence-based care coordinated with other treatments and of minimal complexity. Patient and family must feel empowered to influence decisions about care and treatment. They must be asked what they want.
- Nurse attitudes to serious wounds, often seen by patients in a nurse's non-verbal communication and body language, will influence the patient's own attitude and self-esteem. The practitioner's approach with aims such as 'wound healing', implies that any outcome other than total wound healing is failure. Apart from being unrealistic and demoralizing for the patient, it prolongs the uncertainty and denies the patient an opportunity to adjust and move on. Some wounds never heal and others, once healed, require treatment such as compression therapy, which may continue indefinitely.
- Mangan (1996) – dealing with the grieving process – recognized that wounds change the patient's body integrity. People need concrete and specific information to reduce uncertainty and to understand what is happening.
- The nurse is ideally placed to understand and respond to the challenges faced by individuals living with a wound, and their families. The professional relationship and rapport should develop to enable the practitioner to view the issues from the person's perspective and act appropriately. The aim should be to recognize and support coping strategies. Facilitation may enable people to use the resources in ways which allow more effective coping to take place.
- Edwards (1997) states that listening to patients and providing psychological support is an important step to healing the whole person. In a study involving patients with head and neck cancer, patients reported that even when counselling was available, the counsellors had not listened and tended to have set

solutions to what they perceived the patients' problems to be. The patients wanted someone to listen, and to try to understand their feelings and what they were going through.

- Practitioners should make every effort to facilitate healthy family functioning. Family participation is important. Perhaps the most meaningful and effective source of comfort and consolation for the patient when they most need it is their family. Family members are more likely to reinforce professional advice if they understand the implications. Talking and listening to family members, and getting their perceptions, will enable the practitioner to educate family members so that they feel more aware, involved and supported.

- Effective pain management is essential. Pain undermines everything from the patient's confidence in the healthcare service to their ability and motivation to cope with their situation. The family may be affected similarly, which compounds the patient's ordeal.

- Neil & Munjas (2000) suggest that the practitioner should share with the patient even the smallest improvement in the condition of the wound. Feedback to patients and their family should focus on improvement rather than worsening.

- The relationship between social support and compliance with treatment has several implications for practitioners. This includes aftercare and the prevention of the recurrence of leg ulcers, particularly in older people. Motivation to self-care and compliance with preventative treatment is necessary in the absence of frequent support from the nurse. This has implications for working with other agencies to ensure that wider social needs are met when nursing withdraws.

- A sensitive approach, ensuring that any social or recreational activities offered are relevant to the person, is required. Inappropriate arrangements that impose social contact and are organized without full negotiation with the patient could merely exacerbate feelings of loneliness and isolation.

REFERENCES

Bandura A 1982 Self-efficacy mechanism in human ageing. American Psychologist 37:122–147

Bandura A, Taylor C B, Williams S L et al 1985 Catecholamine secretion as a function of perceived coping self-efficacy. Cited in: Robotham A, Sheldrake D 2000 Health visiting. Specialist and higher level practice. Churchill Livingstone, London

Becker M H 1974 The health belief model and personal health behaviour. Slack, New Jersey

Bowlby J 1980 Attachment and loss: loss, sadness and depression, vol. 111. Basic Books, New York

Cox C L 1986 The interaction model of client health behaviour. Application to the study of community based elders. Advances in Nursing Science 9(1):40–57

Davies B, Oberle K 1990 Dimensions of the supportive role of the nurse in palliative care. Oncology Nursing Forum 17(1):87–94

Dealey C 1994 The care of wounds. Blackwell Science, Oxford

Edwards L 1997 Preventing the recurrence of leg ulceration. Journal of Community Nursing 13(11):34–35

Endler N S, Parker J D A 1990 Multidimensional assessment of coping: a critical evaluation. Journal of Personality and Social Psychology 58:844–854

Eysenck M W 2000 Psychology: a student's handbook. Psychology Press, Hove, UK

Franks P J, Moffatt C J 1999 Quality of life issues in chronic wound management. British Journal of Community Nursing 4(6):283–289

Keeling D, Price P, Jones E, Harding K G 1997 Social support for elderly patients with chronic wounds. Journal of Wound Care 6(8):389–391

Magnan M A 1996 Psychological considerations for patients with acute wounds. Critical Care Nursing Clinics of North America 8(2):183–193

Miller P J, Wikoff R 1989 Spouses psychosocial problems, resources and marital functioning following myocardial infarction. Progressive Cardiovascular Nursing 4:71–76

Morse J M, O'Brien B 1995 Preserving self: from victim, to patient, to disabled person. Journal of Advanced Nursing 21:886–896

Neil J A, Barrell L M 1998 Transition theory and its relevance to patients with chronic wounds. Rehabilitation Nursing 23(6):295–299

Neil J A, Munjas B A 2000 Living with a chronic wound: the voices of sufferers. Ostomy Wound Management 46(5):28–38

Phillips T, Stanton B, Provan A, Lew R 1994 A study of the impact of leg ulcers on quality of life: financial, social and psychologic implications. Journal of the American Academy of Dermatology 31:49–53

Ritter S A, Tolchard B, Stewart R 1995 Coping with stress in mental health nursing. In: Carson J, Fagin L, Ritter S (eds) Stress and coping in mental health nursing. Chapman and Hall, London

Rosenstock I M 1991 The health belief model: explaining health behaviour. In: Glanz K, Lewis F M, Rimer K (eds) Health behaviour and health education theory, research and practice. Jossey-Bass, San Francisco, p 39–62

Rotter J B 1966 Generalised expectancies for the internal versus the external control of reinforcement. Cited in: Sarafino EP, Health psychology. John Wiley, New York

Selder F 1994 Life transition theory: the resolution of uncertainty. Cited in: Neil J A, Barrell L M 1998 Transition theory and its relevance to patients with chronic wounds. Rehabilitation Nursing 23(6):295–299

Seligman M E P 1975 Helplessness: on depression, development death. Freeman, San Francisco

Worden J W 1991 Grief counselling and grief therapy, 2nd edn. Routledge, London

Ethical issues

19

Mick Smith

CHAPTER CONTENTS

INTRODUCTION

Wound care, like other aspects of health care, throws up innumerable ethical problems for practitioners, and many of the moral issues that arise are matters of intense debate. They involve questions about 'patient autonomy', the 'duty of care', the 'just allocation of resources', and so on. But in the context of wound care these questions take on very particular forms that have important implications for those healthcare professionals involved. Although wound care as a topic may seem to lack something of the philosophical immediacy and popular currency of the heated debates around issues like euthanasia, abortion or genetic engineering, it too frequently entails choices that may be considered as matters of life-or-death (Glover 1988). Even in less dramatic circumstances, decisions taken about the treatment of wounds frequently affect the long-term quality of life of the patients concerned.

We all make decisions about what we deem to be the right or wrong course of action for us to follow every day of our lives. Many of these decisions are relatively trivial, but some are not. Non-trivial decisions are usually those that may have important effects on the lives and well-being of others. In such cases it often seems that we need to do rather more than just follow our feelings about what is right, we might also need to be able to justify our decision and our actions to others, including, of course, those affected by them. This in turn means that we need to be able to compare and contrast our decisions with those that have been, or might have been, taken by others in similar circumstances. It is this need that gives rise to ethical theories, frameworks for thinking about moral issues that have been developed to both explain and provide guidance about what is right or wrong.

There are, however, two main problems for those starting to think about how to make, explain, or justify their ethical decisions: first, is the variety of theoretical frameworks available, and second is the fact that different frameworks often seem to give contradictory answers as to what is 'right'. Part of the reason that theories contradict each other stems from the fact that each framework has been developed in particular historical and social circumstances to give voice to concerns that sometimes seemed to be overlooked or dismissed by the available alternatives. An ethical theory is not like a mathematical formula that will allow you to reach an incontrovertible answer about an issue. And although we often speak of 'applied ethics', this doesn't mean that the theories concerned can be applied to medical issues in any straightforward way. Ethical theories will not treat our moral condition in anything like the way that applied medicine treats our physical condition. Rather, it is best to think of these theoretical frameworks as providing different languages within which we can express and debate our concerns.

ETHICAL FRAMEWORKS

Debates in medical ethics commonly take place within and between four key theoretical frameworks centring on 'virtues', 'rights', 'utility' and 'care'.

Virtues

Virtue ethics, as the name suggests, concerns itself with the personal character traits – the virtues – that we expect of someone in respect of their role within society, or sometimes more generally in their role as a human being. Virtue ethics has a long history that can be traced back to ancient Greece. As Alisdair MacIntyre (1993) has noted, many early societies, like those of Homeric Greece (700 to 900 BC) had 'a well-defined and highly determinate system of roles and statuses'. Everyone had a fixed role, as a warrior, a nobleman, a peasant, and so on. Each role had a 'prescribed set of duties and privileges' and everyone had 'a clear understanding of what actions are required to perform these and what actions fall short of what is required' (MacIntyre 1993, p 122). From this perspective, you are what you do, and each role is associated with a set of virtues, those characteristics that epitomize the expectations associated with that role. Thus a good nobleman might be expected to be 'brave', 'skilful' and 'successful' in peace and war. If the nobleman lost too many battles then he simply wasn't to be counted as a good nobleman.

Today's society is much more fluid and people can often occupy a number of quite different and contrasting roles. However, insofar as we do frequently define ourselves in terms of our job, for example as a doctor or a lecturer, then we are still expected to fulfil certain duties and recognize appropriate virtues. Thus Florence Nightingale (1820–1910) set out a number of virtues she deemed necessary to be a good nurse, including: 'truthfulness; obedience; punctuality; observation; sobriety; honesty; quietness; devotion; tact; loyalty; sympathy; humility' (Sellman 1997). Of course, listing virtues in this way is by no means unproblematic. Is honesty always a virtue? Should you always tell the patient the whole truth even when a 'white lie' might aid their recovery? And although most people would agree that its best for nurses not to be drunk on duty, Nightingale's list obviously reflects certain presuppositions about nurses (and women's) place in society and the hospital ward that are characteristically Victorian. And is humility really an appropriate virtue for today's healthcare professionals, given their specialist training and knowledge about particular aspects of patient care?

Getting agreement about just what should count as a virtue is therefore more difficult than it might initially seem. But the language of virtue ethics has some advantages in allowing us to identify certain character traits that we might want to cultivate as people who want to be successful in fulfilling our roles as carers (Box 19.1).

Box 19.1 *Virtue ethics*	Which of the virtues deemed appropriate for nurses by Florence Nightingale are still relevant today and why? Which of them is most important? Are there other virtues that might be particularly relevant for those involved in wound care? Are these virtues specific to nursing or would they be applicable to healthcare professionals in general?

Rights Discourses on 'rights' arose much more recently during the social upheavals that marked the birth of the early modern period (Tuck 1977). In their simplest form, rights theories argue that every person has a natural right to certain freedoms and/or treatment simply because they are human. These 'natural rights' theories, usually founded on particular conceptions of human nature, give explicit recognition to each individual as an autonomous being and posit a radical form of equality between them. The purpose of a rights theory is to set out a series of basic liberties that each person must enjoy in order to be fully human and to protect individuals against anyone who seeks to restrict or usurp these liberties. Liberty itself is often spoken of as a natural human right as, of course, is the right to life itself. Such rights are supposed to be immediately obvious to all (self-evident) and because they are part and parcel of what it is to be human they can neither be surrendered by those that have them (they are inalienable) nor annulled by others (they are indefeasible). Thus Immanuel Kant (1724–1804) declared that '[t]here is nothing more sacred in the wide world than the rights of others. They are inviolable ... His right should be his security; it should be stronger than any shield or fortress' (Kant 1983). Kant believed that each right entailed a corresponding *duty*, an obligation on the part of others to respect those rights.

Rights play an important part in many aspects of contemporary life. They are enshrined in international agreements like the United Nations Universal Declaration on Human Rights, Article 25 of which includes a right to appropriate medical treatment (Dembour 1999). They also provide the foundation for many governments' constitutions. For example, the US Bill of Rights guarantees, amongst others, the right to life, liberty and property, to freedom of speech and assembly, to keep and bear arms, and to trial by jury. But this raises other issues because, as many people have pointed out, many of these rights are far from self-evident. Nor can a right to keep a rifle or stand trial in front of a jury be counted as 'natural' because such things are relatively recent 'cultural' inventions. The fact that rights are supposed to be absolute and irrevocable also causes problems. Does someone's right to liberty mean we can't force him or her to have treatment even if they are carrying a dangerous communicable disease such as tuberculosis? Some rights also seem to conflict with each other; for example, in certain circumstances a person's right to property in the form of a medical patent might jeopardize another person's right to life (Box 19.2).

Box 19.2
Rights theory

A new antibacterial agent is found to be highly effective in reducing the level of postoperative infections. However, the agent contains a number of volatile chemicals that have been associated with health risks for those experiencing regular exposure over long periods of time. Do patients have a right to insist that medical staff use this agent? How might this affect the rights of the medical staff who risk exposure?

Such problems have led many people to condemn the whole notion of rights. The utilitarian philosopher Jeremy Bentham (1748–1832) famously referred to the doctrine of natural rights as 'rhetorical nonsense – nonsense on stilts'. Bentham, a lawyer, thought talk of rights a 'terrorist language' that, by placing limits on government, acted to 'excite and keep up a spirit of resistance to all laws – a spirit of insurrection against all governments' (Bentham 1824). He argued that rights couldn't be natural or God-given; they couldn't exist prior to government but could only be granted by government, and government had to be placed on a rational and secular basis. His principle of utility was meant to do precisely this.

Utility

Bentham defines utility as 'that property in any object, whereby it tends to produce benefit, advantage, pleasure, good or happiness, (all this ... comes to the same thing) or (what again comes to the same thing) to prevent the happening of mischief, pain, evil, or unhappiness' (Bentham 1948). In other words, utilitarianism simply argues that everyone wants to be happy and therefore that anything that increases the general level of happiness is good and anything that decreases it is evil. According to this viewpoint, an action should be judged in terms of its consequences in producing the greatest happiness for the greatest number. This is very different from Kant, who argued that doing one's duty was imperative irrespective of the consequences. For example, for Kant it was *always* right to tell the truth, for Bentham its rightness would depend upon whether it made people happier – a difference that might have obvious implications in terms of patient care.

None the less, utilitarianism does seem to capture something in terms of our intuitions about what counts as 'right' or 'wrong'. Healthcare professionals are certainly encouraged to promote the well-being (happiness) of others and to refrain from doing them harm (Hendrick 2000). For example, these principles, referred to as beneficence and non-maleficence respectively, are placed at the very beginning of the United Kingdom Central Council (UKCC) for Nursing's Code of Professional Conduct (UKCC 1992). But it is not always clear just what such principles entail. How far we should go out of our way to help others, and at what cost to ourselves? Because we might always do that little bit more, the principle of utility would seem to place an almost infinite burden on us to be beneficent. Bentham himself argued that whereas we should legislate to ensure people's probity and non-maleficence, the extent of our beneficence should be largely a private matter left up to the individual. Unfortunately, this distinction hardly seems appropriate for cases where people have a professional duty to care for others.

Utilitarianism might then be regarded as a kind of 'moral accountancy' that tries to quantify the costs and benefits of an act (or the introduction of a rule) in terms of happiness rather than money. It doesn't deal in moral absolutes but enables one to speak about the ethical 'trade-off' between different courses of action, and for this reason often seems directly relevant to those running institutions like hospitals, who must make decisions about the allocation of limited resources. For example, a utilitarian would want to weigh the benefits of a novel surgical procedure or a more effective drug for pain relief against the cost of diverting resources from other patient services and the consequent suffering this might cause.

Unfortunately, things are never simple. Gauging someone's happiness or the degree of pain they are suffering is extremely difficult, and in calculating the consequences of our actions we need to make (potentially fallible) judgements about the duration, intensity and future trajectory of the pleasure/pain we might cause. Because we can't predict the future, our actions might have repercussions quite at odds with our expectations and even actions guided by the very best of intentions may thus come to be judged immoral with the benefit of hindsight (and vice versa). Utilitarianism also fails to give the individual the kind of absolute protection guaranteed by rights. If all that matters is the greatest happiness then we can imagine many scenarios where it might be deemed right to sacrifice one individual for the benefit of others (Box 19.3).

Box 19.3 **Utilitarianism**	A trial of two new drugs for the treatment of severe burns shows that 'Euphorix' considerably reduces the level of pain felt by patients but has little effect on recovery rates. The second drug, 'Despondate', markedly improves chances of survival but has side-effects that make some patients chronically and severely depressed. The hospital's budget is fully committed and only one drug can be bought. Can the use of these drugs be justified on utilitarian grounds and, if so, which should the hospital purchase?

Care Many of the debates surrounding rights-based and utilitarian theories can seem very abstract. Proponents of both are concerned to maintain an emotional distance from actual cases, claiming that only rational criteria must be used to adjudicate matters of right and wrong. Some, like psychologist Lawrence Kohlberg, have argued that the ability to employ this kind of abstract moral reasoning is indicative of having reached moral maturity (Kohlberg 1984). During childhood, Kolhlberg argues, we move from an egocentric (selfish) perspective through stages where we simply follow conventional moral norms and finally to stages where we, as individuals, can understand and employ moral principles like 'justice' or 'utility' to think through moral problems for ourselves. But feminists like Carol Gilligan have challenged this universal model of moral development, arguing that the evidence does not support it and that it employs an inherently masculine model of the moral self (Gilligan 1982).

Gilligan, at one time one of Kohlberg's co-workers, noticed that whereas boys often came to speak about ethical issues in terms of abstract principles, girls usually concerned themselves with particular practical contexts and on explicating personal relationships. For Kohlberg this was simply a sign of girls' moral immaturity but Gilligan suggests that it is Kohlberg's linear model of development that is wrong. Girls speak in a different (not a less developed) moral voice because, unlike boys, they are socialized into occupying predominantly 'caring' roles in society. They thus come to have a different ethical perspective on the world, one that focuses on developing and maintaining personal relations with others and recognizing mutual responsibilities. This 'ethic of care' requires that we get closer to others rather than theoretically distance ourselves from them, that we think of them as members of a network of personal relationships rather than as abstract bearers of rights or bundles of desires. An ethic of care does not seek to be impartial – it is not coldly rational – but emphasizes emotional involvement in particular contexts in terms of sympathy, compassion, fidelity, love, trust, and so on, all of which require a more or less intimate knowledge of the person concerned (Sherwin 1995).

The idea of an ethic of 'caring for' others might seem to have numerous advantages for those employed as healthcare professionals, not least of which is the fact that its practical orientation takes precedence over any theoretical considerations. It also seems highly compatible with a patient-centred approach (Bale & Jones 1997). There are, however, some drawbacks. Discourses of rights and utility at least attempt to treat people in similar circumstances in similar ways; they encapsulate notions of equality and justice. But we all know that personal relationships are seldom egalitarian and that we always know more about and respond more positively to some people than others. Although there may be many moral (and therapeutic) advantages in fostering an empathic relationship with one's patients, an ethics of care might result in some people being unfairly treated. Nor does it sit well with what is often regarded as a requirement for a certain professional detachment. Too much empathy with one's patients might actually make it more difficult to provide them with the treatments they require if, for example, procedures are particularly painful or distressing. Lastly, an uncritical application of Gilligan's thesis might actually operate to perpetuate gender stereotypes in nursing because it might (wrongly) seem to suggest that women are more suited to caring professions than men (Box 19.4).

Box 19.4 *Ethics of care*	A patient who has been suffering from a chronic leg ulcer for more than 2 years is admitted to an understaffed hospital ward. To what extent should the nursing staff on this ward try to understand (or even become personally involved in) the patient's social circumstances and to what degree, if any, should their knowledge of these circumstances affect the way in which the patient is cared for? If the patient was found to have avoided prior treatment because she suffers from a social phobia (American Psychiatric Association 1994) should she be offered a private room, taking into account the extra drain on staff resources this entails? Is a decision like this entirely context dependent, as Gilligan seems to suggest, or are there principles or rules that should govern taking such decisions?

Proponents of each of the frameworks we have examined would argue that the problems associated with them are not insurmountable. However, it does seem that no one ethical framework provides a language suitable for thinking through all the potential moral issues we might meet. Indeed, this multiplicity of different moral discourses might actually be advantageous, because they provide alternative ways of expressing and addressing moral issues. This moral pluralism may be important precisely because, despite what they might claim to the contrary, moral theories are never neutral formulae for determining right from wrong. Rather, the choice of moral theory will actively contribute to shaping what we understand as the important ethical aspects of any situation by emphasizing certain issues, care, rights or justice at the expense of others. For this reason too it is important to understand something of each framework's underlying presuppositions and their limitations. In the next section we will turn to examining their relevance to two topics of special relevance to healthcare professionals, the autonomy of the patient and the responsibilities of the carer.

PATIENT AUTONOMY AND PROFESSIONAL RESPONSIBILITIES

We all like to think of ourselves as being free to decide about important issues that might affect the course of our lives. We value our autonomy, which we associate with 'free will' and 'self-government' but also with taking personal responsibility for our decisions. In this way, the ideal of autonomy is closely linked to morality and has a key role in ethical theories. Both rights-based and utilitarian frameworks presuppose that the individual is capable of making rational decisions for him-/herself. Both also believe that it is absolutely vital to respect the autonomy of others. As we have seen, rights are designed to safeguard people's liberty and guarantee that they have everything necessary to develop and maintain themselves as autonomous individuals. People are deemed to have a right to education or health care precisely because to lack these is to restrict their freedom in important respects. Similarly, utilitarians like John Stuart Mill (1806–1873) have regarded 'liberty' as an integral and necessary part of attaining happiness.

Informed consent   Because wounds can be defined in terms of an injury to our bodily integrity, their treatment might justifiably be regarded as helping to maintain the patient's autonomy (Rumbold 1993). However, things are not quite so simple because people may not always want the treatment on offer. For Mill, the individual's liberty to do as he or she wished was absolute and 'the only purpose for which power can be rightfully exercised over any member of a civilised community, against his will, is to prevent harm to others. His own good either physical or moral, is not a sufficient warrant' (Mill 1995). In the context of wound care this means that it is necessary to obtain patients' consent for all medical procedures affecting them and that, when consent is denied, treatment cannot proceed, even if the patient will suffer as a result. Placing an absolute value on autonomy thus rules out all those forms of 'paternalism' where medical professionals might deem that they know what is in the patient's best interests and act against the patient's wishes.

The idea of informed consent plays a key role in medical ethics. Failure to obtain consent prior to treatment can count as an assault (Mason et al 1994). Informed consent should mean much more than just getting a signature on a consent form, which some have argued 'often amounts to little more than an empty ritual enacted to satisfy the letter of the law' (Yeo et al 1996). This, of course, raises the question of what exactly counts as giving one's consent. It is generally accepted that this should include at least the following:

- the patient is fully *informed* of the medical condition, the treatment options available, any risks associated with treatment and the consequences of rejecting treatment
- patients have the *capacity* to understand the information and to use it to make a rational decision for themselves
- the patient is not coerced but makes the decision *voluntarily*.

We will now deal with each of these issues in turn.

Providing information

There must be a genuine attempt to provide patients with the, often quite detailed, knowledge they require to make a decision. Providing such information in a jargon-free manner can be a real test of the carer's communicative competence. It also requires truthfulness on the carer's part, although guidelines often stress that this doesn't necessarily mean full disclosure, especially if a patient doesn't want to know the risks (Hendrick 2000, p 33). Failure to provide sufficient information about 'substantial risks' can, however, constitute negligence on the part of the carer.

Ensuring understanding

It is not enough to simply provide information; it is vital to make sure that the patient has understood its implications, which leads us to the second point. In some circumstances patients may be incapable of giving their consent. They may be unconscious or be deemed to lack the capacity to understand and make rational decisions about their treatment, for example if the patient is a young child or someone who is suffering from a serious mental illness. In such cases, and especially in emergencies, the courts have tended to support a limited degree of paternalism, usually on the grounds that such people are not, in any case, fully autonomous (Hirsch & Harris 1988). However, many of these decisions have been made on a case-by-case basis because it has proved very difficult to produce comprehensive definitions of patient competence. Some children are very mature for their age; some people suffering mental problems are only incapacitated some of the time, and so on. Thus, even if we accept an absolute right to refuse consent it is by no means clear who counts as an autonomous individual.

Voluntariness

Finally, consent must be given voluntarily. The difficulty here is that patients can experience a wide variety of pressures to accept or decline treatment. Once in care there may well be institutional pressures to comply with accepted norms and practices, patients may find that their decisions are swayed by the interests of friends or relatives, the drugs prescribed may affect their judgement, and so on.

CONCLUSION

All of these issues suggest that the ethical questions, like those of consent and autonomy, are by no means straightforward. Indeed, the very idea of autonomy is problematic because no person is an island – everyone from the moment of their birth is influenced in numerous and very fundamental ways by the society that surrounds them. Our ethical values too are a part of, and party to, these societal influences. Thus there are inevitably cultural as well as individual differences about what we count as right and wrong. This is especially the case in a society like our own that experiences rapid and continual changes in almost every field. Each new discovery seems to raise new ethical problems, some of which challenge our notions of the good life and even (in cases like genetic engineering and reproductive technologies) the idea of what it is to be properly human. Because the frameworks we have developed to speak of ethics all make some presuppositions about human nature, they too are caught up in these debates. That is why they should not be regarded as neutral formulae that can be applied to a situation but as languages that open our thought to different perspectives on life. This means that thinking about ethics is never easy, but then, when so much is at stake, it really shouldn't be.

Activity 1
Informed consent

Case 1
A 16-year-old is admitted in an unconscious state with severe self-inflicted burns as part of a political protest. On regaining consciousness in hospital she refuses to consent to any further treatment although she is made aware that failure to take antibiotics may lead to potentially dangerous infections. She seems perfectly lucid and aware of the implications of her decision. Should she be treated against her will?

Case 2
A 75-year-old diabetic man with terminal cancer and a life expectancy of six months has developed a rapidly spreading infection in his right foot. The patient has been showing some signs of senility. He is told that without surgical intervention he may die from septicaemia in a matter of days. He is also informed that while under general anaesthetic the surgeon may need to amputate his leg. The patient declines to sign the consent form. What should medical staff do?

Case 3
A 25-year-old woman, recently paraplegic following a riding accident, has developed a deep grade IV pressure ulcer since returning home. Her home has been specially adapted and she is cared for by a female friend who has to continue in paid employment and is therefore absent from the flat for more than nine hours a day. The patient refuses all help offered by community nursing and social services. Where do the responsibilities of the primary health care team and social services staff end? Who decides?

REFERENCES

American Psychiatric Association 1994 DSM IV: diagnostic and statistical manual of mental disorders, 4th edn. APA, Washington DC

Bale S, Jones V 1997 Wound care nursing: a patient-centred approach. Baillière Tindall, London

Bentham J 1824 Anarchical fallacies. In: Bowring J (ed) Bentham's works: vol 2. Russell and Russell, New York, p 489–543

Bentham J 1948 A fragment on government and an introduction to the principles of morals and legislation. Blackwell, Oxford, p 126

Dembour M 1999 Medical care as human right: the negation of law, citizenship and power? In: Kohn T, McKechnie R (eds) Extending the boundaries of care. Medical ethics and caring practices. Berg, Oxford

Gilligan C 1982 In a different voice. Harvard University Press, Cambridge, MA

Glover J 1988 Causing death and saving lives. Penguin, Harmondsworth, UK

Hendrick J 2000 Law and ethics in nursing and health care. Stanley Thornes, Cheltenham

Hirsch S R, Harris J (eds) 1988 Consent and the incompetent patient: ethics, law, and medicine. Gaskell, London

Kant I 1983 Lectures on ethics. In: Norman R T (ed) The moral philosophers: an introduction to ethics. Clarendon, Oxford

Kohlberg L 1984 The psychology of moral development: essays on moral development, 2. Harper and Row, San Francisco

MacIntrye A 1993 After virtue: a study in moral theory, 2nd edn. Duckworth, London, p 122

Mason J K, McCall Smith R A 1994 Law and medical ethics, 4th edn. Butterworths, London, p 219

Mill J S 1995 On liberty. Cited in: Honderich T (ed) The Oxford companion to philosophy. Oxford University Press, Oxford, p 569

Rumbold G 1993 Ethics in nursing practice, 2nd edn. Baillière Tindall, London, p 199

Sellman D 1997 The virtues in the moral education of nurses: Florence Nightingale revisited. Nursing Ethics 4(1)

Sherwin S 1995 Feminist and medical ethics: two different approaches to contextual ethics. In: Jecker N S, Jonsen A R, Pearlman R A (eds) Bioethics: an introduction to the history, methods, and practice. Jones and Bartlett, Boston, p 184–189

Tuck R 1977 Natural rights theories: their origins and development. Cambridge University Press, Cambridge

UKCC 1992 Code of professional conduct. UKCC, London

Yeo M, Moorhouse A, Dalziel J 1996 Autonomy. In: Yeo M, Moorhouse A (eds) Concepts and cases in nursing ethics, 2nd edn. Broadview, Peterborough, Ontario

FURTHER READING

General

MacIntyre A 1997 A short history of ethics. Routledge, London

Norman R 1983 The moral philosophers: an introduction to ethics. Clarendon, Oxford

Wain K 1997 The value crisis: an introduction to ethics. University of Malta Press, Msida, Malta

Theoretical frameworks

Heckman S J 1995 Moral voices, moral selves: Carol Gilligan and feminist moral theory. Polity Press, Cambridge

Held V 1995 Justice and care: essential readings in feminist ethics. Westview, Boulder, CO

MacIntyre A 1993 After virtue: a study in moral theory. Duckworth, London

Mill J S, Bentham J 1987 Utilitarianism and other essays. Penguin, Harmondsworth, UK

Smart J C C, Williams B 1990 Utilitarianism, for and against. Cambridge University Press, Cambridge

Medical ethics

Elliot C 1999 Bioethics, culture and identity. A philosophical disease. Routledge, New York

Hendrick J 2000 Law and ethics in nursing and health care. Stanley Thornes, Cheltenham

Kohn T, McKechnie R 1999 Extending the boundaries of care. Medical ethics and caring practices. Berg, Oxford

Pence G E 1998 Classic works in medical ethics: core philosophical readings. McGraw-Hill, Boston, MA

CHAPTER 20

Practice development and the role of the advanced practice nurse (APN)

Janice M Beitz

CHAPTER CONTENTS

INTRODUCTION

Advanced practice nurses (APNs) are a unique group of healthcare professionals theoretically and practically suited to both the highly specialized expert practice required by patients with wounds and the broadly based requirements of the organizations that serve them. APNs are expected to carry out their professional roles as expert clinical practitioner, educator, consultant, researcher and leader/manager/change agent. However, the full performance of the role has been problematic for some time for a variety of healthcare system and legal reasons.

This chapter analyses the roles of APNs as they pertain to wound care and contrasts them to care delivered by specialist level practitioners. A brief historical and international perspective is followed by an examination of selected issues affecting the future of wound care practice. Finally, the many actual and potential contexts for practice available to wound-care APNs are discussed. Resources for wound care and advanced and/or specialized wound care practice are also included, and these supplement the sources given in Chapters 1 and 4.

ISSUES AFFECTING THE CAPABILITIES OF WOUND-CARE APNS

The following case study exemplifies some of the issues affecting the full capabilities of wound-care APNs (Box 20.1).

Box 20.1
Case study of the
APN's role

Elizabeth is an American APN who graduated from a Clinical Nurse Specialist (CNS) Master's of nursing programme focusing on adult health and illness. In addition, she attended an accredited wound, ostomy, continence (WOC) nursing education programme (post-Baccalaureate specialty education) that offered graduate level credits. She is quadruple-board-certified in the three WOC specialties and as an adult CNS. Furthermore, she has completed doctoral level preparation in education.

Because of her extensive education and significant clinical experience in caring for persons with chronic wounds, Elizabeth has developed an active consulting business. In her home state (where she is formally recognized as an APN with Medicare provider reimbursement capability), she can be consulted both by physicians and by other health specialists from hospitals, subacute facilities, and extended care facilities to recommend and order care for her patients. She frequently drives across the state line to a nearby major metropolitan area with a large percentage of elderly patients (a matter of seven miles). Because that State does not recognize CNSs as APNs, Elizabeth can neither assess patients nor order their care as an independent practitioner. Her patients suffer from suboptimal continuity because she must depend on busy attending physicians with very large practices, or their Baccalaureate-educated physician assistants (neither of whom have assessed the patient) to order care. The irony of the mismatch and disconnect inherent in a restrictive practice environment does not escape Elizabeth for its inefficiency, waste of clinical expertise and anachronistic structure.

Questions for critical analysis
- What is some of the critical information in this scenario?
- What additional information is necessary?
- What problems in client care derive from this situation?
- What are some possible options for eradication/amelioration of the problem?

BACKGROUND AND HISTORICAL ISSUES

Today, nurses are providing contemporary wound care at specialist and advanced practice levels throughout the world. For a number of historical and sociocultural reasons, the vast majority is being delivered at specialist level. The dichotomy between the two levels is one of regulatory mandates, legal responsibilities, educational preparation and scope of practice (Table 20.1). However, there is an acknowledged overlap between the two levels. Indeed, it would be virtually impossible to provide advanced practice nursing-level wound care without first having extensive knowledge of and experience in specialty wound care (Beitz 2000, Gray 1994). In practice, some individuals prefer to practise wound care at specialty rather than advanced practice level (Bryant 1993).

Advances in nurse education provision

The practice level of wound-care nursing is heavily dependent on the historical development and societal context of nursing education in respective nations, and on the emerging needs of patients. For example, in the US, nurses can become eligible for licensure and registration as professional nurses by attending 2- or 3-year hospital-based diploma programmes, 2-year associate degree, or 4-year

Table 20.1

Distinguishing advanced practice and specialty practice nursing in the US

Characteristic/skill	Advanced practice level	Specialty practice level
Educational level	Master's	Baccalaureate
Autonomy	Expanded	Limited
Setting	Primary, acute, chronic	Variable (often acute care)
Management of health concerns	Comprehensive prescriptive privileges	Requires physician order
Interdisciplinary interface	Nurse to physician	Nurse to nurse
Diagnostic reasoning	Major emphasis	Less complex processing

Baccalaureate degree programs. Consequently, wound, ostomy, continence (WOC) nursing (formerly enterostomal therapy (ET) nursing) was originally open to nurses with all levels of education. However, since 1983, a bachelor's degree has been required for entry into specialty practice by the WOC Nurses Society (WOCN 1998).

Analogously, as the numbers of master's programmes in nursing grew in the US, the number of advanced practice practitioners who were interested in wound care also proliferated. As patients' needs intensify in the future, the number of APN wound specialists is also likely to expand sharply. To aid this move to advanced practice, several Wound, Ostomy, Continence Nursing Education Programs (WOCNEP) have begun to offer graduate credit for the specialized education (WOCN 2001).

A change has also occurred internationally. In the UK, nursing education has evolved from hospital-based diploma preparation to 3-year university diplomas or 3- or 4-year university degrees. Consequently, many older nurse clinicians who specialize in wound care are prepared with widely different levels of basic nursing education. Similarly, Australian and New Zealand nursing education evolved from 3- or 4-year hospital diploma programmes to 3- or 4-year university degrees. The same educational disparity affects the ET (WOC) nurses (especially older ones) who have practiced in those countries for years (Lusk et al 2001). However, younger Australian and New Zealand nursing graduates who enter ET (WOC) programmes will have a minimum of bachelor's education (Thompson & English 1996). In general, the minimal international expectation for WOC nursing education in other countries is that students are registered nurses with some postgraduate experience (and not necessarily a BS or BA) (Faller 1996).

THE NATURE OF ADVANCED PRACTICE TODAY

The origin of the term 'advanced practice nursing' is not known. It was not used in the American healthcare literature before 1985, although the four roles experienced in the US existed far before that time (Bigbee 1996, Gray et al 2000).

Advanced practice nursing is defined as clinical practice with the essential characteristics of specialization, expansion and advancement:

- Specialization means limiting one's focus to a part of nursing.

- Expansion refers to the acquisition of new practice knowledge and skills (including those that overlap the traditional boundaries of medical practice).
- Advancement includes both specialization and expansion and is characterized by the integration of theoretical, research-based and practical knowledge that is acquired in graduate nursing education (American Nurses Association 1995, 1996).

APNs today have at least a master's degree in an area of specialty, extensive supervised practice during their educational programme, and ongoing clinical interactions. The care they provide is based on comprehensive nursing theory and involves advanced assessment and intervention skills (Doughty 2000). Many of the same interventions used by specialist-level wound-care nurses are also common to APN practice because the advanced practitioners build on the extensive knowledge and experience of specialty practice.

In the US, advanced practice nursing has evolved into four roles: nurse anaesthetist, nurse midwife, clinical nurse specialist (CNS) and nurse practitioner (NP). The two latter roles relate specifically to the current discussion in that within advanced practice nursing, both NPs and CNSs most commonly deliver chronic wound care. All four types of APN roles have advanced-level certification available from the American Nurses Credentialing Center (ANCC) or other specialty organizations (AACN 2001).

Nurse anaesthetists provide anaesthesia-related care in acute and outpatient settings. Nurse midwives manage women and newborns perinatally. CNSs have traditionally functioned as expert bedside clinicians and patient advocates in the acute care (hospital) setting with ill clients. Their practice includes patient and staff education, research utilization and dissemination, consultation, direct clinical care and implementation of population-based care (National Association of Clinical Nurse Specialists 1999). CNSs often target the care of specific nursing populations like critical care, orthopaedic and geriatric patients.

More recently, the National Association of Clinical Nurse Specialists (NACNS) has altered the description of the CNS role to describe its functioning not as subroles but within 'spheres of influence': patient/client, nursing personnel and organizations/networks. The CNS designs care for a particular patient population of interest through education, consultation and evaluation of interventions. Identification of practice patterns and outcomes management processes is crucial for any CNS to achieve organizational goals (NACNS 1999). A sample system-wide goal may be to decrease nosocomial pressure ulcer incidence and prevalence.

Conversely, nurse practitioners (NPs) have traditionally been found mainly in primary-care settings with a care focus on one healthy or mildly ill patient at a time. NPs may work with special groups of people like adults, geriatric persons or children, or take a lifespan approach (family NP). However, a growing number of NPs now function in acute-care settings with the critically ill, and even as CNSs are developing and managing community-based disease management programmes targeting such disorders as congestive heart failure and chronic wounds (Dailey & O'Brien 2000).

The beginning of the convergence of CNS and NP roles has probably occurred because of the common core of essential knowledge acquired in graduate nursing education (Sechrist & Berlin 1998). Both types of practitioner learn about strategic planning, financial issues, research methods, outcomes assessment, population-based thinking and advanced pathophysiology, pharmacology and physical assessment. However, research suggests that the two roles will stay distinct in the US for the foreseeable future (Lincoln 2000). As the four roles eventually evolve, the focus of care of most nurse anaesthetists, nurse midwives and nurse practitioners will be the provision of direct patient care for one patient at each interaction. CNSs will more commonly administer indirect care to patient groups through the roles of educator, expert clinician, consultant and researcher (Doughty 2000).

One role component with which many NPs have less involvement is that of researcher (assessing outcomes and quality improvement); this is present more in CNS practice. Lancellot (1996) describes her role as a wound-care CNS when coordinating a bench-marking project for pressure-ulcer care in several healthcare organizations in a health alliance group. Because of her work and her colleagues' research analyses, medical centres in the alliance with 'best practices' in the prevention and treatment of pressure ulcers were identified, creating enormous public relations strengths for these facilities.

Why are APNs so valuable to contemporary health care in the US and around the world? The past four decades have taught that health promotion, disease prevention and early intervention are cost effective in the long run for most medical conditions (O'Flynn 1996). Multiple healthcare-related studies and literature sources have suggested that critical reflective thinking, self-directed learning, leadership skills and cultural competence with diverse populations are vital to improve health care in the twenty-first century (Brady et al 2001, Pew Health Professions Commission 1995). APNs demonstrate these skills because they are emphasized in graduate nursing education with a strong focus on caring for diverse, often underserved, patients (Vezeau et al 1998).

When compared with specialty-level practice or even expert nursing practice, the primary and unique aspect of advanced practice nursing is its autonomy. Multiple examples of autonomous wound-care advanced practice activities exist in the literature. Morris describes the actions of a rehabilitation and wound-care APN (CNS) who developed a wound-care programme for a home care agency (Morris 1999). She functioned as clinician (direct caregiver), teacher (informed mentor and formal staff educator), researcher (a quality assurance project developer), consultant (programme design adviser and developer of a resource manual), manager (overseer of product vendor relationships and product purchases), and leader (activator of the wound-care committee she developed). Her professional autonomy permitted the full fruition of the development of the wound-care programme.

Dailey and O'Brien (2000) describe similar CNS activities but advance them to include a comprehensive chronic wound-care disease management model wherein selected care foci (e.g. congestive heart failure, diabetes care) become centres of excellence (COE). The leadership role enacted by the wound-care APN is based on the 'pillars of care management':

- stratifying the population
- using evidence-based guidelines
- good clinical management
- thorough data collection and outcomes measurement.

Dailey and O'Brien (2000) suggest that wound-care APNs are key to marketing the quality of their care to actual and potential customers. They can create educational brochures that use evidence-based guidelines or best practices, provide expert seminars and educational programmes, develop care pathways personalized to disease processes and the home care agency, and provide critical liaisons to local nursing education programmes for information sharing about key areas of practice, skill preparation and knowledge. In addition, CNSs can be deeply involved with the use of innovations such as telemedicine and electronic communication as enacted for home wound care.

Some consequences of licensing and credentialing in the US

A special note must be made about licensing and credentialing of APNs in the US. Nurse practitioners and other APNs must function within the guidelines of a particular State's regulations for AP nursing practice because they must be licensed within the State(s) in which they deliver care. Some States may require APN-level certification by national examination as an additional requirement, besides Master's education. However, lack of standardization across the nation exists. For example, an APN with full scope privileges (i.e. prescriptive privileges, third-party reimbursement and hospital-admitting privileges) may lose them by relocating to a different locale. The lack of a national standard is a significant barrier to full utilization of AP nursing skills in any specialty (Sherwood et al 1997). The practical consequences of this were illustrated in the case study in Box 20.1.

SPECIALTY NURSING AND WOUND CARE

In the US and internationally, most nurse clinicians deliver acute and chronic wound care at specialty level. However, specialization in nursing is not a phenomenon related just to wound care. Specialty level practice is heavily present in the US, with more than 30 extant nursing specialty organizations (Benner 1999).

Many forces are driving the proliferation of specialization in nursing around the world: expansion of the knowledge base, social and technological advances, and the escalating costs of health care are just a few. The shift to primary care and prevention is also transforming health care internationally (Flanagan 1998a). In an excellent overview, Castledine (1998) categorizes these driving forces as those external to nursing itself including:

- increased complexity of care
- changing health needs of populations
- structural changes in the healthcare system
- new technologies
- delegation by the medical profession
- consumer demand

and forces internal to nursing as including:

- development of nursing science
- extension of boundaries of nursing care
- development of more post-Baccalaureate curricula
- paralleling of medical specialties
- a search for more financial recognition and autonomy.

As in the past, modern nurses are adapting to the changing context of health care by extending their scope of practice to new roles and responsibilities.

Nurse specialists who are not APNs do not generally have the legal or ethical freedom to practice the fuller scope permitted by AP nursing preparation. They do, however, practice full-scope specialized wound care. Sample activities may include the direct delivery of clinical care, monitoring statistics, product evaluation processes and staff development education. They generally do not have the advanced pathophysiology, pharmacology and comprehensive assessment skills to order topical care or prescribe medications independently.

Nurses who wish to specialize as wound, ostomy, continence nurse clinicians must attend one of several Wound, Ostomy, Continence Nurses Society (WOCN) accredited programmes in the US. Entry requirements include: a Baccalaureate degree, active registered nursing licensure, and previous and current clinical experience (WOCN 2001). Following didactic and preceptored clinical practice experience, graduates are eligible to complete a national certification examination in WOC nursing (at specialty, not advanced practice level) to validate their specialist role. The WOCN Certification Board does not have an advanced practice level of wound care certification available for possible participants, although the need for this has been suggested. The literature strongly supports that WOC/ET specialist nurses help provide quality wound care while minimizing the expenditure of healthcare dollars, including avoidance of skin breakdown litigation related to pressure ulcers (Kaufman 2000).

Other avenues to recognized wound specialization for nurses and other allied healthcare professionals in the US exist. For example, the American Academy of Wound Management (AAWM) offers a certification examination to persons who wish to demonstrate theoretical understanding of specialized wound-care practices (AAWM 2001).

Wound certification as proposed by the AAWM recognizes competency in wound care by allowing successfully certified people to demonstrate essential knowledge for comprehensive wound care. The examination by its nature does not evaluate psychomotor skills. Three levels of AAWM certification exist: diplomate status (requires doctoral degree and at least 2 years of wound care clinical or research experience); fellow status (requires masters level education and 2 years of wound care clinical or research experience) and clinical associate (requires bachelor's education or licensure as a registered nurse or physician assistant) (AAWM 2001).

A COMPARISON OF ADVANCED PRACTICE NURSING AND SPECIALTY-LEVEL WOUND-CARE NURSING

Generally speaking, the differences in educational preparation and scope of practice are the greatest dissimilarities between AP nursing and specialty-level wound-care nursing. Although some clarity has developed, more work is necessary to delineate roles, responsibilities and abilities between AP nursing and specialty-level wound practitioners. Sadly, research to show how each level of nurse clinician is independently able to best effect quality care for acutely and chronically wounded patients is lacking. In addition, the small number of APN wound-care clinicians makes comparisons difficult. Consequently, differences in outcomes obtained are elusive and can at best be speculated upon at this time in WOC nursing history. Most importantly, what is not known about varying levels of practice cannot be managed effectively to patients' greatest benefit.

The international scene for specialized versus advanced practice wound care is unstructured because advanced practice nursing is evolving around the world. The UK is an exemplar of where levels of practice in wound care are in transition. The major impetus for resolution is the same force driving the American healthcare scene: achieving the most appropriate and effective use of economic and healthcare resources (Humphris 1999). More than a decade ago, Cooper pointed out that wound-care specialization, and especially advanced practice wound care, evolved out of the need for organized, theory-driven, coordinated wound management (Cooper 1990). That need has only deepened in the ensuing years.

Nursing specialization in the UK in the last 20 years has expanded across a wide range of practice areas. British 'nurse specialists' function in such diverse areas as inflammatory bowel disease, nutrition, breast care, diabetes, and wound care (the last called tissue viability specialists). As in the US, the focus of care of tissue viability specialists (TVSs) is primarily on those persons with chronic, non-healing wounds. The TVS role requirements have proliferated as changes in healthcare services and needs demand increased efficacy.

TVS nurses perform clinical, educational and quality assurance roles similarly implemented by their Baccalaureate-educated WOC nurse counterparts in the US. Their duties include audit (assessment) of current practices and outcomes, implementing standards of care, enacting staff education, measuring the appropriateness of specialist referrals and evaluating the impact of continuing education (CE) days (Newton 1999, p 52). Clinical interventions for wounds, pressure ulcers and leg ulcers include wound assessment, topical therapy, Doppler assessment, conservative sharp debridement and compression therapy. Prescriptive authority and ordering of treatments is not included in their autonomous practice.

A relatively recent survey (Flanagan 1997) suggests that the evolution of these TVSs has been 'rapid and haphazard' (Flanagan 1998b, p 649) because the TVS nursing role is not standardized across the UK. Results show that the TVS appointment was new for 90% of the respondents. Consequently, they had few professional nursing role models. Six percent held masters degrees and 28% were Baccalaureate prepared; however, 39% had no special academic qualifications, even though they agreed that continuing education was critical. Only 34% had completed a nursing board specialty course in tissue viability (wound care and physiology). Their three main reported responsibilities were leg ulcer care, pressure ulcer prevention and general wound management.

In discussion, Flanagan suggests that in the UK the precise meaning of titles such as 'nurse specialist' and 'nurse practitioner' is often taken for granted, with accompanying confusion (Flanagan 1996). The majority of UK nurse clinicians uses the title 'clinical nurse specialist' to describe their role, but do not have commensurate graduate level education.

Humphris (1999) proposes that nurse specialists' outcomes must be evaluated in terms of quality, access, education and economy. However, this suggested evaluative framework ignores a critical point. Are these nurse specialists educated with a Master's degree (often called second degree in the UK) or not?

Several studies have attested to the efficacy of the 'specialist nurse' but do not attempt to fully clarify the educational preparation or the scope of practice of the nurse subjects (Nightingale et al 2000). Outcomes assessment of professional practice can deteriorate into an 'apples versus oranges' comparison, yielding spurious data and false interpretations with neither advanced- nor specialty-level practitioners receiving their fair and just analyses.

British nurses are also engaging in the role of nurse practitioner. The clinical practice of the NP remains unregulated, unstandardized and heavily dependent on local forces (Hicks & Hennessy 1997). The United Kingdom Central Council (UKCC) for Nursing, Midwifery, and Health Visiting has pushed for clarification of the role and requisite education of CNS and NP, although no full consensus has yet occurred (UKCC 2001).

In a cogent analysis targeting 'higher level of practice' problems, Woods (1997) explains the confusion occurring over role titles in the UK. After describing the four APN roles as delineated in the US, she presents the various terms proposed for use in the UK and makes comparisons: nurse practitioner, clinical nurse specialist, nurse consultant and nurse clinician. In the UK, NPs and CNSs have widespread variance in the level and type of preparation. Nurse consultants and nurse clinicians (proposed role titles that do not exist as such in the US) are expected to be prepared at least to Master's degree level. Given her proposal, some similarities exist between the CNS (US) and the nurse consultant (UK) and the nurse practitioner (US) and nurse clinician (UK).

In the past decade, the UKCC has more clearly specified broad standards for specialist education and practice, and standards for advanced education and practice are still in process (UKCC 2001, Woods 1997). In 1994, the UKCC defined for the first time the nature of specialist nursing practice. The abilities that were described included such things as the ability to demonstrate higher levels of clinical decision making, monitoring and improving standards of care, skilled professional leadership, clinical audit and research, and the teaching and mentoring of colleagues. There was no mention of educational preparation, although the Council suggested a clear difference between practising within a specialty and *being* a nurse specialist (Flanagan 1998, p 304).

Since then, a change has been implemented to raise standards for specialty nursing. The UKCC's Standards for Post-Registration Nurse Education define the minimum academic level of study leading to the qualification of specialist practitioners as first degree (similar to a Baccalaureate degree) (Flanagan 1996).

DEMONSTRATING COST EFFECTIVENESS

Despite the differences and similarities, a major area in which all APNs and specialist nurses in Europe, the UK, Australia and the US are facing constant scrutiny is the focus on cost effectiveness. Both levels of practitioner must demonstrate cost effectiveness and clear, measurable, positive outcomes with their patient populations. One of the challenges facing nurses in this endeavour is that extant research studies mix operational definitions of clinicians' educational preparation and expertise and fail to control multiple possible intervening variables (Flanagan 1998a). Another major challenge is the relative paucity of good psychometric evaluative methods and instrumentation. This latter deficit hampers a meaningful analysis of the efficacy of both specialist and APN wound-care clinicians.

Validated assessment instrumentation

The efficacy of advanced practice nursing has been evaluated by various assessment instruments and by targeting indices such as patient satisfaction or wound healing. The accuracy of such evaluation depends heavily on the instrumentation used. Selecting the 'right tool for the right task' is crucial (Buus-Frank et al 1996). Unfortunately, no valid and reliable instrument that focused specifically on wound-care effectiveness as enacted by APNs (or specialist nurses) could be identified by this author. Multiple instruments are available to analyse the impact of practice enacted by nurse practitioners, clinical nurse specialists, nurse anaesthetists and nurse midwives, but they are either generic or target another area of clinical practice specifically.

A brief review of the literature reveals some of the gaps and dilemmas extant in the realm of wound-care evaluation. Byers & Brunell (1998) submit that any user of an evaluation instrument or measurement device should use specific selection criteria. These include: significance (relevant to consumers and useful), range (assesses the scope of practice adequately), quality (documented reliability and validity) and feasibility (cost effective and able to truly capture the population of interest) (Byers & Brunell 1998, p 298).

Humphris (1999) suggests a possible framework in her posited approach to evaluation of nurse specialists. She includes the format of dimension, perspectives and measures. Dimensions include such issues as quality, access to care, education of patients and economy of care. Perspectives include the views of patients, the public and professional stakeholders. Measures include choosing and using data that can be adequately collected and that truly measure the role of nurse specialists.

Hicks & Hennessey (1997) describe a survey that was performed of nurse practitioners in the UK. The valid and reliable instrument surveyed training needs for the NPs and their common clinical activities but did not evaluate or assess their efficacy in practice.

In a different area of specialization, Buus-Frank et al (1996) described the development of an instrument measuring evaluation of the neonatal nurse practitioner role. The tool format is clear and comprehensive and foreshadows a similar future instrument that could be developed for the APN role and wound care specialization. Several others have developed instruments related to CNS or APN practice (Levitt et al 1985, Peglow et al 1992, Prescott et al 1981). However, they are general analyses of selected APN subrole components and do not address wound care per se.

In an excellent overview of APN outcomes measurement, Kleinpell-Nowell & Weiner (1999) scrutinized the various outcome indicators used in nursing research to measure the efficacy of APN practice. These issues included care-related issues (cost, length of stay, morbidity, time spent with patients) patient-related issues (patient satisfaction, access to care, stress levels, knowledge, blood glucose levels) and performance-related issues (quality of care, completeness of documentation and time spent in role components). They also note that pressure-ulcer prevention and wound healing were measured as research outcomes but not in published APN research. Clearly, it is now time to analyse the efficacy of APNs in affecting the quality of wound-care delivery. The first step is the development of a psychometrically sound measurement method or instrument. A second component is a study designed to evaluate chronic wound care with specified levels of practitioners and strict control of intervening factors.

THE CARE SETTING

Nurses and other healthcare clinicians deliver wound care in a variety of settings. Up until the 1990s, most nurses provided specialist and advanced practice wound care in the hospital setting. However, healthcare reform in the US and cost consciousness around the world are changing options for practice settings for wound-care clinicians.

Although a good proportion of specialist nurses (e.g. WOC nurses) still practise in the acute-care setting, a large shift has occurred whereby they are heavily represented in home care; more rapid discharge means that patients with more serious wounds are seen earlier in the care continuum at home.

Another major setting for wound-care delivery is extended-care and/or skilled nursing facilities. The largest percentage of chronic wound patients is seen in the elderly population and, as this group is burgeoning world-wide, it is understandable that wound-care nurses of both levels would increasingly serve in this setting.

In the US, both APNs and specialist nurses are delivering care in these settings. In some practice partnerships, APNs follow patients from clinic or office to the hospital with an exacerbation and then back to home or office care when improvement occurs.

Another setting that is evolving quickly for care of chronic wound patients is specialized wound-care clinics. APNs often supervise and/or collaborate with other care providers in these ventures where such advanced techniques such as hyperbaric oxygen therapy (HBOT), growth factors and electrical stimulation can be introduced into the plan of care and monitored meticulously. Some wound clinics have both specialist and advanced practice wound-care nurses working together with differing responsibilities.

Around the world in such countries as Canada, Australia, New Zealand and Israel, advanced practice nursing roles are gaining momentum (Hawkins & Thibodeau 2000). It is almost certain that a large proportion of these clinicians will care for persons with chronic wounds. How these advanced practice nursing clinicians will ultimately be utilized will depend heavily on legal issues and developing needs of patients.

CONCLUSIONS

Many factors that will affect the practice of wound care for all levels of practitioners are emerging. Cost-control issues, the enlarging elderly population, increasing diversity of ethnic and racial groups, and societal expectations for the best in healthcare-related technology will drive significant changes. It is likely that specialist, and especially APN, wound-care nurses will enjoy enhanced practice opportunities. Nurses who are versatile in care delivery and who can expertly use electronic communication and research findings will prosper (Beitz 2001, Kerstein et al 1998).

The 'new millennial nurse' (Beitz 2000, p 62) for chronic wound care will probably require advanced physical assessment skills, prescriptive authority (especially for topical therapy), computer-based data management and communications, use of alternative therapies and the 'upstream thinking' of population-based epidemiological risks for disease. As APN students are learning these skills today, specialist nurses around the world may be preparing themselves for the future of health care by completing a graduate degree.

Because wound-care nursing is part of the healthcare system, and any system is a product of the political, sociological, economic, cultural and demographic trends of the time, as societal needs intensify, the changes in wound-care nursing expectations and preparation will also evolve. The future of chronic wound care is likely to be challenging but highly rewarding for those nurses who position themselves to provide comprehensive, cost-effective, high-quality wound care at specialist and advanced practice levels in a variety of delivery settings.

REFERENCES

American Academy of Wound Management (AAWM) 2001 Application for board certification. AAWM, Washington, DC. Online. Available: www.aawm.org/certification

American Association of Colleges of Nursing (AACN) 2001 Certification and regulation of advanced practice nurses. Online. Available: www.aach.nche.edu

American Nurses Association (ANA) 1995 Social policy statement. ANA, Washington DC

American Nurses Association (ANA) 1996 Scope and standards of advanced practice registered nursing. ANA, Washington DC

Beitz J 2000 Specialty practice, advanced practice, and WOC nursing: current professional issues and future opportunities. Journal of Wound, Ostomy and Continence Nursing 27(1):55–64

Beitz J 2001 Overcoming barriers to quality wound care: a systems perspective. Ostomy/Wound Management 47(3):56–64

Benner J 1999 Guide to specialty certification. In: Springhouse Publications. Nursing 99 career directory. Springhouse Publications, Springhouse, PA, p 20–23

Bigbee J L 1996 Historical and developmental aspects of advanced practice nursing. In: Hamric A, Stross JA, Hanson C H (eds) Advanced practice nursing: an integrative approach. W B Saunders, Philadelphia, p 3–24

Brady M, Leuner J, Bellack J et al 2001 A proposed framework for differentiating the 21 Pew competencies by level of nursing education. Nursing and Health Perspectives 22(1):30–36

Bryant R 1993 ET nursing: advanced practice, specialty practice – or both? Journal of Wound, Ostomy and Continence Nursing 20(6):229–230

Buus-Frank M E, Conner-Bronson J, Mullaney D et al 1996 Evaluation of the neonatal nurse practitioner role: the next frontier. Neonatal Network 15(5):31–40

Byers J F, Brunell M L 1998 Demonstrating the value of the advanced practice nurse: an evaluation model. AACN Clinical Issues 9(2):296–305

Castledine G 1998 The future of specialist and advanced practice. In: Castledine G, McGee P (eds) Advanced specialist nursing practice. Blackwell, London, p 225–232

Cooper D 1990 The surgical clinical nurse specialist in a tertiary setting: establishing a subspeciality in wound care. In: Sparacino P, Cooper D M, Minarik P A (eds) The clinical nurse specialist: implementation and impact. Appleton-Lange, Norwalk, CT, p 181–209

Dailey M, O'Brien K 2000 Clinical nurse specialists: key to improving outcomes in home care. Home Health Care Management & Practice 12(3):32–42

Doughty D 2000 Integrating advanced practice and WOC nursing education. Journal of Wound, Ostomy and Continence Nursing 27(1):65–68

Faller N 1996 ET nursing education: a global perspective. In: Erwin-Toth P, Krasner D (eds) Enterostomal therapy nursing growth and evolution of a nursing specialty worldwide. Halgo Inc, Baltimore, p 87–97

Flanagan M 1996 The role of the clinical nurse specialist in tissue viability. British Journal of Nursing 5(11):676–681

Flanagan M 1997 A profile of the nurse specialist in tissue viability in the UK. Journal of Wound Care 6(2):85–87

Flanagan M 1998a Education and the development of specialist practice. Journal of Wound Care 7(6):304–305

Flanagan M 1998b Factors influencing tissue viability nurse specialists in the UK: 1. British Journal of Nursing 7(11):649–657

Gray M 1994 Specialty practice and the allure of advanced practice. Journal of Wound, Ostomy and Continence Nursing 21(4):133–134

Gray M, Ratliff C, Mawyer R 2000 A brief history of advanced practice nursing and its implications for WOC advanced nursing practice. Journal of Wound, Ostomy and Continence Nursing 27(1):48–53

Hawkins J W, Thibodeau J A 2000 Advanced practice roles in nursing. In: Hawkins J, Thibodeau J A (eds) The advanced practice nurse: issues for the new millennium. Tiresias Press, New York, p 1–41

Hicks C, Hennessy D 1997 The use of a customized training needs analysis tool for nurse practitioner development. Journal of Advanced Nursing 26(2): 389–398

Humphris D 1999 A framework to evaluate the role of nurse specialists. Professional Nurse 14(6):377–379

Kaufman M W 2000 The WOC nurse: economic, quality of life, and legal benefits. Nursing Economics 18(6):298–303

Kerstein M, van Rijswijk L, Beitz J 1998 Improved coordination: the wound care specialist. Ostomy/Wound Management 44(5):42–53

Kleinpell-Nowell R, Weiner J 1999 Measuring advanced practice nursing outcomes. AACN Clinical Issues 10(3):356–368

Lancellot M 1996 CNS combats pressure ulcers with skin and wound assessment team (SWAT). Clinical Nurse Specialist 10(3):154–160

Levitt M K, Stern M B, Becker K L et al 1985 A performance appraisal tool for nurse practitioners. Nurse Practitioner 10(8):28–33

Lincoln P E 2000 Comparing CNS and NP role activities: a replication. Clinical Nurse Specialist 14(6):269–277

Lusk B, Russell L, Rodgers J, Wilson-Barnett J 2001 Preregistration nursing education in Australia, New Zealand, the United Kingdom, and the United States of America. Journal of Nursing Education 40(5):197–202

Morris K 1999 Role of the rehabilitation advanced practice nurse in home care. Home Healthcare Nurse 17(5):323–325

National Association of Clinical Nurse Specialists (NACNS) 1999 Statement on clinical nurse specialist practice and education. NACNS, Glenview IL

Newton H 1999 Improving wound care through clinical governance. Nursing Standard 29:51–56

Nightingale A J, Middleton W, Middleton S, Hunter J 2000 Evaluation of the effectiveness of a specialist nurse in the management of inflammatory bowel disease (IBD). European Journal of Gastroenterology and Hepatology 12: 967–973

O'Flynn A I 1996 The preparation of advanced practice nurses. Current issues. Nursing Clinics of North America 31(3):429–438

Peglow D M, Klatt-Ellis T, Stelton S et al 1992 Evaluation of clinical nurse specialist practice. Clinical Nurse Specialist 6(1):28–35

Pew Health Professions Commission 1995 Health professions education and managed care: Challenges and necessary responses. Center for the Health Professions, San Francisco

Prescott P A, Jacox A, Collar M, Goodwin L 1981 The nurse practitioner rating form. Part I: conceptual development and potential uses. Nursing Research 30(4):223–228

Sechrist K R, Berlin L E 1998 Role of the clinical nurse specialist: an integrative review of the literature. AACN Clinical Issues 9(2):306–324

Sherwood G D, Brown M, Fay V, Wardell D 1997 Defining nurse practitioner scope of practice: expanding primary care services. The Internet Journal of Advanced Practice Nursing 1(2):1–13. Online. Available: www.ispub.com/journals/IJANP/Vol/N2/scope.htm

Thompson J, English E 1996 ET nursing education in Australia. Journal of Wound, Ostomy and Continence Nursing 23(3):130–133

United Kingdom Central Council for Nursing, Midwifery, and Health Visiting (UKCC) 2001 The PREP handbook. Online. Available: www.ukcc.org.uk

Vezeau T M, Peterson J W, Nakao C, Ersek M 1998 Education of advanced practice nurses serving vulnerable populations. Nursing and Health Care Perspectives 19(3):124–131

WOCN Society 2001 WOCN-accredited professional education programs. Journal of Wound, Ostomy and Continence Nursing 28(3):27A

Woods L P 1997 Conceptualizing advanced practice nursing practice: curriculum issues to consider in the educational preparation of advanced practice nurses in the UK. Journal of Advanced Nursing 25(4):820–828

Wound, Ostomy, Continence Nurses Society 1998 WOCN 30th anniversary opening session commemorative program. The Wound, Ostomy and Continence Nursing Society, Laguna Beach, CA

Wound, Ostomy, Continence Nurses Society 2001 WOCN accreditation policy and procedure manual. The WOCN Society, Laguna Beach, CA

FURTHER READING

Ackermann M H, Norsen L, Martin B et al 1996 Development of a model of advanced practice. American Journal of Critical Care 5(1):68–73

Blackley P 1996 Future trends in ET nursing internationally. In: Erwin-Toth P, Krasner D (eds) Enterostomal therapy nursing: growth and evolution of a nursing specialty worldwide. Halgo, Baltimore, p 1–12

Byers J F 1998 Demonstrating the value of the advanced practice nurse: an evaluation model. AACN Clinical Issues 9(2):296–305

Castledine G 1998 Clinical specialists in nursing in the UK: the early years. In: Castledine G, McGee P (eds) Advanced specialist nursing practice. Blackwell, London, p 3–54

Davies B, Hughes A M 1995 Clarification of advanced nursing practice: characteristics and competencies. Clinical Nurse Specialist 9(3):156–160

Gooch S 2000 Prescribing: the role of the tissue viability nurse. NT Plus 96(36):19–20

Greco K E 1995 Regulation of advanced nursing practice: part one – second licensure. Oncology Nursing Forum 22(8):35–38

Hutton D J 1997 The clinical nurse specialist in tissue viability services. Journal of Wound Care 6(2):88–90

Junkin J 2000 Promoting healthy skin in various settings. Nursing Clinics of North America 35(2):339–348

King B 2000 Prescribing the role of the tissue viability nurse. NT Plus 96(36):19–20

Krasner D 1996 ET nursing and wound care: embracing the challenge. In: Erwin-Toth P, Krasner D (eds) Enterostomal therapy nursing – Growth and evolution of a nursing specialty worldwide. Halgo Inc, Baltimore, p 135–144

McGee P 1998 Specialist and advanced practice: issues for research. In: Castledine G, McGee P (eds) Advanced specialist nursing practice. Blackwell, London, p 87–92

McGee P 1998 Specialist practice in the UK. In: Castledine G, McGee P (eds) Advanced specialist nursing practice. Blackwell, London, p 135–154

McGee P 1998 Advanced practice in the UK. In: Castledine G, McGeeP (eds) Advanced specialist nursing practice. Blackwell, London, p 177–184

Mendez-Eastman S 1999 A glimpse at the specialty of wound care. Plastic Surgery Nursing 19(2):67–73

Robinson S 1996 Advancing home care nursing practice with an ET clinical nurse specialist. Home Healthcare Nurse 14(4):269–274

Sieloff C L, Di Carlo B L, Killeen M B, McDermott S D 1994 A unique perspective on advanced practice nursing. Nursing Connections 7(4):39–44

Spencer-Cisek P, Sveningson L 1995 Regulation of advanced nursing practice: part two – certification. Oncology Nursing Forum 22(8):39–42

WEB-BASED RESOURCES

Multiple quality resources for wound care and advanced practice and specialist nursing are available online. No differentiation of web-page quality, integrity, veracity, etc., is presented. These evaluative decisions are left to users.

Name of organization/journal/ network	Web address (all have http as prefix)
Agency for Healthcare Research and Quality (formerly the Agency for Healthcare Policy and Research)	www.ahcpr.gov/
American Academy of Dermatology	www.aad.org
American Academy of Nurse Practitioners	www.aanp.org
American Academy of Wound Management	www.aawm.org
American Association of Critical Care Nurses (AACN Journal)	www.aacn.org/aacn/jrnlci.nsf
American Burn Association	www.amerburn.org
American College of Nurse Practitioners	www.acnp.org
American Physical Therapy Association	www.apta.org
Association for the Advancement of Wound Care	www.aawc1.org
Australian Wound Management Association	www.awma.com.au/main.html
Canadian Association for Enterostomal Therapy	www.caet.ca
Canadian Association of Advanced Practice Nurses	www.caapn.com
Canadian Association of Wound Care	www.cawc.net
Centers for Disease Control	www.cdc.gov
Cochrane Collaborative	www.cochrane.org

**WEB-BASED
RESOURCES**
—*continued*

Name of organization/journal/ network	Web address (all have http as prefix)
Dermweb (Dermatology Source)	www.derm.ubc.ca
European Pressure Ulcer Advisory Panel	www.epuap/menu.htm
European Tissue Repair Society	www.etrs.htm
Food and Drug Association (FDA) of the United States	www.fda.gov
Health Care Financing Administration (HCFA) of the United States	www.hcfa.gov
National Association of Clinical Nurse Specialists	www.nacns.org
National Association of Pediatric Nurse Practitioners and Nurses	www.napnap.org
National Institute for Diabetes and Diseases of the Kidney	www.niddk.nih.gov/
National Library of Medicine (United States)	www.nlm.gov
National Lymphedema Network	www.lymphnet.org
National Organization of Nurse Practitioner Faculties	www.nonpf.com
National Pressure Ulcer Advisory Panel (NPUAP) of the United States	www.npuap.org
Southern Australian Wound Management Association, Inc	www.wound.sa.edu.au/
Tissue Viability Society (United Kingdom)	www.tvs.org.uk
United Kingdom Central Council	www.ukcc.org.uk
Wound Care Communication Network	www.woundcarenet.com/science.htm
Wound Foundation of Australia	www.vcp.monash.edu
Wound Healing Society	www.whs.org
Wound, Ostomy, Continence Nurses Society	www.wocn.org
Wound Repair and Regeneration (Journal)	http://wizard.pharm.wayne.edu/wrr/WRR.htm
World Wide Wounds (Electronic Wound Care Journal)	www.worldwidewounds.com

INDEX